70405

ankins, Robert W.

Management accounting
for health care
organizations.

.95

	DATE	

Management Accounting for Health Care Organizations

Tools and Techniques for Decision Support

Robert W. Hankins, PhD
Associate Professor
Xavier University
Cincinnati, OH

Judith J. Baker, PhD, CPA
Executive Director of the Resource Group, Ltd.
Dallas, Texas

JONES AND BARTLETT PUBLISHERS
Sudbury, Massachusetts
BOSTON   TORONTO   LONDON   SINGAPORE

World Headquarters

Jones and Bartlett Publishers	Jones and Bartlett Publishers	Jones and Bartlett Publishers
40 Tall Pine Drive	Canada	International
Sudbury, MA 01776	2406 Nikanna Road	Barb House, Barb Mews
978-443-5000	Mississauga, ON L5C 2W6	London W6 7PA
info@jbpub.com	CANADA	UK
www.jbpub.com		

Library of Congress Cataloging-in-Publication Data

Hankins, Robert W.
  Management accounting for health care organizations : tools and techniques for decision support / Robert W. Hankins and Judith J. Baker.—1st ed.
     p. ; cm.
  Includes bibliographical references.
    ISBN 0-7637-3225-7
   1. Health facilities—Accounting. 2. Health facilities—Costs—Accounting. 3. Health services adminis-tration. 4. Managerial accounting.
   [DNLM: 1. Health Services Administration—economics. 2. Costs and Cost Analysis—methods. 3. Decision Support Systems, Management. W 84.1 H241m 2004] I. Baker, Judith J. II. title.
   RA971.3.H25 2004
   362.1'068'1—dc22

                                                                                    2003026943

Publisher: Michael Brown
Associate Editor: Chambers Moore
Production Manager: Amy Rose
Associate Production Editor: Renée Sekerak
Marketing Manager: Joy Stark-Vancs
Manufacturing Buyer: Therese Bräuer
Art Creation: Smolinski Studios
Composition: Modern Graphics
Cover Design: Kristin E. Ohlin
Printing and Binding: Malloy, Inc.
Cover Printing: Malloy, Inc.

Printed in the United States of America
08 07 06 05 04   10 9 8 7 6 5 4 3 2 1

This book is dedicated to those who have
chosen to spend time and effort toward improving
the wellness of our communities and the efficiency of
our health care system.

CONTENTS

PREFACE

This book is intended to give those who seek to manage health care organizations the foundation they need to assure that their organization produces information that will support their responsibility to make decisions. It focuses on decisions that involve choices among alternatives. Because the primary objective of such choices is to assure financial viability within a competitive environment that is demanding quality services and products, much of the content concerns costs. It can also serve as an introductory text for those who wish to concentrate in the areas of information systems in general and industrial engineering applications in health care.

The text assumes that costs are incurred in performing activities that must happen in order to produce outputs. It stresses those activities as the underlying cause of costs. Tools and Techniques for Decision Support. Writing the book was motivated by the happy meeting of an academic who had been teaching management accounting in graduate programs for health care organizations and a consultant who had been working in that area for some years. The thrust of our effort is to help managers understand how information is used, the determinants of information that is needed, the appropriate approaches to collecting data with which to generate that information, and effective ways to communicate that data to those who need and want it.

A basic objective is to improve the organization's ability to understand the relative cost of different intermediate services, care protocols, and services/products for which it is paid, in order to make wise choices among them. Traditional inventory cost calculations evolved for financial reporting purposes whereas, Medicare costing procedures are designed for reimbursement purposes.

The book also covers some common types of cost-dependent decision models and the necessity of using information based on accurate measurement of variables other than cost.

For readers who have not recently studied financial accounting and statistical inference, there are appendixes in the back of the book. Understanding the material in these appendixes will prepare readers to be able to understand text material using concepts from those subject areas.

We are very interested in any comments readers might have to improve the content or usability of this book. We hope it is a help in improving managers' abilities to make quality decisions.

Robert W. Hankins, PhD
Associate Professor
Department of Health Services
Administration
Xavier University of Cincinnati
Cincinnati, Ohio

Judith J. Baker, PhD, CPA
Executive Director
Resource Group, Ltd.
Dallas, Texas

ABOUT THE AUTHORS

ROBERT W. HANKINS, PhD

Professor Hankins received a bachelor of science in electrical engineering from Duke University, an MBA from The Ohio State University, and his doctorate in business administration from the Kenan-Flagler School of Business of the University of North Carolina at Chapel Hill. Over the past 20 years, he has taught management accounting and financial management in the Department of Health Services Management at Tulane University's School of Public Health and Tropical Medicine and in the Department of Health Administration at Southwest Texas State University. He is currently an associate professor of health administration at Xavier University in Cincinnati. Prior to teaching, he served as a U.S. Air Force officer holding both staff and command positions in technical support organizations.

Professor Hankins has published in journals such as *Medical Care, Socio-Economic Planning Sciences, Healthcare Information Management*, and the *Texas Journal of Rural Health*. He has been a principal investigator for a Health Care Financial Administration cooperative agreement project, a reviewer for the Academy of Management and the Southern Management Association, and a speaker for seminars held by organizations that include the American Public Health Association, Texas Public Health Association, Operations Research Society of America, American College Health Association, and the Health Care Financial Management Association as well as private professional education groups. His teaching and research is centered on the identification, generation, and presentation of information for decision making.

JUDITH J. BAKER, PhD, CPA

Judith Baker received her bachelor of science in business administration from the University of Missouri, Columbus; a master's in human and organization systems

xv

from the Fielding Institute, Santa Barbara; a master's in liberal studies from the University of Oklahoma, Norman; and her doctorate from the Fielding Institute. She is a full-time health care consultant and a partner and executive director of the Resource Group, Ltd., in Dallas, Texas. Her clients include providers, manufacturers, and suppliers across the spectrum of health care delivery organizations. She is a nationally recognized health care costing and payment authority. She provides support for and training about new payment methods and has extensive experience in cost reporting. As a Centers for Medicare and Medicaid Services (CMS) subcontractor, she consults on new programs and validates cost report databases used for CMS rate-setting purposes. Her work focuses on health care costs, prospective payment systems, resource utilization indicators, and related knowledge management. She holds adjunct or assistant professorships at Texas Women's University and the University of Rochester's School of Nursing.

Dr. Baker is editor emeritus of the *Journal of Health Care Finance*, (Aspen Publishers, 1995–2002), an author of an array of books and articles on cost accounting and payment systems, including *Activity Based Costing and Activity Based Management for Health Care* (Aspen Publishers, 1998), *Prospective Payment for Long Term Care 2000–2001* (Aspen Publishers, 2000), *Cost Accounting for Healthcare Organizations* (McGraw Hill, 1999), and coauthor of *Healthcare Finance: Basic Tools for the Non-Financial Manager* (Aspen Publishers, 2000).

1   Background

Before discussing specific management accounting processes and outputs, it is useful to look at management in general, what managers should accomplish, and the role of information in managers' work.

Chapter 1 contains an overview of these topics, a formal definition of management accounting, and the reasons that management accounting should now go beyond its traditional focus on costs. Because the purpose of management accounting is to assist decision makers, Chapter 2 discusses the process of making decisions and factors affecting the usefulness of information systems in producing effective decisions. These discussions are to set the stage for examining specific items of information with which management accountants are concerned, and the processes used to identify and manage them.

ACCOUNTING AND MANAGEMENT

LEARNING OBJECTIVES

After studying this chapter, students should be able to:

1. Define accounting and differentiate between management accounting and financial accounting.

2. Discuss general organization functions, for which managers are responsible.

3. Explain the role of decision making in management and discuss general categories of information needed to support health care managers' decision responsibilities.

4. Explain the basic differences between for-profit and not-for-profit health care delivery organizations and their information needs.

ACCOUNTING DEFINED

The American Accounting Association has defined *accounting* as "the process of identifying, measuring, and communicating economic information to permit informed judgements and decisions by users of the information."[1] Interestingly, the definition does not limit the form of the information to dollar amounts; it simply says "economic information." This opens accounting to the measurement of a wide range of variables. Additionally, the definition does not specify who the users will be. This implies that accounting should serve a wide array of decision makers.

The individuals whom accounting should serve can fall into two groups. First is the organization's management, ranging from the board of directors and executives to operating personnel who manage specific production and support activities. Second is the people outside the organization who are interested in the organization's performance and viability, such as investors, creditors, regulators, and union officials. These are people who must make decisions about their relationships with the organization. In trying to generalize accounting practice to meet the needs of different categories of users, two approaches have evolved.

The first has been called the "decision-model" approach. This approach develops normative measurement procedures and aggregated values to serve various users. It does this by computing numbers whose derivation is consistent across organizations. The rules for these computations constitute generally accepted accounting principles (GAAP). Because the decision makers know the rules used to compute the reported numbers, they can adjust these numbers as they think appropriate for their specific decisions. The other approach has been called the "decision-maker" approach. Here, specific types of decision processes are analyzed to understand how the decision is made, what variables are considered, and how measures on these variables can be aggregated to support each specific type of decision.[2] The difference between these two approaches can be illustrated in the problem of setting the value of an existing piece of equipment. The decision-model approach states the value of all equipment at its depreciated historic cost. Using the decision-maker approach, a manager attempting to decide on replacing a piece of equipment might use its current salvage value.

It is probably safe to say that as one looks inside an organization, a greater variety of information users makes more types of decisions than are made by accounting users outside the organization. The difference is between macrolevel decisions about the organization and the greater volume of microlevel decisions within the organization. This book will first, and primarily, address the role of accounting in supporting managers of the organization for which the accounting is being done. It will then relate this purely management accounting to financial accounting, which is done to assist people outside the organization. Before discussing information and measurements needed in decision processes that managers use, it is helpful to view the general situations that require managerial decisions.

THE WORK OF MANAGERS

The study of managerial work originally focused on the responsibilities that managers must assume. Managers are responsible for assuring that adequate planning, organizing, staffing, leading, and controlling happen within their organization.[3] In the 1970s, management study began to focus on what managers actually did to assure these functions were performed well.[4] A great deal of study about what management is and what managers do occurred in the last half of the 20th century. The results of this study can be summarized by saying that managers go through continual iterations of communicating, making decisions, and then communicating decisions. The specific processes involved in these cycles depend on an array of factors. This book is primarily concerned with the information that managers at various levels within health care organizations should have in order to make the decisions they must make, how that information can be acquired, and how it should be presented. The discussion of managers' work begins by describing the basic functions for which managers are responsible.

Planning

Classic American management thought assumes that an organization has objectives it is attempting to obtain. Typically, these can be expressed in a pyramidal hierarchy with a general, overreaching objective at the top. This objective is supported by more detailed objectives that must be met on the way to it.[5] The broad objective is often referred to as the *organization's mission*. The basic approach toward achieving the mission is frequently referred to as the *organization's strategy*. Recently, much has been written about forming basic objectives and planning strategy. Processes for doing this have primarily been derived from the study of businesses working in market economies. Classic theory assumes that someone has looked at society and determined that it desires (or needs) something it does not have. The decision is made to supply the need. Supplying such needs becomes a business organization's mission. The organization may already exist and choose to add this mission to its existing product (or service) line, or a new organization may be created to fill the need. In business terms, the society to be served is called the *market*, and each need is referred to as a *market opportunity*.

STRATEGIC PLANS   Strategies have classically been considered long-term approaches or processes used to achieve the mission of the organization. Planning has been described as "thinking about the future," "action laid out in advance," "the design of a desired future and of effective ways to bring it about," and "the conscious determination of courses of action designed to accomplish purposes."[6] Mintzberg implies that planning can be thought of as making decisions in consideration of the future in attempts to control the future. He adds that the decisions referred to here are interrelated: "drawn together into a single, tightly coupled process so that they all can be made (or at least approved) at a single point in time."[7] Strategy is established by approval at a point in time of decisions to integrate a broad array of future activities.

In the 1960s, large quantities of resources were dedicated to strategic planning. This involved determining a mission and planning long-term sequences of activities leading to its accomplishment. This planning was frequently done in strategic-planning departments by professional planners. Their specific duties were to articulate the organization's mission and objectives and to lay out the organization's future activities. These activities were usually based on highly sophisticated analyses and stated in a strategic plan with a 5- to 10-year life. By the mid-1980s, many of these strategic-planning departments were found valueless and dismantled. The reason for the change was that, in many markets, the outside environment was changing too rapidly and too unpredictably to allow accurate forecasts of market needs or available technology over so long a period. Concurrently, strategic plans became controlled by professional planners. Organization managers who understood the markets and appropriate technology lost the power to manage the activities for which they were responsible. Organizations realized that strategic planning was not a task to be accomplished at set intervals based primarily on planning techniques. Effective strategy is determined by markets for products and available production technologies. Rather than annually producing new 5-year plans, strategies should be revised when changes in markets and technologies demand a change in the approach to meeting the mission. These changes are best predicted and understood by managers dealing with the organization's markets and the technologies that support them. This evolution in thinking about strategy and strategic planning is explained in detail by Henry Mintzberg.[8]

Although an organization should have a general strategy for attending to its market, deciding on strategy is more complicated than that implies. First, many organizations have more than one market. For instance, a hospital may have as its mission "To enhance the health of all the people in our regional community and to provide high-quality care in a compassionate and efficient manner."[9] Its general strategy may be to establish facilities that are capable of providing primary care health support activities to patients in any age group within no more than 15-minutes travel time and to provide tertiary care services in all medical and surgical specialties within no more than 1-hour travel time from its clients. In this case, providing cardiovascular care would be part of its mission. This would require that a strategy also be established for the delivery of the multitude of interventions involved in cardiovascular care. The point here is that when the intent is to accomplish a broad mission over a long period of time, strategy also takes on a pyramid structure of component strategies that support the mission. Setting each strategy demands information about the relevant markets and technologies.

As an example, suppose you are part of the executive management team of a large pharmaceutical company. Your company has become aware of the potential need to address the AIDS pandemic. You believe you have the capability to produce drugs that will be effective in radically slowing the progress of human immune viruses and delaying the onset of AIDS for undetermined amounts of time. Also assume that the general mission statement is that of one large pharmaceutical firm: "We will become the world's most valued company to patients, customers, colleagues, investors, business partners, and the communities where we work and live."[10] The mission statement then gets more specific in a statement of purpose: " . . . we dedicate ourselves to humanity's quest for longer, healthier, happier lives through innovation in pharmaceutical, consumer, and animal health products."[11] With such a mission and purpose, the first strategic decision would be whether to address market needs related to AIDS; then a technical strategy for producing and testing the drugs must be established. Assuming that drug development is successful, the company must establish a strategy for serving the market and producing a profit. Several alternative marketing strategies are available. Four of these would be to:

1. Assume that poor nations will be supplied funds to purchase the drugs and, therefore, produce and sell at established world market price so as to maximize world profits.
2. Assume that poor countries will not be able to pay more than the cost of producing the additional drugs they will use. The strategy could then be to set adequate prices in industrialized countries to earn adequate profits and

assume that there will be no accounting contribution from sales in poorer countries.

3a. Assume that poorer countries will not be able to pay any price. A strategy could then be to give the drugs to poor countries, capitalize on the public relations value of the contribution, and gain adequate revenue from sales in richer countries to cover all costs and an adequate profit.

3b. Or—market only in societies that can pay a price yielding adequate profit, because management believes inadequate distribution systems and internal corruption in poor nations would simply waste the resources used to supply them while reducing surpluses available for continued research.

Selecting an appropriate strategy in this oversimplified decision situation calls for information from a wide array of sources, such as market analysts, political analysts, distribution specialists, lawyers, medical researchers, pharmacological specialists, production specialists, and cost accountants. If early estimates about relevant variables indicate that none of the strategies would produce viable results, the basic objective should be abandoned. This means that setting objectives is, in itself, a planning activity. Note that some of these information sources are outside the organization, some are at high levels within the organization, and some are at lower levels within the organization. This means that information collection and use must involve systems to transmit the need for information and individual items of information across various organization boundaries. The breadth of this information need is determined by the variety of activities needed to meet the objective. Therefore, early questions to be answered include what activities must be accomplished in order to successfully provide significant pharmaceutical relief to the AIDS pandemic and what information will be needed to assure that these activities are performed efficiently and effectively. An important point here is that the information needed by managers cannot be determined until the activities essential to obtaining the organization's objectives are determined.

OPERATIONAL PLANS   *Operational plans* are specific, preestablished sequences of actions to reach specific short-term objectives. Operational planning deals with specific activities necessary to meet the production needs of a set time frame under an existing strategy. The operational planning cycle has come to be the annual business cycle, and the operations plans are the basis for annual budgeting. Operations plans are built on projections of production needed to meet sales plans for the operating period. Budgets for the period can then be derived from an analysis of the activities needed to achieve the planned sales and estimates of the cost of resources needed for those activities. An extremely important fact in considering strategic and operations planning is that both begin with the market. Equally important, planning must be based on analysis of the activities necessary to reach the objectives. Much of this book will deal with analyses of these activities and the cost of the resources needed to complete them.

Organizing

The production and distribution of wellness interventions, as with many other products, requires a great variety of skills and specialized equipment. The expertise to apply these skills cannot be had by a single person. Hence, the industry has specialization; the necessary skills are distributed among groups of people who make up the organization. Organizing concerns deciding how these people (and the resources they use) are grouped and linked so as to maximize efficiency across all the activities needed to accomplish the organization's mission. *Staffing* is the process of selecting specific people to fill positions within the organization. Specialization is a consideration because it is usually both effective and efficient to have the work of people using similar skills coordinated and supervised by a person highly competent in using those skills. The nature of long-term assets needed is a consideration for similar reasons. As an example, surgeons apply similar knowledge and skills and use the same long-term assets (those in a surgical suite). It is logical for the management of surgical activities to be under a single person, such as the chief of surgery. This manager is the focal person for one set of activities, among many, that may be required to care for a patient—that is, the surgical procedures. The concept of organization based on the advantages of specialization needs little explanation today. However, an optimal organization structure for a specific organization is not obvious and may differ greatly in different situations. For example, should all surgical patients be placed in a completely surgical ward after leaving the recovery room? Under what conditions is this, or is this not, practical or efficient? If follow-up care for surgical patients is not managed by surgical specialists, who should manage the ward, and how should it be staffed? In somewhat the same vein, because addressing different illnesses uses different diagnostic tests and treatments that use different, specialized high-tech equipment, should management of these processes be grouped by the illness (cardiological, pulmonary, oncological, etc.) or by the technology applied? Are high-tech radiological diagnostic procedures for cancer patients better managed by radiologists or an oncologist? Dividing people and assets into modules to permit the desired quality of performance at adequate levels of efficiency is the rationale for departmentalization within the organization.

Producing a specific output generally requires integrating the activities of various departments. In a hospital, the treatment of a patient requires activities by administrative, diagnostic, medical, radiological, surgical, nursing, dietetic, and other personnel. To treat the patient effectively and efficiently, these activities must be managed. The effectiveness and efficiency of treatment is dependent both on the quality of the specialized activities and the quality of the coordination among the specialists. From the standpoint of the patient, the treatment is the integrated application of all the activities necessary to effect a cure. From a clinical perspective, understanding the case involves understanding the clinical activities applied to the case. From an economic perspective, understanding the case involves understanding the resources demanded by the activities needed to care for the patient. The implications of these facts in producing adequate cost data for management decisions is a primary subject of this book.

Leading

When managers make decisions whose implementation involves other people, the activities required of these people and any constraints that must be placed on their freedom to act must be communicated to them. Additionally, managers must communicate with members of their organization and generally conduct themselves in ways that motivate people to work cooperatively toward the organization's mission. Effective leadership is the subject of literature in the field of organization behavior. Accounting is not deeply involved in leading, but because parts of the system used to communicate information derived from management accounting data is also used to communicate directives, management accountants must become aware of problems caused by this joint use. For accountants, procedures for reporting information to its users are frequently intertwined with leading and leadership.

Controlling

Robert Anthony stated that "management control is the process by which managers influence other members of the organization to implement the organization's strategy."[12] The control function is needed at all levels of management. Anthony goes on to differentiate task control as " . . . the process of assuring that specific tasks are carried out effectively and efficiently."[13] At either level of detail and specificity, the control function involves seeing that the objectives of plans are realized. When they are not, control initiates the process of revising the objective, the plan, or the quality of process performance. Variables affecting economic implications involve volumes of outputs, the technologies applied in their production, the integration of production and distribution activities, their costs, and the revenue derived from sales. Management accounting is deeply involved in accurate measurement of these variables and communicating the control information derived from them.

DISCUSSION QUESTIONS

1. What are the differences between the content and use of management, as opposed to financial accounting?
2. What are the differences between "decision-model" and "decision-maker" approaches to determining measurements to support management decisions?
3. Why are accounting measurements more important to planning and controlling than to organizing and leading?

4. What is the difference between a mission and a strategy?
5. What is the relationship between markets and organizations' missions?

NARROWING THE MANAGEMENT ACCOUNTING ARENA

In fundamental ways, all activities of an organization affect its economic situation. According to the American Accounting Association's definition given in the first paragraph of this chapter, accounting should involve measuring and communicating information about all activities. Doing this would necessitate a wider array of skills than accountants, or any other specialists, could handle. Accounting's focus tends to be on information derived through quantitative measures, though the quantities are not limited to dollars.

Among necessary quantitative measures, those related to potential demands for services and the share of those demands that the organization can expect to acquire are generally left to marketing specialists. Marketing also assumes responsibility for estimating prices the market can be expected to pay. Estimates for the prices the organization must pay for the resources it uses are generally left to purchasing and personnel managers, though the use of these estimates in activity analysis is the work of accountants. Clinical information on the effectiveness of protocols is generally measured by clinical specialists. Again, this measurement by nonaccountants may be transmitted to accountants in order that the relative efficacy of protocols can be compared to their relative cost.

As information systems are increasingly used to integrate more types of data, accountants are becoming more involved with clinicians and computer support experts in designing decision support systems. For instance, analyzing the availability and cost of capital funds is the work of the finance staff and banking consultants. Measuring the amount of capital needed uses the efforts of management accountants. The dividing line between accounting and financial management is less well-drawn than this division implies. Both specialists use dollar amounts as a common denominator, and, quite often, both sets of activities are under the direction of a chief financial officer (CFO). In small organizations, some people may be involved in both types of work. This all means that management accountants must maintain close coordination and open communication channels with other activities within the organization.

Because much of the information used in the control function is dollar denominated and produced by management accounting, reporting information for control purposes has traditionally fallen to management accountants. However, when this information indicates the organization is not moving toward its objectives as planned, deciding on corrective action demands information on why this is happening. It is valuable for managers to know that problems exist. Information to indicate why they exist is of even greater value. Therefore, optimal management information includes both the degree to which objectives are being reached and the state of activities necessary to reach them.

EXPANDING MANAGEMENT ACCOUNTING BEYOND MONEY MEASUREMENT

The survival of economic organizations, with the exception of not-for-profit organizations that are continually provided charity or grant capital, depends on revenue. In a for-profit organization, revenue provides the inflow of cash that leads to the ability to pay obligations, create retained earnings for reinvestment, and pay dividends to owners. If revenue does not provide adequate earnings before interest and taxes, cash from prior capitalization will run out. At this point, the organization is not able to pay its expenses, modernize, or expand to meet competition. Because it is unable to meet current creditor or equity holders' demands for return on their investments, it will generally be unable to raise more cash and will become bankrupt. Not-for-profit organizations with inadequate revenue will also become unable to meet existing obligations and will need additional injections of equity from charity or grants. Their ability to get this cash depends on the level of support from their community. This, in turn, depends on the degree to which the community believes it is being served by the organization. Continual injections of capital into nongovernment, not-for-profit health care organizations are relatively small and relatively rare. This is the reason that in health care, the financial management of for-profit and not-for-profit providers is much the same. In most cases, they both depend on revenue for survival.

Adequacy of revenue depends on the costs it must cover. These include the costs of modernization and expansion as well as operating expenses. To the extent that operating expenses are reduced, a given level or revenue will provide more money for modernization and expansion. The absolute amount of revenue earned depends on the quantity of services sold and their prices. These, in turn, depend on the market's demand and its perception of the quality of the services provided. These things can be measured by such variables as market share, patient satisfaction, and payer satisfaction. These are lagging variables, in that they are the result of past management action, and their amounts reflect historical conditions. Managers also need measurement on variables that cause improvement in these lagging variables. These are called *leading variables* and indicate the degree to which service providers are doing what is necessary to assure high-quality care, low expenses, customer satisfaction, and its resultant high revenue. As an example, a hospital may find that it has a 13 percent share of the emergency room business in its drawing area, and it may be using only 30 percent of its emergency room capacity. Patient satisfaction surveys might indicate that waiting times for services are thought to be too long, and the competing hospitals have better reputations for prompt attention. Waiting time should become a measure of quality of service. As it is shortened, emergency room revenue can be expected to climb. Waiting time is therefore considered a leading, quantitative measure for management control. Its measurement would become a task for management accounting. Reports that contain such leading indicators, as well as lagging money measurements of performance, are referred to as *balanced score cards*. The concept of balanced score card reporting is discussed in some detail in Chapter 16.

DISCUSSION QUESTIONS

1. What types of measurements are generally considered the responsibility of management accounting? Why?
2. What is the primary difference between lagging and leading variables associated with revenue?
3. Why should measurements of leading variables be reported to management in addition to common lagging variables which are currently in financial statements?

FOR-PROFIT AND NOT-FOR-PROFIT OBJECTIVES

One difference between health care and most other societal needs is that the health care industry has both for-profit and not-for-profit producers. In the for-profit (business) arena, providing a product is not the organization's basic objective—it is the means to the basic objective. For a business organization in a market society, the basic objective is profit. This is why not-for-profit organizations are often called *nonbusiness organizations*. To understand differences in the information needs of for-profit as opposed to not-for-profit organizations in health care, we should look more closely at this difference in objectives.

A market society uses the price-profit mechanism as its primary means of answering its fundamental economic questions: What shall we produce? What resources (including people) and technologies shall be used in production? And, who will get the things produced? The mechanism assumes that people will pay a price for products up to the amount at which they would get more benefit from spending their money on something else. A business organization can, therefore, make a profit only if it produces things that people value more than other products they can buy for the same amount of their money. To be successful, a for-profit organization must understand what markets want produced and the value the markets place on those things. If this is the case, the needs and desires of the members of society can be met through businesses' pursuit of profit.

An assumption in operating a market economy is that all members must have money with which to buy. Obviously, if some people do not have adequate amounts of money, they cannot purchase needed products at any price. If the society feels certain products—for instance, a given level of health care—should be available to everyone, there are three ways to furnish such things to those who cannot pay. The products can be produced for them by a not-for-profit organization, bought for them by a charity or government-funded organization, or given to them through charity from its for-profit producers. Health care is provided to medically indigent people by all three of these methods. However, whichever approach is used, people with money pick up the cost of care for people without money. This occurs through (1) providers charging higher prices than necessary to those who can pay in order to cover the costs of those who can't, (2) charitable contributions by people with money to organizations that produce or fund care for indigents, and (3) the government taxing those with the ability to pay in order to fund care for those who lack the ability to fund themselves.

There are two other key assumptions needed in order for a market economy to serve a society well. The first is that the buyers understand the relative benefits of all the products available and know the prices of these products. This is called the *perfect-knowledge assumption*. It allows buyers to make appropriate choices in spending limited funds among alternative products. The second is that, for each product available, there are many suppliers attempting to increase their revenue by selling a better product at the same price or the same product at a lower price than their competitors. This could be called the *competition imperative*. If these assumptions are operating, competition among producers attempting to sell to well-informed customers controls prices and promotes improvements in both products and services.

Whether a health care organization is a profit-seeking business or a not-for-profit entity, it must acquire funds in quantities great enough to pay for the resources it uses, including the periodic cost of new equipment needed to maintain modern medical practices. This means that managers of either type of organization must make decisions about the products desired by the market and the sources of money to buy the resources needed to produce those products. (For our purposes, both goods and services produced for sale will be called *products*.) Classic management theory has tended to flow from the study of for-profit businesses. It therefore focuses on sales revenue as the primary source of continuing funding. Money capital to meet large, periodic needs can be acquired by debt or the sale of equity to stockholders, but the price of this capital (interest on debt and profit on equity) must be paid from future revenue. Because revenue comes from sales, establishing strategy focuses on alternative ways to gain levels of sales necessary to survive among competitors. Not-for-profit care deliverers are at a disadvantage with respect to acquiring new capital; when debt and donations from charity or government or private grants are not available, they have no ability to raise private ownership equity. To the extent that additional injections of capital from government and charities are not available to not-for-profit care deliverers, they are dependent on debt and revenue. If they have borrowed beyond their debt limit, they must compete for this revenue with other not-for-profit and for-profit providers. The result of this financial reality is that not-for-profit care deliverers must make the same types of decisions that for-profit businesses must make in establishing their mission, selecting strategies, and budgeting from operational plans. This means that they also have the same demands for information to support the same types of decisions.

Though not-for-profit organizations are not required to bear the cash expense of taxes paid by for-profit care providers, governments have increased the enforcement of their obligations to meet tax responsibilities by providing unreimbursed services to their communities. However, not-for-profit providers do have a distinct advantage in the amount of revenue they can keep because they do not have to suffer cash outflows to pay the cost of their equity capital through dividend distribution. The primary difference in the information needs of not-for-profit care deliverers is information needed to secure equity capital from charity and direct community inputs and information needed to maintain their tax-free status.

DISCUSSION QUESTIONS

1. Why is the financial management of a not-for-profit health care organization essentially similar to that of a for-profit provider?
2. From question 1, in what ways do its financial pressures differ?

Conclusion

Health care deliverers are currently under severe financial pressure. The purchasing power of large third-party payers gives those payers unprecedented control of revenue. To a great extent, deliverers of care have become price takers rather than price setters. This means that care-delivering organizations' control over their revenue primarily rests in managing the volume of their sales. At any volume of sales, potential profit—even if the goal is simply to break even—is tied to costs. Costs occur from the use of resources in the activities necessary to deliver care. In responding to needs for care, there are usually alternative actions available. Efficient care delivery is produced when the lowest cost alternatives that produce acceptable quality of care are selected. Choosing these alternatives requires information on the quality of their outcomes, activities they involve, and the resources they consume. Assuring the financial survival of health care organization, therefore, depends to a large extent on the effectiveness of the organization's use of internal information to make sound decisions about activities leading to market success. Access to equity capital that can assure long term viability demands this success.

KEY POINTS

- Accounting involves identifying, measuring, and communicating economic information to support decisions.
- Financial accounting supports decisions that people outside the organization make about their relationship with the organization.
- Management accounting supports decisions that are made within the organization by its managers.
- Decision-model approaches to generate information use predetermined, normative methods to identify variables and measure them, such as GAAP.
- Decision-maker approaches to generate information analyze specific decision-makers' models to isolate and measure the variables used in those models.
- Managers' work involves assuring that planning, organizing, staffing, leading, and controlling functions are performed within the organization.
- Planning involves setting sequences of actions needed to reach objectives.
- Determining a mission involves finding a product or service that is needed by society and could be supplied by the organization.
- Strategic planning involves setting a general approach for accomplishing a stated mission.
- Setting objectives involves determining specific ends that must be accomplished in order to fulfill a mission.
- Setting goals involves establishing measures that indicate that missions or objectives have been accomplished.
- Operational planning sequences specific activities that are to be done in order to meet specific objectives within an operating period, usually a year.
- Organizing involves setting a structure of work and resource units through which to accomplish plans.
- Staffing involves selecting specific individuals for specific roles within the organization's structure.
- Leading involves motivating the organization's members to work together to accomplish the organization's mission.
- Controlling involves assuring that the organization is reaching its objectives and revising objectives and/or plans as appropriate.
- Decisions made in performing these functions all demand that information be used in an appropriate decision model.
- Measurements related to the demand for products and the selling prices of products are usually left to marketing personnel.
- Measurements related to resource prices are usually left to purchasing and personnel managers.
- Measurements related to resource utilization and costs are made by management accountants.
- Measurements from accounting, marketing, purchasing, and personnel activities must be integrated to support managers' decisions. This is usually the responsibility of management accounting.
- Generally, both for-profit and not-for-profit health care organizations depend on revenues and cost control to maintain their viability. Therefore, financial management and management accounting are much the same in both types of organizations.
- For-profit organizations have the advantage of access to owners' equity.
- The efficiency of for-profit organizations'

service to society is tied to the validity of the perfect knowledge assumption and the competition imperative.

- Not-for-profit organizations are expected to "pay" taxes through community service. They are usually not under equal pressure to pay for their equity capital.
- Market success for businesses can be measured in profit. For not-for-profit organizations, it can be measured as ac-

counting surpluses and the degree to which the organization furnishes unremunerated services to its community.

- The key point is that viability is dependent on efficient performance, which depends on high-quality management decisions. These, in turn, require effective decision models and good information.

EXERCISES

EXERCISE 1
It might be said that the development of managers begins with the process of the aspiring managers learning to manage themselves. Before discussing identifying, measuring, and presenting information to support the management of a health care delivery organization, consider the role of basic management functions in managing the activities necessary to prepare oneself for an entry health-services management position.

Assume you are such a person.

1. For each function, briefly state the activities that will be involved as your preparation proceeds.
2. What information will you need in

order to (1) plan your preparation, (2) organize the resources for the activities that will be involved in the process, (3) motivate (lead) the activities of others related to your mission, and (4) control your preparation process. Make a list of the information items needed to support each of the four management functions.

EXERCISE 2
Divide the information items you have listed in Exercise 1 into those best presented in terms of dollars and those best presented in other units of measure.

REFERENCES

[1] American Accounting Association. *A Statement of Basic Accounting Theory* (Sarasota, FL: American Accounting Association, 1966), p. 1.
[2] ———. *Statement on Accounting Theory and Theory Acceptance* (Sarasota, FL: American Accounting Association, 1977), p. 10.
[3] Koontz, Harold, Cyril O'Donnel, and Heinz

Wehrich. *Management* (New York: McGraw-Hill, 1984), p. 64.
[4] Mintzberg, Henry. *The Nature of Managerial Work* (New York: Harper & Row, 1973), Chapter 2.
[5] Keeney, Ralph and Harold Raiffa. *Decisions with Multiple Objectives: Preferences and Value Trade-*

offs (New York: John Wiley and Sons, 1976), Chapter 2.

[6] Mintzberg, Henry. *The Rise and Fall of Strategic Planning* (New York: Free Press, 1994), p. 7.

[7] Ibid., p. 11.

[8] Ibid., Chapter 3.

[9] About Health Alliance, U Mass Memorial Health Alliance, www.healthalliance.com (accessed October 5, 2003).

[10] About Pfizer, Pfizer, Inc., www.pfizer.com/pfizerinc/about/mission (accessed October 5, 2003).

[11] Ibid.

[12] Anthony, Robert. *The Management Control Function* (Boston: Harvard Business School Press, 1988), p.34.

[13] Ibid., p. 37.

CHAPTER 2

MANAGEMENT ACCOUNTING AND INTERNAL DECISION MAKING

DECISION CHARACTERISTICS

Because our focus is on providing information in support of management decisions, it may be helpful to discuss some elements of the decision-making processes. In taking the decision-maker perspective, we define the term *decision* broadly, taking the approach that decision analysis is composed of processes in which an individual decision maker contemplates a choice among actions. Because there are many ways decisions can be classified, we will consider classifying them by two characteristics that relate to accounting inputs. The first is the degree to which the problem and the decision process are well specified. The second is the spectrum from routine to nonroutine.

Specificity

The specificity of the problem deals with how much is known about the problem environment: what is going on, what variables are important to a good solution, how the variables affect each other, how they can be analyzed, and what the criteria are for choosing a solution. Management accounting is made easier when the problem and the variables that should be considered in solving the problem can be well specified.

Routineness

Routine decisions are made in frequently recurring instances of the same basic problem. Examples include the daily staffing of a ward or clinic, the amount of cash to leave in checking accounts, the amount of a specific supply to reorder, and whether or not to contact a physician when a patient's signs change. With routine decisions, the basic problem is familiar, but decisions may change because of changes in the circumstances within which the current problem exists.

Other types of decisions occur infrequently. Examples include whether to set a new strategy, to add or drop specific services, to buy specific "big-ticket" long-term assets, to attempt to change management culture, or to use in-service versus off-installation contract training (and to what extent). Making nonroutine decisions tend to take on characteristics of a project. They usually address a specific issue about which there is little precedence. These decisions can affect the organization for an extended period of time.

DISCUSSION QUESTIONS

1. In what ways are the characteristics of specificity and routineness related?
2. What factors tend to lower the specificity of a problem?

DECISION MODELS

Decision makers use special kinds of models and procedures in their decision making. These procedures may be loose in term, and only partially specified, but guide the decision maker's behavior. As Mintzberg points out, "The brain must use some procedure—some higher order program—to react to any stimulus."[1] It is important to realize that the proper starting point for designing an information system is understanding the array of decisions that people within the organization must make, and the way they make them. This is not a trivial task. For management accountants, a critical step is to determine what information the decision maker seeks in making each type of decision. The more one deviates from well-structured, routine decisions, the harder this becomes. If the decisions are routine, the organization has probably evolved standard decision processes for which the information requirements are well known. As one moves to less-specified, periodic problems, the decision processes become more manager specific. It then becomes the job of management accountants and information-system managers to ferret out the information needs of the managers' decision models. This will be discussed later. The following further explains decision processes and information demands in general.

A great amount of research has been done on the basic approaches people use to make decisions. Essentially, this literature treats decision and choice as synonymous terms.[2] It also contends that decisions involve making choices among alternatives. James March points out that rational decisions, or choices, are based on the answer to four questions:[3]

1. What are the results sought?
2. What is the set of alternative actions possible?
3. What will be the results of each alternative action?
4. What rules will be used to select the alternative chosen?

Certain outcomes are desired when solving problems. These results have specific criteria on which their quality is evaluated. In deciding whether to add a product line, some of these criteria might be the extent to which the new services would improve community health and produce revenue. Also, the incremental cost to provide it and the extent to which the product line would increase use of other product lines are criteria.

Such criteria for evaluating an alternative define *attributes* of the decision outcome. In making decisions, people select among alternatives by evaluating the alternatives on the attributes they are seeking. Research has shown that people tend to follow certain approaches or models when doing this evaluation.[4] These models have associated *choice rules* for picking from among alternatives. Different people in different situations use different types of models. The combination of decision models, attributes, and choice rules used for the decisions faced by an organization determine the information that the organization must manage. This will be evident as some commonly used models are discussed.

When facing routine problems, the real problem is quickly isolated; it is recognized as it occurs. Through past experience, the decision maker formulates a model (an organized approach) for selecting among alternative actions that could solve the problem. When faced with less-routine problems, the results of the selected action must have certain levels of an array of specific attributes. The decision model must guide the decision maker in considering and integrating these attributes. A common example from everyday life may be helpful. Suppose that you, a graduate student, have had your car die. It is unrecoverably "dead." You must now solve your personal transportation problem. Because you have been brought up with the American transportation bias, you see no choice but to buy another car. You have thousands of alternative cars available—how do you choose among them? The first thing you do (consciously or unconsciously) is list the attributes your car must have. A possible set includes being inexpensive and efficient to operate, or an acceptable color, style, and size, as well as having adequate power and handling characteristics.

Some of these attributes are obviously conflicting. In most cases, the bigger, the better handling, and the more powerful the car, hence, the higher the price and operating cost. Such conflicts create significant decision problems. Several types of decision models have been found in common use. The type of model used depends on the importance of the decision, its complexity, and the time available in which to make the choice among alternative solutions.

Noncompensatory Models

Noncompensatory simply means that the choice rule does not allow for a high score on one attribute to compensate for a low score on another. Consider three commonly used noncompensatory models.

CONJUNCTIVE MODELS When using conjunctive models, one looks at all relevant attributes in conjunction with each other. For a solution to be chosen, it must pass the test of acceptance on each attribute. This type of rule obviously assumes that measures of the attributes exist (enter management accountants). In applying a conjunctive rule, thresholds are set for the measure of each attribute. For an alternative to be selected, it must meet or exceed each threshold. Going back to the example of a graduate student buying a car, the following could be the thresholds for each attribute:

Price: < $8,000
Efficiency: > 25 mpg
Rated better than average on maintenance cost by *Consumer Reports*
Color: White, red, or metallic gray
Style: Sport coupe
Size: Intermediate or larger
Power: 0 to 60 mph in < 8 secs
Handling: Better than average, as rated by *Consumer Reports*

In applying the conjunctive choice rule, the student would buy only the car that met all of these thresholds. If more than one car passed the tests, the thresholds on the most-wanted attributes can be increased. This continues until only one car is left.

If one car does not meet all the thresholds, the decision maker must

- Decide which attributes can tolerate a lower threshold until one car does meet them all.
- Expand the search for cars from which to buy.
- Expand the search for other ways to meet the personal transportation needs.

The choice rule is to select the action that meets the thresholds finally set for each attribute.

DISJUNCTIVE MODELS Disjunctive rules are simpler and generally yield less satisfactory decisions. With them, attributes are also selected and thresholds set for each one. However, with disjunctive models, the choice rule is to simply select the alternative that meets the most threshold requirements.

LEXICOGRAPHICAL MODELS Like the models already discussed, lexicographical models demand the selection of attributes to be considered and a measurement on each attribute. However, this type of model does not use thresholds. Instead, it demands that the decision maker prioritize the attributes from most important to least important. The choice rule is rather simple. Consider the most important attribute first. If an alternative exceeds all others on the measure of that attribute, it is selected. If more than one of the alternatives tie, then the process moves to the second most important attribute and picks the alternative among the previous ties, with the highest score on the second most important attribute. If there is a tie at the second level of screening, the process goes on until only one alternative remains.

Compensatory Models

Compensatory models allow trade-offs among attributes. In the car example, the buyer could trade more power for less efficiency or accept less than their favorite color in order to get the style preferred. This is done by using scalar measures and attaching weights to the attributes. Weights can be attached in various ways. Again, look at the example of purchasing a car. An acceptable level for all the attributes that are measured could be set using a ratio or ordinal scale. For instance, say that 18 miles per gallon (mpg) is a good reference point for evaluating fuel economy. Fuel economy could be weighted by awarding three points for every mile per gallon over 18 and subtracting three points for every mile per gallon under 18. Therefore, a car getting 23 miles to the gallon would be awarded 15 points for fuel economy ($[23 - 18] \times 3$). One getting 15 miles to the gallon would be awarded -9 points ($[15 - 18] \times 3$). Similarly, the buyer could use 12 seconds from 0 to 60 mph as the reference for power. Decide instead to award four points for every second under 12 and subtract two points for every second over 12. If the car under consideration accelerated to 60 mph in 14 seconds, it would get a weighted power score of -4 ($[14 - 12] \times [-2]$). When the attribute is measured using a nominal scale, as would be the case in considering the color, simply attach a weight to each color. The weight reflects the relative preference. For instance, assign eight points for white, four points for red, and two points for metallic gray. All other colors would get no points or negative points.

The relative weights given to different attributes depend on how the relative importance of the attributes are rated. If a white car is desired, weight white as 200 points. These 200 points would swamp all the other weights, and the buyer would be assured of picking a white car if one is available. Similarly, if power is most important, award 100 points for every second under 12 seconds on the zero to 60 mph attribute. The specific set of weights used depends on the preferences of the decision maker, or more rationally, on the relationships among the attributes considered and the overall outcome desired. The choice rule is to select the action with the highest total score. To develop a good compensatory model, the problem must be understood quite well. If the problem is understood and the time is available to work out a compensatory rule, it should give the decision maker a better solution than would a noncompensatory rule.

Notice that compensatory rules take on the form of mathematical formulae. If they are used on frequently recurring problems in which the decision maker routinely measures the attributes of the alternative solutions, they lend themselves nicely to computerization. Also notice that to use a computer to solve such problems (make such choices) on short notice, the measures of the attributes must be in a readily accessible database. Notice, too, that for a computer solution to be available on short notice, the decision model, and the appropriate measures for its attributes, must have been determined ahead of time.

DISCUSSION QUESTIONS

1. What are the relationships among decision models, decision attributes, measurements, and choice rules?
2. What makes compensatory decision models generally produce better decisions than noncompensatory models?
3. What are the advantages of noncompensatory decision models?
4. When must a nominal variable be given ordinal or ratio measures?
5. How does management accounting relate to decision processes?

INFORMATION SYSTEMS

Management accounting measurements are of no value unless they furnish the information needed for managerial decisions as they occur. Using management accounting, therefore, demands an information system that can provide the appropriate information in usable form to the appropriate decision maker at the proper time.

Appropriate Information

We will later, in some detail, address the relationship between the nature of a problem, its solution, and the information sought. Now, we simply point out that appropriate information is the information needed to make the decision at hand and solve the problem being addressed. This means that *the decisions that must be made constitute the starting point for information-system design.* System design should not, as is frequently done, begin with a listing of information that is currently available. One of the great advantages of the support that computers can give to information systems is the quantity of data and analysis programs that can be continuously stored and rapidly disseminated to specific users. However, this capability can be a mixed blessing. It can lead to a great quantity of inappropriate information flowing to decision makers. Quite possibly, the greatest cause of good information not being used is that it is lost in a sea of unwanted or redundant messages.

Usable Form

Because decision makers are looking for specific items of information to use in their decision processes, the system should provide those items in quickly understandable formats. To be most effective, the formats should show only that for which the decision maker is looking.

Appropriate Recipient

One reason that decision makers using reports from their information system must wade through the sea of messages inappropriate for their needs is that the reports contain information for people other than the one who must make the specific decision at hand. A good system allows decision makers to rapidly "pull out" what they need, undiluted by what they do not need.

Proper Timing

It is human nature when one discovers a problem to immediately want all the information that may be useful in its solution. This is feasible to varying degrees, depending on the nature of the needed information. At the other extreme, information that is received after the time at which a decision must be made is useless to that decision. The ability to get adequate amounts of appropriate information in time to apply it to a specific decision depends on several factors. First is the awareness of an appropriate decision model and the information it uses. This is the result of previous analyses of the types of decisions that will be demanded, and storage of the data relevant to them. If the information is not in the system, timeliness is dependent on the speed of information search procedures. Timeliness also depends on the ability of the decision maker to rapidly call for and receive the appropriate information from the system.

Daily staffing of a ward illustrates the concepts just discussed. The demand for nurses on a given day depends almost entirely on the number of patients on the ward and the patients' demands for nursing interventions. Therefore, the problem is fairly well specified. Projected ward census and patient acuity data can be measured and put into a database. Each night there is a need to make the staffing decision for the following day; therefore, the staffing problem is routine. Early each morning, a nursing administrator can access the database and call in the number of supplemental nurse-pool personnel needed for the coming day. The decision that must be made is the reason for having the census and acuity measures, the database and communication system, and a software model for computing the number of nurses needed from the data provided. The starting point for designing this system is the need for efficient staffing decisions on a daily basis. This decision is emphasized as the starting point because, all too frequently, organizations have bought sophisticated computer and telecommunications equipment, added some "slick" software, and then asked themselves, "How do we want to use this stuff?"

DISCUSSION QUESTIONS

1. What should be the starting point of designing an information system?
2. What components should an effective information system have? What resources and tools are necessary?
3. What are the characteristics of a good information system? What specific failures can occur if they do not exist?

INFORMATION SYSTEMS AND THE DECISION ENVIRONMENT

Providing appropriate measures for decision makers, therefore, involves four basic steps:

1. Determine the types of decisions managers make and the models they use to make them.
2. Identify the independent variables in these models.
3. Get measurements of these variables.
4. Report the measures to the appropriate managers.

Aside from the problems involved in valid and reliable measurement, general problems that complicate managers' decision making exist in human thought processes and the environment in which decisions are made. These problems complicate management accounting.

Decision-Maker Problems

Research into human mental processes and capabilities of decision makers has discovered phenomena that limit an individual's ability to make effective decisions. This research shows that there are bounds on people's rationality.[5] In addressing problems, people tend to depend on their personal experience and acquired biases to determine solutions. They frequently do not adequately search for other possible approaches. The graduate student car purchasing problem gives an example. It may be that leasing is a rational alternative to purchasing. Or, it could be that using public transportation for routine travel on most days and renting a car for other trips is as convenient and, over time, cheaper than purchasing. However, a bias toward car ownership prevents considering these alternatives. Biases can also cause a lack of comprehensiveness in attention to specific consequences. Again, with reference to a car purchase, a bias toward ownership may have the buyer considering the increased per-mile cost of renting a car but not considering the cost of garaging and parking cars they own.

People also seem to have significant limits on their ability to process information that is available. One is the inability to mentally manipulate more than two or three variables concurrently. Models that consider too many variables can confuse as well as help. As a result, managers may try to simplify decision situations by eliminating variables they believe do not have a material effect on outcomes. This can lead to incomplete and badly misspecified decision models. Planners may not consider the increased traffic flow associated with a new hospital as a significant variable in planning its location and later find that objections from residents block obtaining a building permit. Decision makers may also break a complicated problem into a sequence of more simple problems. This can cause solutions to the individual problems to be optimized at the expense of the quality of the solution to the general problem. For instance, in attempting to increase profitability, a clinic may schedule patients for early arrival in order to reduce un-billable physician and equipment time. However, the resultant waiting times might cause patients to seek care elsewhere. Another tendency in complicated situations is to develop overly simple *rules of thumb*. These are easy to apply but may produce solutions that are far from optimal. An example would be to always purchase the lowest priced supplies, despite the fact that periodic late delivery may cause expensive work stoppage or litigation.

These weaknesses in human decision making are compounded by any lack of understanding or specification of the problem. Decision makers may not understand what attributes of actions taken will solve the problem at hand. When they do understand the decision attributes that should be sought, they may not understand what actions will produce those attributes. Any shortcoming here reduces the possibility of the decision model being valid and effective. If the model is not valid, at least some of the variables and relationships it uses will be inappropriate. Collecting and reporting data on these variables will be of no help to the organization. The cost of the related management accounting efforts will be wasted. Effective and efficient management of information that supports managers is therefore dependent on managers themselves, management accountants, and information technology specialists. Just as important, it is dependent on close relationships and communication among these three groups of people. Management accountants cannot support managers well until they are made aware of the decision models the managers' use and the variables within those models.

DISCUSSION QUESTIONS

1. What human characteristics limit managers' decision-making ability?
2. How can information system design help managers to overcome or compensate for these human characteristics?

Decision-Environment Problems

Thus far, we have implied that management accounting can support decision makers by

- working with them to understand their decision models
- isolating the variables used in those models
- measuring those variables
- storing the measurements and models
- assuring that this information is transmitted in easily understood forms to the decision makers when they need it

Much information system literature implies that decision support and information systems are computer- and electronic-communication systems. For routine decisions, after decision models are established, this is often the case. However, for many major decisions, equating information systems with computers and electronic communications is too simplistic. Thomas Davenport, in his work with corporate executives, has found that ". . . most executives rely on verbal information as their most important source."[6] He points out that "managers tend to get two-thirds of the information they use from human sources—most of that through face-to-face conversations, the rest from telephone conversations. The other third is structured information, most of which comes from documents about the external environment, from market research reports to industry magazines, and the *Wall Street Journal*."[7] This indicates that the concept of an information system must extend well beyond the computer and electronic-communication system, which is often referred to as the *information tech environment*. Davenport emphasizes that knowing *how* people create, distribute, understand, and use information is essential to information system structure and operation. This demands that ". . . communications with those who will be affected must be broad, frequent, and ongoing."[8]

The basic tasks needed to have information support managers' decisions must be considered as parts of a continuing process involving structures and activities that promote determining information requirements, capturing information and knowledge, distributing it, and using it. Davenport emphasizes an additional dimension of information systems, which he calls *information ecology*. It involves understanding the culture, behavior, and work processes, as well as the politics of the organization. These factors affect how people create, understand, distribute, and use information. Information ecology focuses on the correct use of appropriate information as the central objective of an information system. Failure to attend to the ecological dimension is as disastrous to the success of an organization as having inadequate computer- and electronic-communication systems. Davenport contends that attention to strategic approaches to information uses, internal political effects on information availability, organization and culture-based attitudes about what information is useful, and how it should flow are as important to the support of management as the computer or communications technology used. In fact, the information-technology portions of the information system cannot add value to the organization unless the information ecology has been addressed.

DISCUSSION QUESTIONS

1. What are the differences in emphasis between information technology and information ecology perspectives on decision making and decision systems?
2. Which should be considered first?
3. What negative effects result if each is not considered?

This book will begin by concentrating on the effects of cost on the operating decisions of organizations providing health care. It will focus on the flow of resources (hence, costs) into the activities necessary to achieve and maintain good health within the populations served by those organizations. Well-specified, continuing operations will be addressed first, and an array of accepted general models for using management accounting information in common types of decision situations will be covered. Later, decision models for less routine, ad hoc decisions will be evaluated. The use of this information shall be related primarily to planning and controlling. The final chapters will address isolating and finding useful information, as well as the content and structure of useful reports.

CONCLUSION

For good decisions to be made, problems should be understood to the degree that a decision process or decision model could be established. The variables in the model must then be defined. Measures on these variables must be made, and they must be available when decisions are needed. When the decision can be computerized, the decision model and the data on its variables can be brought together, and the resultant output can be communicated to the appropriate decision maker through the application of computer-supported information technology. However, the environment in which decisions are demanded frequently does not allow creation and application of electronic information technology. In these situations, the management accounting must also provide support to determine information needs and sources, as well as measurement and presentation. It is important to realize that problem analysis, decision-model formulation, management accounting, and information system design and operation cannot be separated. They are all essential components of management decision making. As a corollary, the academic areas of accounting, decision theory, management science, and electronic-information systems are fundamentally inseparable.

As economic considerations are applied to decisions, it is essential that the revenue and cost implication of each alternative be understood. The revenue estimates generally come from the marketing staff. Cost estimates are the responsibility of management accountants. The *relevant costs* are the costs of all the activities that must be performed if the alternative being analyzed is implemented. These activities probably occur in a variety of units, or departments, throughout the organization. Management accounting, therefore, must be based on an analysis of activities needed to reach any objective in question and the resources demanded by those activities. This, in turn, demands cross-departmental information flows that parallel the flow of activities from separate departments to the organization objectives. Management accounting frequently takes a primary role in analyzing and documenting activity flows because they form the foundation of cost analysis as well as the road map for coordination.

KEY POINTS

- Problems with high specificity are more easily modeled and supported by management accounting.
- Routine problems lend themselves to computer-supported solutions more efficiently than nonroutine problems.
- Decision makers tend to have specific approaches, or models, they use in making decisions. These involve specific variables and opinions about the relationships among them.
- Solutions are intended to produce identified attributes that indicate the quality of the solution.
- Measures of the solution attributes and choice rules allow selection among alternative solutions available.
- Compensatory decision models allow making trade-offs among various attributes to reach an overall best solution.

- Information systems should provide acceptable access to appropriate information in usable forms and in a timely manner.
- Information is appropriate when it is what the decision maker needs and is unencumbered by material that is not needed.
- Information should be presented in a form in which the desired information is quickly understood.
- Information must be available to the decision maker before the decision must be made, which means that approximate measures of appropriate information delivered on time are superior to more accurate and comprehensive information that is late.
- Human limits on mental processes should be considered when providing information to decision makers.

- Consideration of how people create, distribute, understand, and use information is essential to effective information systems. The aggregate of factors affecting these things is referred to as *information ecology.*
- Information systems must include mechanisms to monitor the information ecology and understand decision models used, as well as computer and electronic communication systems.

- Creating effective management information systems demands cross-disciplinary coordination of skills and cross-departmental communication. Responsibility for the content of the output of these systems is a joint responsibility of management decision makers and decision-system personnel.

EXERCISE

You are relocating to a city of 800,000 population in a different state. You are, therefore, looking for a place to live and will, of course, make a choice among the alternatives available.

1. List the attributes of living facilities that you believe are relevant to your choice.
2. State the measure you would use to quantify the degree to which each attribute is met by each alternative.
3. Are there any differences among the importance of the different attributes?

If there are, explain how you would handle them in making your choice.
4. Do you believe you have a well-specified decision situation? Explain why or why not.
5. Which type of decision model (of those discussed in the chapter) do you believe is most appropriate for this situation? Explain why.
6. What would be your choice rule?

REFERENCES

[1] Mintzberg, Henry. *The Nature of Managerial Work* (Englewood Cliffs, NJ: Prentice Hall, 1973), p. 135.
[2] Slovic, Paul, Baruch Fischoff, and Sarah Lichtenstern. "Behavioral Decision Theory." *Annual Review of Psychology* (1977): p. 10.
[3] March, James G. *A Primer on Decision Making* (New York: Free Press, 1994), pp. 2–3.
[4] Slovic, Paul, Baruch Fischoff, and Sarah Lichtenstern. "Behavioral Decision Theory." *Annual Review of Psychology* (1977): p. 18.

[5] March, James G. *A Primer on Decision Making.* (New York: Free Press, 1994), pp. 8–22.
[6] Davenport, Thomas H. *Information Ecology: Mastering the Information and Knowledge Environment* (New York: Oxford University Press, 1997), p. 27.
[7] Ibid., p. 98.

2 Costs and Costing

We shall now look more closely at techniques for determining how cost information can be used to improve decisions, what costs should be measured, and how they can best be measured. Chapter 3 explains the different perspective taken in viewing costs, and defines an array of cost categories. Appendix 3 explains how to make the important quantitative differentiation between fixed costs and variable costs. Chapter 4 then discusses the general types of health care products whose costs should be understood and gives an example of a relatively simple costing analysis to support a product-pricing problem. Chapter 5 defines levels of activities, their relationship to activity centers within organizations, and the concept of cost drivers. It then describes following the flow of institutional level overhead costs to products. The appendices to the chapter explain two approaches to charting the flow of costs to specific outputs. Chapter 6 discusses cost flows into production centers, costing specific products, and the use of transfer prices to create pseudo profit centers. Chapter 7 summarizes the preceding material by presenting examples of the analysis and charting of cost flows to specific centers and services or products. Chapter 8 then covers methods for isolating overhead activities whose costs should be followed and finding the drivers of these activities.

The purpose of Part II is to explain how accuracy of cost information can be optimized by analysis of the activities that cause costs to be incurred and the processes involved in the ABC approach. The final chapter in this section, Chapter 9, explains procedures managers can use to design and implement ABC systems.

LEARNING OBJECTIVES

After studying this chapter, students should be able to:

1. Define and explain the significance of

cost objects	direct and indirect costs	direct material	direct labor
traceable costs	fixed and variable costs	mixed costs	unit cost
full cost	absorption costs	product-direct costs	center-direct costs
production costs	incremental costs	marginal costs	selling costs
period costs	discretionary costs	administrative costs	relevant costs
sunk costs	committed costs	joint costs	standard costs

2. Explain the interaction between fixed-cost and variable-cost resources and the importance of differentiating them.

3. Explain the concept of marginal cost, its difference from variable cost, and its importance in decision making.

4. Explain the fixed-cost problem.

5. Explain the inappropriateness of the term true cost.

6. Explain the confusion between costs and charges in health care management.

7. Perform a cost-behavior analysis.

GENERAL CONSIDERATIONS

One point that will be stressed in this book is that the appropriate amount of cost associated with an activity or product depends on the type of decision that is being made. There are many perspectives from which the cost of a thing can be viewed. Discussion of some of these perspectives and some definitions should be helpful at this point.

The general term *cost* is used for the amount of money exchanged for an object or service obtained. It is the sum of these historical amounts that becomes the accounting valuation of a specific activity or product. In the case of a trading (buying and selling) organization, the cost of a traded item becomes the item's inventory value (used in the balance sheet) and turns into the *cost-of-goods-sold* expense when the item is sold. When moving from a trading organization to producing organizations, the concept of the cost of goods sold follows. The advantage of this perspective is that when the item is sold, we can use this value as one of the expenses associated with the sale. However, arriving at the cost of a specific item produced is much more difficult and inexact than in a trading organization, where each item is valued at the amount paid for it. Producing organizations consider the cost of an item produced as the sum of the costs of all the resources put into it.

DEFINITIONS

The following terms are commonly used to illustrate different perspectives on costs.

Cost Objects

The terms *cost object* and *cost target* are frequently used as general designation for the thing whose cost is to be understood. The cost object could be a department within the organization, an activity within a department, a product or a service produced by one department for use by another, or a product or service produced for sale outside the organization. Because outputs of health care organizations can be both tangible products and services, these terms are used almost synonymously; that is, a service is considered a product when the differentiation is not important.

Production Costs

Production costs refer to costs incurred to produce an output for sale. It is important to realize that the models for "costing" output were developed largely by firms manufacturing material goods—that is, physical things. Traditionally, production costs have been those incurred in the factory, as opposed to other parts of the organization.

Direct Costs

Let us use handmade shoes as an example. It is relatively easy to measure the quantity of leather, thread, nails, glue, inner-sole material, heels, and other materials used in a pair of shoes. One can actually see the flow of these materials into each pair of shoes and can observe how much of each is used on one pair. One can also measure the time spent by different types of labor on each pair. Because the price paid for each type of material and labor is known, the cost of resources that are directly traceable to the product can be computed. These cost elements have traditionally been divided into two categories: direct material and direct labor.

Indirect Costs

Other types of costs that must be incurred by the organization in order to manufacture shoes include rental of buildings and equipment, salaries of supervisors who do not work directly on the shoes, janitorial services in the factory, heating, and lighting, and the like. In most cases, these costs cannot be physically traced to units of each product, or if they can, the cost of tracing is more than the value of the information. These types of costs are called *indirect costs,* or *production overhead costs* when they are related to manufacturing processes. The terms *indirect cost* and *overhead* are used synonymously.

Two subcategories of overhead exist: fixed and variable.

Fixed Overhead. For an accounting period, *fixed production overhead* is composed of costs that must be paid whether or not the organization produces anything. They are the same amount for a period over a great range of production quantities. Fixed costs often become fixed through some sort of contract. For instance, equipment rent must be paid whether or not the equipment is used. Similarly, salaried employees are paid whether or not there is work for them during each "working" hour.

Variable Overhead. In addition to fixed production overhead, there is also *variable production overhead*. This category contains indirect costs elements whose total during an accounting period increases as output increases. An example is lubricants. Company management does not keep track of (trace) how much machine lubricant is used in producing each pair of shoes, but they do know more lubricant is used in periods of high production. Variable overhead is expressed as the average increase in overhead as production increases. It can be measured in dollars per unit of production. Note that because direct labor and direct material costs are measured by the amount of these resources traced to a unit of production, these two cost categories can also be expressed in dollars per unit of output. Therefore, three categories of variable production costs exist: (1) direct labor, (2) direct materials, and (3) variable overhead. Each can be expressed in dollars per unit of output. They can be summed to get a total variable manufacturing cost per unit of output. If this cost for each type of product made is multiplied by the quantity of each product and these amounts summed, the organization's total variable production cost for an accounting period can be determined.

JOINT COST A *joint cost resource* is one that must be purchased in order to produce any or all of a number of products. A classic example is a pig. To produce hams, bacon, pork shoulders, tenderloins, or pigs' feet, a pig must first be purchased. The problem is determining how much of the price of the pig should be considered a cost of producing hams as opposed to pigs' feet. To determine a cost for each product, there must be a system established for distributing the cost of the pig (the joint cost) among the rather different products derived from it. Another example is a barrel of crude oil. Its cost must be divided among products varying from extremely light lubricants to kerosene, to the foundation for petroleum-based fertilizers. Various ways to distribute joint costs will be discussed later.

BALANCE OF FIXED COSTS VERSUS VARIABLE COSTS

The relative amounts of fixed and variable cost resources used in production has shifted greatly over the past 40 years. This is especially true in health care delivery. During this period, the capabilities of medical equipment have increased dramatically. The cost of this increasingly sophisticated equipment has also risen dramatically. Concurrently, the wages of nurses and other salaried clinicians have increased. This labor is usually a fixed cost because quantities of these clinicians must be available to cover normal caseloads. If organizations attempt to arrange employment contracts that pay this labor only when needed, the best-qualified people usually will not accept the instability and lack of employment security such arrangements cause. Providers then lose the best people. If the organization's locale has adequate numbers of highly skilled workers who do not want full-time work, it might be able to create nurse and technician pools that allow the organization to call in extra workers when demand for them exceeds normal expectations. The use of nurse pools was quite popular in the 1980s. Their popularity has diminished somewhat because of related continuity of care and in-service training problems. It may also be possible to contract with outside agencies when additional labor is needed, as opposed to maintaining an internal part-time labor pool.

These changes in the nature and relative cost of resources have changed the health care delivery industry to one with much greater fixed than variable costs, primarily because of the expanding use of expensive, high-tech equipment and expensive labor, which is essentially a fixed cost. The management implications of the change will be discussed in later chapters.

OVERHEAD COST BEHAVIOR

When an organization incurs overhead costs, it frequently cannot differentiate the variable portion from the fixed. For instance, a certain amount of electric power is used to simply keep the production facility open. Power to light, heat, or air condition and to run certain support equipment is necessary, regardless of output level. Yet as output increases, total power consumption for the period will increase because usage of electric production equipment will increase. However, it might be that only one electric utility bill is received for the period. Cost elements that have both a fixed and a variable component are referred to as *mixed costs*. Because managers need to differentiate between fixed and variable amounts, it is desirable to discover what the variable cost per unit of such mixed cost elements is. Such determination is known as *cost-behavior analysis*. Here, behavior means behavior of total cost for a period relative to the period's level of output. Cost-behavior analysis technique is covered in the appendix to this chapter.

PRODUCT-DIRECT VERSUS CENTER-DIRECT COSTS

A few additional remarks about the traceability of costs are necessary. *Traceable* means that the resource causing a cost can be visually or physically traced to the cost object in question. Machine lubricants are an example. We have discussed that lubricants are not traced directly to the product (in our example, shoes). However, they are traceable to the shoe shop, where they are used. Similarly, in a hospital, the head nurses' salaries may not be traceable to specific patients, but they are traceable to the wards that each nurse manages. Conversation frequently occurs about costs that are traceable to a department, but are not further traceable to a specific product made in the department. These costs are considered direct to the producing center, but indirect to the products.

UNIT COST

Management frequently wants to know what it costs to produce a single unit of a specific product, such as a particular laboratory test. This is usually not as simple as it sounds.

The fixed costs present a problem. The total of variable production costs for a period is the total variable cost per unit summed over the units produced. Fixed costs, however, are naturally expressed as dollars per period. To find a fixed cost per unit of output, one must divide the period's fixed cost by the quantity of the unit's output during that period. Therefore, fixed cost per unit of output depends on how many units are output in the period. This is an extremely important fact when attempting to estimate future product costs.

There are two ways of looking at unit cost: either full or variable. The *variable production cost* of an item is the sum of the costs of its direct inputs and variable production overhead costs. For financial accounting purposes, the Financial Accounting Standards Board (FASB) dictates that all the costs of *manufacturing* an item be included in its finished-goods inventory value. This amount is referred to as the *full cost of manufacturing*. The full cost of an item includes its variable production cost and a "fair share" of fixed production overhead costs. Computing the full cost necessitates distributing the fixed overhead costs of the production activities among the items produced. Full cost is sometimes referred to as the *absorption cost,* because the full cost of all items produced absorbs the fixed production cost into the cost of the finished goods. Note that for financial accounting, only the fixed cost associated with production activities are included in the full-cost amount. General management and administrative costs, along with the costs of selling and distributing the product, are not.

Summary of Production Costs

Costs that occur through the use of resources in production activities are referred to as *production* or *manufacturing costs,* even though they may not be directly traceable to individual units of the products manufactured. (Note that production costs, in the case of health care, produce services rather than material things.) Those that are not traceable to the products are called *indirect production costs,* or *production overhead.* These indirect costs can be either fixed or variable, depending on the way they are incurred. In all, there are two basic, overlapping perspectives from which production costs can be viewed: direct versus indirect, and variable versus fixed. The full cost of a product is the sum of costs demanded to complete all the activities involved in its production. Each of these component activities will probably incur cost from each of these two dimensions.

Selling and Administrative Costs

There are many costs incurred outside production activities. These have to do with general administration, marketing, selling, and distribution. Examples of administration costs are the chief executive officer's salary and the costs of running the personnel department. Examples of selling costs are the costs of advertising and a salesperson's salary. (The health-care industry usually refers to marketing costs and not to selling costs.) Research and development costs are also included in this category. Examples of distribution costs are the costs of packaging orders and shipping them to customers and the costs of a pharmacy department packaging the prescribed dose and delivering it to the patient. In providing products to the market, these costs are just as relevant to sales revenues as production costs. They reduce the surplus gained from sales revenue, just as production costs do. Therefore, they are just as important to economic decisions as production costs are. When these costs are not traced to specific products. Instead they are considered costs of the period in which they are incurred, rather than the period in which the item manufactured is sold. They are, therefore, called *period costs.*

DISCUSSION QUESTIONS

1. What are examples of direct costs, as opposed to indirect costs, in operating a dental clinic?
2. Among the indirect costs in the dental clinic, which are fixed and which are variable?
3. In a hospital diagnostic radiology center, what costs would be direct to product, and which would be direct only to the center?

4. In a hospital or clinic, what are examples of specific production costs, as opposed to selling and administrative costs?

MARGINAL COSTS

The distinction between full and variable cost is extremely important to management decision making. Remember that fixed production costs are incurred for a period of time whether or not the resources purchased are used. Because these costs are involved regardless of the production level, they are frequently irrelevant to decisions about production levels. As production increases, these costs will not increase unless the output quantity increases to the point that additional fixed costs elements must be incurred. Conversely, if production decreases, these costs do not go away; they are fixed for an accounting period. Therefore, the additional cost of increasing production during that period is the variable cost of the increase, not the full cost. Likewise, the savings from reducing production is the variable cost of the reduced output.

With reference to increases in production levels, the additional production cost of the changed quantity is the *marginal* (or *incremental*) cost of the change in the quantity produced. Marginal cost is the additional cost brought on by a change in operations or the additional cost resulting from an operating decision. These are the *relevant costs* for a decision at the margin. Similarly, marginal savings are the savings resulting from an operating decision. Management focuses on marginal costs and savings because rarely is there a situation in which one starts from scratch, or a situation in which there are not already fixed costs.

Management, therefore, is usually more concerned with marginal or incremental costs than with full cost. With reference to product costs, this means managers are frequently more interested in variable costs than full cost. Because direct costs are rather easily measured, the primary problem in isolating variable product cost is in separating variable from fixed overhead costs and then determining whether some fixed overhead costs are marginal to the specific change being analyzed.

It is important to maintain a distinction between variable and marginal costs. Variable costs are always marginal. That is, if production increases, the costs increase by the variable cost of the added production. However, some fixed costs may also be marginal costs in some situations. If the output increases radically, the company may exceed the capacity of the current production facility. In this case, some facilities would have to added. For example, suppose a company is considering whether or not to enter a new contract to provide certain services for a particular employer's health program. For the price charged, the employer must cover all additional costs of providing the service. Revenue in excess of these additional costs will add to the organization's surplus.

Obviously, variable costs, such as supplies and medicine, needed to provide each service are part of this additional cost. If the additional services will force the company to lease additional equipment and hire more salaried employees, these fixed costs are also marginal to this decision and should be added to the variable costs to find the minimum price that will not lower the organization's financial performance. Though these equipment and labor costs are fixed with reference to each service provided, they are marginal to the contract. They are costs the company does not have, but will incur, when it enters this contract.

An important additional consideration is that once the fixed costs of the expansion incur, and if production later reduces to levels that existed before the expansion, the company does not get rid of the new fixed-cost elements until it can change the contracts under which the company acquired them. In the short run, fixed costs are not easily eliminated. However, a company must be careful not to overemphasize the "fixed" in fixed cost. A manager should never be resigned to fixed costs that are not productive. Fixed cost can be eliminated. The question is, how rapidly? The amount of time necessary to rid an organization of a fixed cost depends on how it is incurred. For instance, a cost under a rental contract can be eliminated when the contract expires. The depreciation expense on an owned asset may be avoided by selling the asset. How much of the cost will be avoided depends on how close the selling price is to the purchase cost net of depreciation. The ability to eliminate unnecessary salaries depends on the nature of the related labor contracts and the long-run organization behavior implications of frequently expanding and contracting one's labor force.

COMMITTED COSTS

Costs that cannot be changed, usually because of a contractual obligation to pay, are referred to as *committed costs*. Within an accounting period, fixed costs are committed.

SUNK COSTS

Sunk costs are already paid and cannot be recovered, regardless of future actions. These are usually associated with long-term assets that have not been fully depreciated but are of no future use. An example would be the cost of equipment that was purchased recently but has become technologically obsolete. In this case, new equipment must be bought to satisfy the clinicians who no longer will use the old technology, regardless of the fact that it is still operating. If the old equipment cannot be sold at current book value, the undepreciated cost is not relevant to decisions about replacing it. That cost is unrecoverable no matter what is done; it is sunk.

DISCRETIONARY COSTS

Costs which, if incurred, will not affect the operation of the organization within the current accounting period are called *discretionary*. An example could be certain types of training or facility renovation. Though they may not be necessary in the short run, usually they must eventually be sustained.

DISCUSSION QUESTIONS

1. What makes a cost relevant to a specific decision?
2. What are the relationships between marginal, variable, committed, sunk, discretionary, and relevant costs in a decision situation?
3. In deciding whether to open an outreach clinic as part of your health care system, specify some costs that would be in each of the previous listed categories and explain whether or not they are relevant to the decision to open the outreach clinic.

STANDARD COST

A *standard cost* is the amount a cost ought to be. It assumes a specified level of efficiency, known prices for the resources used, and the degree to which fixed costs are utilized. Standard costs are used to estimate the cost of future activity. They are also used after an operating period to compare cost performance to that which was planned. This is fundamental to the control process, which will be discussed in detail later in this book.

TRUE COSTS

Frequently, people refer to the *true cost* of a production output. This implies that there is a single value, though perhaps difficult or impossible to measure, for a unit of the output. The term true cost should be avoided. The amount of cost relevant to a specific decision is usually dependent on the environment and other variables specific to that decision. A simple example should make this apparent. Consider the cost of a specific surgical procedure. A large part of that cost is the cost of the surgical facilities used— a fixed-cost resource. Therefore, the cost of a specific operation on a specific patient will depend on how frequently that facility is used. The cost of an operation to a provider cannot be known until the level of use of the fixed-cost resources involved is determined. One can compute the *average cost* given a known or projected level of utilization, but it is wishful thinking to state a true cost of a future surgical procedure without additional, speculative information. The need to pay attention to this fact will frequently appear throughout discussions of appropriate cost information for specific decision situations.

COSTS AND CHARGES

In the health care industry, some confusion exists about the terms *costs* and *charges*. The confusion stems from the fact that the Centers for Medicare and

Medicaid Services (CMS) [formerly the Health Care Financing Administration (HCFA)], prior to paying under the current prospective payment system, paid hospitals their *reported cost* for caring for Medicare patients. These costs were computed using a CMS-required procedure. Therefore, for Medicare patients, a hospital's allowed charge to CMS for treating a patient was, generally speaking, its reported cost of treating that patient. (Thus, the Medicare payment was called a *cost-based payment.*) Hospitals had established prices for specific services and kept track of the services and the aggregate of patient charges as services were rendered; hence, the term *fee-for-service* payment. However, hospitals did not know, much less keep track of, the cost of individual services for patients. In this book, *cost* will refer to what a health care deliverer, or provider, pays for the resources needed to perform the activities used to produce a cost object. *Charge* will refer to what an organization bills its payers for a product sold.

An organization's charges are costs only to the payer, not to the provider. This is an important distinction in health care management accounting, because some people substitute charges for cost. This misleading and generally inaccurate practice is called *using charges as a proxy for cost.*

Key Points

- Production costs include direct and indirect costs.
- Indirect costs include both fixed and variable overhead.
- Mixed costs have both a fixed and a variable component.
- Marginal costs occur with reference to the increase of service or product levels.
- Marginal costs are the additional production cost of the changed quantity.
- Incremental cost is another term for marginal cost.
- Committed costs are those that cannot be changed.

- Sunk costs are already paid and cannot be recovered, regardless of future actions.
- Standard cost is the amount a cost ought to be.
- In this book, "cost" will refer to what a health care deliverer, or provider, pays for the resources needed to perform the activities used to produce a cost object.
- In this book, "charge" will refer to what an organization bills its payers for a product sold.
- An organization's charges are costs only to the payer.

EXERCISES

All of us probably have experience with dental care and have observed activities within dental offices or clinics.

1. Based on this experience, list the costs of running a dental facility according to the following cost categories; realize a cost item may fall into more than one category:
   Direct materials
   Direct labor
   Fixed overhead
   Variable overhead
   Operating
   Selling
   Administrative

2. Briefly describe a situation that would lead you to evaluate marginal costs. List the types of costs that would be marginal in that situation. Specify which of these marginal costs would be fixed and which would be variable.

APPENDIX 3 COST-BEHAVIOR ANALYSIS

GRAPHICAL VIEW OF OVERHEAD COSTS

Cost-behavior analysis refers to a process for understanding how total costs change from accounting period to period as the amount of production changes. The existence of fixed and variable components of total cost has already been discussed.

Fixed costs are those that have a set amount for an accounting period, regardless of the level of output. Variable costs are those whose total for a period will increase or decrease if output increases or decreases. If we look at the situation graphically, the fixed cost-to-output relation is as shown in Figure 3A-1. Fixed costs are naturally expressed in dollars per accounting period.

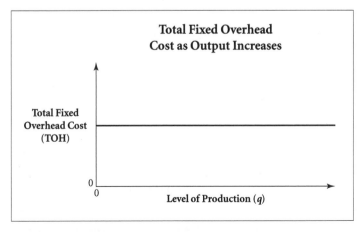

Figure 3A-1   **Total Fixed Overhead Cost as Output Increases**

Total variable overhead costs increase by the variable overhead cost per unit each time an additional unit is produced. If the variable overhead cost per unit is the same, regardless of the rate of output, total variable overhead cost will behave as shown in Figure 3A-2.

Because overhead costs commonly have both fixed and variable components, total overhead cost for an accounting period should behave as depicted in Figure 3A-3. The cost should be the sum of the fixed and variable component at any specific level of production. The figure reflects that at zero production, the overhead cost is the fixed overhead amount. As one produces, the total overhead increases by the variable overhead, per unit, each time a unit is made. Total overhead cost (TOH) for an accounting period can be expressed as the product of variable overhead cost per unit (VOHu) times the number of units produced (q), which computes the total variable overhead (TVOH), plus the fixed overhead cost (FOH). Algebraically:

$$TOH = (VOHu)(q) + FOH \qquad\qquad (1)$$

DISTINGUISHING FIXED FROM VARIABLE COSTS

Cost-behavior analysis is a method for breaking the cost of an activity into its fixed and variable components by analyzing the total cost of the activity over a collection of past accounting periods. Suppose management wants to know how the overhead costs of their clinic vary from month to month when the number of clinic visits per month varies. Historical data are used to determine the fixed and

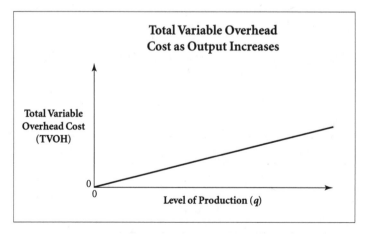

Figure 3A-2   **Total Variable Overhead Cost as Output Increases**

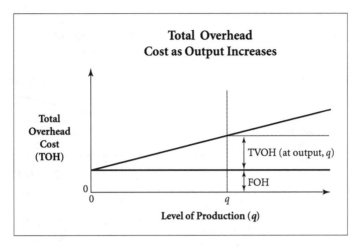

Figure 3A-3 **Total Overhead Cost as Output Increases**

the variable components of the clinic's overhead cost. Total overhead cost for each of a number of past months is plotted against the number of clinic visits in each month. A line can be fit to the data to represent the way total overhead cost varies with clinic visits. Statistically, this is referred to as a *regression line*. (See Appendix B for a discussion of regression analysis.) The point at which this line crosses the vertical axis is the overhead cost when there are no visits (zero on the horizontal axis). This is, by definition, the amount of fixed overhead; that is, the overhead when there is no production. Each visit moves the plot one unit along the horizontal axis and up the vertical axis by the additional overhead caused by one more visit. The slope of the regression line is, therefore, the additional overhead caused by an additional visit, which is the variable overhead per visit. Figure 3A-4 illustrates this.

The algebraic expression of a straight line is:

$$y = b(x) + a \qquad (2)$$

In this situation, the expression is interpreted as:

$$TOH = (VOHu)(q) + FOH \qquad (3)$$

Where: TOH = y = Total Overhead for a month

VOHu = b = Variable Overhead per visit

q = x = Number of visits in the month

FOH = a = Fixed Overhead for a month

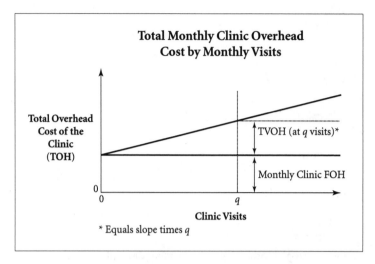

Figure 3A-4   Total Monthly Clinic Overhead Cost by Monthly Visits

Equation (3) can be used to predict overhead cost in the future when monthly visits (workload demand) are forecast. This is a valuable tool in the budgeting process.

THE HI-LO METHOD OF COST-BEHAVIOR ANALYSIS

To use the Hi-Lo method of cost-behavior analysis, graph paper is needed so that the data can be plotted accurately. The analysis involves the following steps:

1. Plot the data on the graph paper with cost on the vertical axis and output on the horizontal axis.
2. Draw a straight line through the data points that best fit the data array. This is the line that gives the lowest aggregate distance from itself to all the data points. This can be called your "eye ball" analysis.
3. Pick two points on the line: one at the higher end, and one at the lower end. These are the "hi" and "lo" points on which your analysis will be based.
4. Find the vertical distance between these points. This is the change in overhead cost as output goes from the low point to the high point.
5. Find the horizontal difference between these points. This is the change in output associated with the change in cost.
6. Divide the change in cost by the change in output. The result is dollars of overhead cost per unit of output. This is VOHu.
7. Then use one of the two points and the prediction equation to find the FOH.

a. TOH = (VOHu)(q) + FOH.
b. Substitute the TOH and q from the Hi or the Lo point, and VOH per unit just computed.
c. Compute the FOH.

An Example Using the Hi-Lo Method

The OurTing Hospital is reviewing the cost of operating its food service section over the past 5 years. The following data have been collected.

YEAR	MEALS SERVED	COST REQUIRED ($)
1988	12,000	200,000
1989	8,000	180,000
1990	25,000	230,000
1991	8,000	190,000
1992	17,000	220,000

The requirements are as follows:

a. Determine the variable and fixed components of cost using the Hi-Lo Method.
b. Calculate the estimated cost of running the section in 1993 if 28,000 meals are served.
c. Is the cost behavior roughly linear? Explain briefly.
d. How would you rate the "fit"? Excellent, good, fair, poor, or no fit? Why?
e. Does your "eyeball" analysis agree with your Hi-Lo analysis? Explain briefly.

Figure 3A-5 is provided to assist you.

a. The Hi-Lo solution is as follows:

Steps 1 and 2: Graph the points.

Step 3: Assume that, from your graph, the Hi point you picked is at 21,000 meals for $225,000; the Lo point is at 8,000 meals for $185,000.

Note: Each analyst will draw a somewhat different line; however, your line should run close to these points.

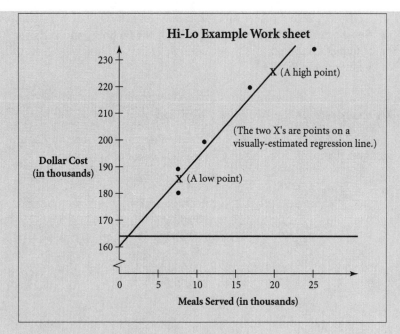

Figure 3A-5   **Hi-Lo Example Work Sheet**

Steps 4–6: ($225,000 − $185,000) = $40,000

(21,000 − 8,000) meals = 13,000 meals

$40,000/13,000 meals = $3.077 per meal, Variable Cost

Step 7: Using the representative Lo point:

Total Cost = (Variable Cost/meal)(q) + Fixed Costs

$185,000 = ($3.077/meal)(8,000 meals) + Fixed Costs

Fixed Costs = $185,000 $24,615 = $160,385

Note: This figure can be checked by confirming it at the Hi point: $225,000 for 21,000 meals.

$225,000 should equal $3.077/meal (21,000 meals) + $160,385.

$225,000 should equal $64,617 + $160,385.

$225,000 = $225,002.

b. At 28,000 meals, the predicted cost would be:

> $$\text{Total Cost} = \$3.077/\text{meal } (28{,}000 \text{ meals}) + \$160{,}385$$
> $$= \$246{,}541.$$
>   c. Yes, the straight regression line falls close to all the data points.
>   d. This nearness to the line can be said to be a good fit.
>   e. In this case, yes, the "eyeballed" regression line goes through the vertical intercept quite close to $160,385, the amount the analysis computed as the fixed cost.
>
> *Notes:*
>   1. If the regression line is extended to the vertical axis, it intercepts the axis very close to the fixed-cost component.
>   2. If you "break" an axis to conserve graphing space, break only the vertical axis and do this only below the intercept point. If these rules are violated, the graphical check of the amount of fixed costs will be incorrect.

The previous example concerned the analysis of overhead costs of food service with reference to the number of meals served. Realize that cost-behavior analysis can be used to separate the variable and fixed components of cost of any mixed cost with reference to any causal factor.

A few comments on interpretation of cost behavior analyses are in order. If, when the regression line is drawn, the data points do not lie close to the line, the line obviously does not represent the variation of total overhead cost with output very well. Statistical jargon for this situation is that the line does not "fit" the data. The worse the fit, the less accurate the predictions will be. Also, keep in mind that the analysis is based on past conditions, and historical data. To the extent that future activity will be different, using a prediction model based on historical data will give inaccurate results. Using new equipment, having changed rental agreements, and changing salary structures caused by using new technology are examples of such a change.

Cost-behavior analysis is an example of the use of the statistical procedure called *simple regression*. (See Appendix B.) If the cost and output quantity data are entered into a computerized statistical regression program, the output will produce the numbers indicated as follows:

a = FOH
b = VOH visit

THE REGRESSION METHOD OF ANALYSIS

Today, many calculators are capable of regressing a total cost on some unit of activity. The general answer is usually given in the format of Equation (2). The regression analysis will also give an R^2 statistic. If this statistic is 1.00, the fit is perfect. This means that the computer program was able to draw a straight line that passes through each of the data points by using the historic data. If the line is near 0, there is no fit. This means that there was no significant relationship between the units of activity and the cost in question during the periods from which the data were collected. This indicates that the model has no predictive value.

The simple regression solution of the OurTing Hospital problem is as follows.

When the data were set into a simple regression calculator model, the output was:

$$a = \$165,262 = \text{Fixed Costs}$$
$$b = \$2.767 = \text{VC/meal}$$
$$R^2 = 0.917$$

This indicated an excellent fit.

This indicates that our Hi-Lo visual-line fitting was good enough to limit the error on the fixed-cost estimate to about 3 percent of the regression (the more accurate approach) solution.

$$(\$165,262 - \$160,385)/\$165,262 = 0.0295$$

The analysis also produces a p< statistic. This statistic relates to the probability that the sample data, used accurately, represent the population from which it was taken. For instance, this analysis of a sample of meals served indicates that the total cost of providing food services varies at a rate of $2.767 per meal. If the reported p< statistic is 0.01, there is a probability of less than 1 percent that there is no relationship between the number of meals served and the total cost of providing meals. High p< values (approaching 1.0) indicate that variables other than the number of meals served are the primary reasons for year-to-year changes in the cost of providing meals, even though the R^2 for the analysis of the sample was high. Simple regression analysis is discussed more thoroughly in Appendix B in the back of this book.

Problems

Problem 1.   Sterile Supplies

The data here have been taken from your instrument-sterilization-unit's cost records. They refer to the monthly cost of producing sterile instrument packs.

Month	Packs Produced	Total Cost($)	Month	Packs Produced	Total Cost($)	Month	Packs Produced	Total Costs($)
January	800	1,400	April	900	1,550	July	300	850
February	500	1,000	May	400	1,000	August	500	1,150
March	700	1,250	June	600	1,250			

Required:

   a. Prepare a scatter graph to analyze the behavior of the total cost of the unit as its output varies. Do an eyeball analysis and state the estimate of the monthly fixed cost of running the unit.

   b. Do a Hi-Lo analysis and state the estimated fixed cost per month and variable cost per pack.

   c. Do your two estimates of the fixed portion of the cost structure agree? If not, why not?

   d. If your estimate of production for September is 720 packs, what is your best estimate of September's cost of operating the instrument-sterilization unit?

Solution:

   a. Plot a scatter graph and estimate regression line. Your line should show a fixed component of cost to be about $490. The rest of this solution assumes the data points taken from the estimated regression line. Your line might not be exactly the same as the one drawn by this analyst.

   b. Hi point: 800 packs for $1,400.
      Lo point: 100 packs for $600.

Variable Cost/pack = ($1,400 − $600)/(800 − 100) packs = $800/700 packs

$$= \$1.143 \text{ per pack}$$

Using the Hi point: Total Cost = (Variable Cost/pack)(q) + Fixed Cost

$$\$1,400 = (\$1.143/\text{pack})(800 \text{ packs}) + \text{Fixed Cost}$$

$$\text{Fixed Cost} = \$1,400 - \$914 = \$486$$

   c. Yes, the two approaches yield answers within reasonable rounding and graphing errors.

   d. Total Cost: Cost = $1.143/pack (720 packs) + $486

$$= \$1,309$$

Problem 2.   Flick Hospital X-ray department

The number of X-rays taken and the total X-ray department overhead costs over the last 9+ months at Flick Hospital are given here.

Month	X-rays Taken	X-ray Costs ($)	REQUIRED:
January	6,250	29,000	1a. Using the Hi-Lo Method, determine the
February	7,000	28,000	formula (algebraic model) for X-ray
March	5,000	23,000	overhead-cost behavior.
April	4,250	20,000	1b. What is the
May	4,500	22,000	(i) Variable-overhead rate
June	3,000	16,000	(ii) Fixed overhead amount
July	3,750	15,000	
August	5,500	24,000	Be sure to show the units for your answers.
September	5,750	26,000	Check figures: VC= $3.87/X-ray
			FC = $ 3,221/mo.

2. What would you expect total X-ray costs to be in a month when 3,900 X-rays were to be taken?
   Check figure: $18,314
3. Does your algebraic model agree with your graphical model? Explain.

Note: Your answers will vary somewhat depending on the degree to which your eyeball line matches the one used in this solution.

Problem 3.   Biomedical Engineering

Accountants believe that because the variable costs of the biomedical engineering (BME) department primarily involve engineering labor, engineering hours (EH) is the driver variable behind cost behavior of the department. Check this out by doing a regression analysis of total BME cost on EH charged to other departments (using the eyeball method). Weekly data are shown for the last 2 months.

Week	1	2	3	4	5	6	7	8	9
Cost ($)	90,000	80,000	95,000	60,000	70,000	75,000	40,000	85,000	105,000
EH	60	50	70	30	50	60	30	60	70

Required:
1. Does the relation between cost and EH appear to lend itself to a linear model? Explain.

2. Use the Hi-Lo (algebraic) Method to determine the weekly fixed cost and variable cost per EH charged to other departments.

Check Figures: VC = $1,187/EH

FC = $16,062/week

Your answer will differ somewhat depending on the placement of your eyeball line.

3. Why is it not good to use the actual high-data points? Explain.
4. Do you feel confident of your estimates using your prediction model TC = FC + VC_{eh} (EH) will give you a good measure of the total cost of running the BME department for a week if you accurately predict the EH for that week. Why or why not?
5. If you expect the BME department to furnish 63 EH to other departments next week, what is your best estimate of the total cost of running the department next week?

    Check Figure: $90,843

6a. How much variable BME department cost would you assign to the overhead pool of a revenue center that used 12 EH in a given week?

    Check Figure: $14,244

6b. How much fixed BME department cost would you assign that revenue center? Why are you having trouble answering this last question?

INTRODUCTION TO COSTING

After studying this chapter, students should be able to:

1. Explain how verb-adjective-noun triplets can define activities that can be aggregated to describe the work of an organization.

2. Explain the three basic schemes for paying for health care services and their relation to defining a health care organization's products.

3. Describe fundamental processes for tracing and allocating resources to activities.

4. Explain appropriate uses of historical cost data in estimating costs for planning purposes.

5. Recognize some ways that inaccuracies can occur from overly simplistic models.

6. Define the primary product of the health care industry, and define and explain the role of intermediate products.

7. Explain the relationship of the capacity issue to the fixed-cost problem.

INTRODUCTION

Health care managers are commonly interested in the costs related to six categories about which decisions must be made:

(1) products
(2) programs or product lines
(3) organization centers (e.g., departments)
(4) specific payers
(5) individual clinicians who order activities and resources
(6) patients and patient populations

We will first focus on costing individual products, and later expand the discussion to the more aggregated cost objects.

Product Costs for Management Decisions

Managers do not manage the past. Instead, they study the past to understand the processes involved in their organization's reaching its objectives and the factors that affect those processes. Managers make decisions about what their organization should produce, the processes (technology) that it will use, the combinations of resources that will be employed in the production, and how the output will be sold and distributed. The cost of providing outputs to its customers is basic to these decisions. The cost of providing an output must be less than the amount people are willing to pay for it, or in most cases, the output cannot be sold without a loss. The cost must also be near the cost at which it can be furnished by competitors, or the organization will be underpriced by competitors and probably lose its customers.

Payment Mechanisms

The first questions about cost that a care provider must ask itself are "What do we produce," or, "what are our products?" The fiscally relevant answer is that an organization's products are those things for which it is paid. A problem is that many care-delivery organizations operate concurrently under at least three fundamentally different types of payment systems, which cause them to have three fundamentally different products. Any other outputs of the organization are public relations or marketing items, but should not be considered products. The three different types of payment systems, or payment mechanisms, include fee for service, prospective payment, and capitation.

Fee for Service

Under this type of payment, the provider is paid separately for each item of service it delivers in the care of a patient. The amount is determined by the cost of the resources used to produce the services. These include items such as drugs, diagnostic tests, surgical procedures, therapy sessions, bed days, and so forth. They are referred to as *billable line items* because each appears on a separate line on the patient's claim form or bill. As discussed earlier, fee for service is the traditional method of paying for health care.

Prospective Payment

Under this system, prices for specific outputs are set ahead of the time care is delivered. The set price is the payment regardless of the amount of resources used to produce the output. When prices are those in a contractually agreed-upon list of fees for services, paying by fee for service takes on a prospective aspect. However, today the term is used for systems that pay a predetermined amount for care of patients in predetermined case categories. The amount of the fee is set ahead of time for each of an array of diagnoses, patient conditions, and/or procedures. Examples of prospective payment groupings include diagnosis related groups (DRGs) for hospital inpatients, ambulatory payment classifications (APCs) for hospital outpatients, and fee schedules such as physician fee schedules. The price received for treating a specific patient depends on the category in which the patient's diagnosis, condition, and/or procedure is classified. In the case of DRGs, the payment is generally not directly related to the specific line items used in the patient's treatment. Payers usually compute the price for cases in a specific category based on averages of the historic cost of such cases.

A similar approach is to pay a specified rate per day of inpatient treatment (per diem) for patients in broader categories. These categories are usually determined by the ward or unit in which the care is given, because different wards or units have different fixed cost and intensities of individual patient care. An example is the difference between average daily costs of care in an intensive care unit, as opposed to a general medical/surgical ward.

Capitation

In a capitated system, the care provider is paid a flat fee to provide a client whatever services are necessary (as prescribed in a contract with the payer) over a defined period of time. Anyone who has bought health insurance has paid for health care in a capitated fashion; only rather recently have care deliverers received payment under a capitated system. Care providers make capitated payment arrangements with payers, such as insurance companies and managed care organizations (MCOs), who contract for the provision of care for large groups of potential patients. For reasons discussed throughout this book, costing to support capitated payments is still rather poorly specified. It pays inadequate attention to interactions among fixed-cost utilization, convenience of access, and efficiency. The payments themselves frequently appear to be the result of the negotiating power differential between the provider and the payer more than the outcome of appropriate and rigorous cost-of-service and benefit-of-service analysis. Capitated payment arrangements put the care deliverer in the position of insuring the capitated population it serves. Care providers usually lack the skills required to manage the insurance functions. Because of financial problems resulting from this weakness, providers are abandoning capitated payment systems. For instance, assume a large multidisciplinary group practice with its own clinics and hospital formed an HMO that contracted primarily with firms in white-collar industries. If that HMO did not adjust its per-member rate when it entered a capitated arrangement with a shipyard, payment for the care demanded would probably be too low and would cause serious financial problems.

IDENTIFYING APPROPRIATE COST

At this point, it is helpful to consider what must be known in order to measure the cost of these three types of products.

Fee-for-Service

For a fee-for-service line item, the cost would be the sum of the direct costs and variable overhead, along with a share of the fixed overhead costs incurred by the activities necessary to produce the service. Because each line item is a salable product, costing under a fee-for-service system involves no more than determining the cost of each service.

Prospective Payment

The cost of the discharge of an inpatient paid under a prospective-payment system would be the sum of the costs of all the line items used in the patient's care. Though this is obvious, a related management problem is not. That problem is negotiating the prospectively set price for a category of patients, as opposed to retrospectively summing the prices of the line items used in the care of a specific patient. To negotiate a prospective price, the manager should know ahead of time the types and quantities of line items that will be needed for each category of patient that might require treatment. The manager must also know how much the activities necessary to produce each of these items will cost. Under a DRG-type system, the provider will be paid the same amount for every inpatient discharged in a particular category. This approach assumes that there will be many discharges in each category. The manager can, therefore, concentrate on the average cost within each category. If the average set of items needed for such patients is known, the average cost could be estimated. The average set of inputs is defined by the protocol of care for each category of patient. This is why much research is currently being done to discover normal, or standard, care protocols for a nearly exhaustive set of patient categories.

Capitation

For capitated contracts, as with prospective payment, care providers should know the cost of the line items they must produce and the usual set of line items that each category of patient will need. However, they also need to know how many of which categories of patients will demand care from among the populations of people they have capitated. This information comes from sophisticated statistical applications, collectively referred to as *acturial science*. The lack of this expertise within care-delivery organizations is the reason for the decline in capitated systems just mentioned.

Summary: Increasing Financial Risk

In this book, the focus is on attempting to understand the cost of the activities needed to treat clients in these three generally used approaches to payment. It should be noted that as one goes from fee for service through prospective payment to capitated-payment systems, more of the uncertainty about the types and quantities of resources to meet the demands of the contracts falls on the provider. Under fee for service, the provider need only control the cost of the individual services it provides. It will be paid a negotiated amount for each of these. Under prospective payment, it must also control the quantity and kind of intermediate products it provides for its patients, because it will receive the same payment regardless of the array of services provided. However, the provider will be paid for each episode of care it furnishes. Under a capitated contract, the provider is also responsible for cost variations caused by the number of people in its capitated groups that present themselves for care. This means that the provider is not paid for each episode of care it provides. Instead, a set amount per period of time for each individual is paid to the provider by the company with whom it contracts to provide care. Each of these changes creates more financial risk associated with variation in physicians' ordering practices, severity of illness of patients, and the quantity and mix of patients seeking care under the payment contract. To control costs, the care provider must measure, understand, and project estimates of these variables.

DISCUSSION QUESTIONS

1. Explain the rationale behind the statement that health care delivery organizations have three different categories of products.
2. Explain why care providers have different levels of risk depending on the category of the product they have contracted to deliver.

FINAL VERSUS INTERMEDIATE PRODUCTS

Earlier, we contended that the basic product of health care is wellness. If this is so, then the health interventions provided by health care providers are not outputs; they are health care inputs. It is not appropriate to refer to a bed day of hospital care as an output of the hospital. No sane person goes to a hospital to enjoy a day's experience in a hospital bed. The appropriate measure of health care output is the wellness of those served relative to their wellness had they not received the care given. The health care industry and policy makers are facing this truth, but results-oriented output measures are extremely difficult to create. Progress in that direction is occurring, but more slowly than managers would like.

Within health care organizations, goods and services are produced as inputs to produce wellness. Though a particular test is an input to a specific patient's care, it is an output of the laboratory. One can speak of these outputs as *intermediate products*, remembering that the final product, wellness, is the output sought by the customer. These intermediate products are the sort of things that have traditionally been billable line items. The actions that must be taken to produce the intermediate products will be called *intermediate activities*. They are the basic building blocks for estimating the cost of meeting the demands of any payment system or the product for which it pays. Estimating the cost of intermediate products is the starting point for more sophisticated costing by care providers.

The Capacity Issue

As discussed earlier, the full cost of a product is composed of two types of cost. The first type, *direct costs*, consists of those that can be directly traced in measured amounts to the product. The other type is *indirect costs*, often called *overhead costs*. Indirect costs are those that must be incurred by the care deliverer, but the amount used in the production of a specific unit of output cannot be directly observed. Such items as utilities, production administration, heating, building depreciation, and equipment rental are examples of costs that are indirect to a unit of a product.

Indirect costs also have two components: variable and fixed. Here we speak of variability with relation to the level of activity in the entity suffering the cost. Cost behavior analysis is used to separate mixed costs into their fixed and variable components. To reiterate, the fixed part of indirect costs is extremely troublesome in determining the cost of a single item. The trouble with fixed costs is that the cost per item depends on how many items were produced during the accounting period. In hospitals, this is so closely related to hospital utilization that it is called the *excess capacity issue*.

An extreme example will illustrate the importance of the excess-capacity problem at the total organization level. Suppose a small clinic has $50,000 of salary, building rental, equipment rental, and miscellaneous contract costs per month. These are all fixed costs because they must be paid whether the clinic sees 30 or 500 patients in a month. If the clinic sees 30 patients, the $50,000 must be assigned to those patients. This creates a fixed cost component of $1,667 per case. If 500 cases are seen, this component drops to $100 per case, or $50,000 ÷ 5000. At 1,000 cases, it drops to $50 per case. Note that if the caseload dropped from a normal volume of, say, 800 cases per month to 200 cases, a nurse may be able to double as the receptionist and cut the monthly fixed costs by the salary of the receptionist. If the caseload was expected to remain low for some time, this would be a rational move. However, fixed costs such as building and equipment rental can usually not be reduced so easily.

Once a fixed cost structure is established by purchases or contracts for fixed cost items, it is usually expensive or impossible to change it quickly. This means that lowest cost per case, or per intermediate product, can only exist when the delivery organization is operating near the capacity for which it was designed. Excess capacity is expensive, especially because estimates show that approximately 80 percent of hospital costs are fixed costs.

DEPARTMENTS AND ACTIVITIES

Identifying and costing the activities leading to the discharge of an inpatient in a specific DRG, at first, seems to be an unacceptably complicated, time consuming, and expensive process. It is always wise to ask if the management information derived from an analysis is worth the cost of the analysis. The ease with which comprehensive activity analysis can be done depends on the degree to which it can be distributed across the organization and how many separate activities are costed. Because specific activities happen in specific departments within an organization, they can be analyzed independently of other departments. A corollary of this observation is that though activities flow in some sequence into any cost objective, each activity can be analyzed separately, and the activities necessary for any specific cost objective can be analyzed concurrently. The people involved in it can analyze each. To analyze activities across an organization, it does, however, need support personnel to:

- Train department personnel on activity analysis and cost measurement.
- Coordinate cross-departmental flows of information and resources.
- Integrate department-cost information into organization-level information.
- Report the resulting information for use by managerial decision makers.

These activities are the domain of management accountants working with information system personnel.

DISCUSSION QUESTIONS

1. Why do we say that most outputs of health care delivery organizations are intermediate, as opposed to final, products? Which product category is closest to being a final product—a billable line item, prospectively paid units of care, or capitated care? Why?
2. What circumstance of production makes capacity management critical to intermediate product cost? Why?

3. If we recognize that activities cause costs to be incurred, why must we analyze departments in order to estimate product costs?

IDENTIFYING ACTIVITIES

We can begin by examining what must be done to determine the cost of producing a specific product by analyzing the cost of visits in a primary-care clinic. Cost refers to the amount that must be spent in order to produce, sell, and distribute the product. This amount is set by what has to be done to complete these three basic activities, what resources must be used, and what those resources cost. Activities can be identified in a verb-adjective-noun triplet, such as "perform a general physical." Resources flow into activities, and activities create products and their associated revenues. More pragmatically, resources are used in activities, and in turn, the outputs from these activities, along with more resources, are used in subsequent activities that eventually lead to providing a billable health care product.

EXAMPLE: A PRIMARY-CARE CLINIC

A physician owning a small primary-care clinic wanted to know whether each of the clinic's four categories of office visits was profitable. He was deciding whether some types of visits should be eliminated because they were unprofitable. Therefore, he needed to know the cost of visits in each category, as opposed to an average cost of all patient visits. The visit categories are defined in the notes accompanying Table 4-1. Each category demanded a standard set of activities, and its price was set by third-party payers. The managing physician began isolating the processes (activities) involved in patient visits. It is useful to chart activities according to who is taking the actions and their chronological sequence. Figure 4-1 is an example of such a chart. The persons or groups accomplishing the activities are listed across the top and the sequential steps are shown down the page. The average time taken for each activity was estimated from experience and is shown on the flow arrows leaving the activity ovals. Costing each category of visit was done using the following steps:

1. Separating fixed from variable costs. The physician-manager understood that fixed and variable cost behave differently from period to period, both in their total and in their effect on the cost of a single visit. He approached cost-behavior analysis rather simplistically by summing the total cost for a year of all the types of cost he believed were variable. He included salaries, supplies, and postage as variable costs. He determined their total cost from the general ledger. He then subtracted the total variable cost for the year from the grand total of costs and considered the difference to be the fixed costs for the year.

Table 4-1 **Cost of Visits by Category with Additional Services**

Visit Category*	Examination ($)	X-Ray ($)	Lab ($)	Consult. Order ($)	Report Process ($)	Pap Smear ($)	Medical Assistant ($)	Total ($)
99212	37.61							37.61
99213	37.61							37.61
99213	37.61			11.04	8.50			57.15
99213	37.61		8.50					46.11
99213	37.61	8.50	8.50					54.61
99213	37.61	8.50	8.50	11.04	8.50			74.15
99213	37.61	8.50	8.50	23.13	8.50			86.24
99214	80.69	Incl.	Incl.					80.69
99214	80.69	Incl.	Incl.	10.85	8.50	Incl.		100.04
99215	109.67							109.67
99215	109.67			11.04	8.50			129.21
99215	109.67			23.13	8.50			141.30
99215	109.67			11.04	8.50	8.50	1.20	137.71
99215	109.67			23.13	8.50	8.50	1.20	149.80

*Notes: 99212 - Self-limited or minor visit with problem-focused history, problem-focused examination, and straightforward medical decision making

99213 - Low-to-moderate severity visit with expanded problem-focused history, expanded problem-focused examination, low-complexity decision making

99214 - Moderate-to-high severity visit with detailed history, detailed examination, moderate-complexity decision making

99215 - Moderate-to-high severity with comprehensive history, comprehensive examination, high-complexity decision making

2. Determining fixed cost allocation. The next step was to determine how much of the costs that were fixed for a year should be allocated to each specific type of visit. He believed that fixed costs were caused primarily by doctors. He, therefore, decided that allocating fixed costs by the amount of time a doctor spends on a visit would assign fixed costs appropriately across visit categories. An intermediate variable was therefore created: "fixed cost per 10-minute block of doctor's time." This variable was computed by measuring the total number of 10-minute blocks of physician time used during the baseline year. The total fixed cost for that period was divided by the total number of physician 10-minute blocks used. The result was that each 10-minute period of a doctor's time was associated with $16.08 of fixed overhead cost. The number of time blocks for a visit category ranged from one to three.

3. Determining variable cost rates. The physician-manager decided that variable cost should be divided into two types: salary and nonsalary. Doctor, medical assistant, and receptionist costs were considered direct costs. Their cost was, therefore, their salary rate times the amount of time that each type of personnel was involved in an activity. Indirect variable

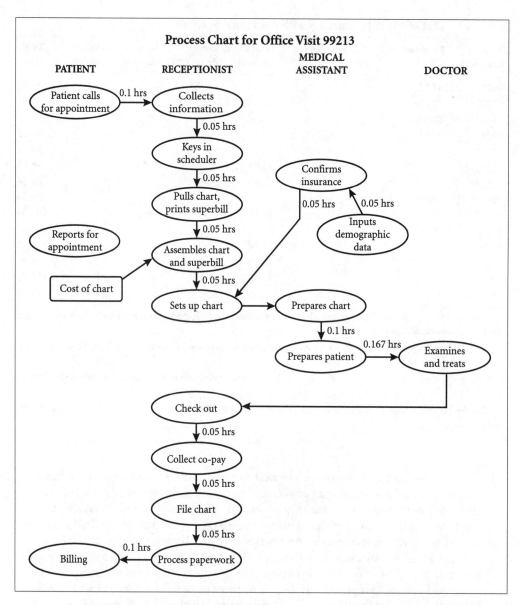

Figure 4-1   **Process Chart for Office Visit 99213**

costs of the practice were computed as the total variable costs less the salary costs. Visits were believed to cause an equal amount of variable overhead regardless of their category. The total nonsalary variable cost for the past year was divided by the total number of visits to get the variable-overhead rate. This came to $3.99 per visit.

4. Determining average cost-per-visit category. Table 4-2 lists the activities demanded by a routine office visit by a new patient and sequences them into four aggregate activities:

1. Schedule the patient ("patient appointment scheduling").
2. Receive the patient ("patient reception").
3. Examine the patient ("examination").
4. Discharge the patient ("patient checkout").

It also shows the cost of the resources used in each activity, the assignment of fixed and variable overhead, and the total cost of all activities required by that category of visit. Similar analyses were done for the other visit categories.

Table 4-1 also shows the total cost of visit categories, with additional activities such as radiological (X-ray) or laboratory testing. The other types of visits and the additional services were analyzed in the same way as the 99213 visit just described. This analysis showed, for instance, that a simple office visit by a return patient that included a laboratory work-up would cost $37.61 + $8.50 = $46.11. Clinic management then compared this cost information with prices offered by payers. With this product-specific analysis, managers could decide which visits were profitable, and which were not.

Management's Interpretations

The physician-manager interpreted the results shown in Table 4-1 as follows:

An office visit for an established patient (99213) could cost me from $37.61 to $86.24, depending on what lab work or X-rays I ordered, or if I requested a consultation. My reimbursement was $38.11 or less. The cost of a brief visit (99212) is the same as for a limited one (99213), but the reimbursement is less. The intermediate office visit (99214) on an established patient cost me from $80.69 to $100.04, and the comprehensive evaluation (99215) cost me from $109.67 to $149.80. Some managed care companies downgraded my services from 99215 to 99213 and paid me $38.11 for what had cost me $149.80. I discontinued comprehensive evaluations of my patients. There is a need to achieve the objective of correct diagnosis and treatment without losing money. This led me to a belief that a new, fundamentally different way of evaluating patients is needed if the physician is to be compensated fairly, the patient is to be treated properly, and the current marketplace is to determine the value of the service.

Table 4-2 **Process Mapping Worksheet**

99213 - Routine visit, new patient

Activities	Direct Cost ($)	+ Allocated by	(Amount)	× ($ Base Cost)	=	Total ($)
1. Patient appointment scheduling						
Collect information		Recpt.time	0.10 hrs.	8.50/hr.		.850
Phone system		# of calls	1/apmnt.	0.18/call		.180
Key into scheduler		Recpt.time	0.05 hrs.	8.50/hr.		.425
Software		Appointment	1	.04/use		.040
Pull chart & start superbill	0.05(form)	Recpt.time	0.05 hrs.	8.50/hr.		.475	1.97
2. Patient reception						
Assemble chart		Recpt.time	0.05 hrs.	8.50/hr.		.425
Confirm insurance		Recpt.time	0.05 hrs.	8.50/hr.		.425
Input demographics		Recpt.time	0.05 hrs.	8.50/hr.		.425
Set up chart	1.50 (chart)	Recpt.time	0.05 hrs.	8.50/hr.		1.925	3.20
3. Examination						
Chart preparation		MA time	0.10 hrs.	12.00/hr.		1.200
Patient preparation		MA time	0.10 hrs.	12.00/hr.		1.200
Examination		MD time	0.167 hrs.	54.00/hr.		9.090	11.49
4. Patient checkout						
Check out patient		Recpt.time	0.05 hrs.	8.50/hr.		.425
Collect co-pay		Recpt.time	0.05 hrs.	8.50/hr.		.425
File chart		Recpt.time	0.05 hrs.	8.50/hr.		.425
Process paper		Recpt.time	0.05 hrs.	8.50/hr.		.425
Bill patient		Clerk time	0.10 hrs.	9.00/hr.		.900
Source	.28					.280
Postage	.34					.340
Supplies	.01					.010	3.23
Total							$19.89
General overhead						
Fixed		MD time block	1	16.08			16.08
Variable		# of patients	1	3.99			3.99
Total							$39.96

> I realized that I needed business intelligence about the insurance companies and how they operate and handle claims. We profiled the various insurance companies, with respect to what they paid for each procedure, and determined our clinical approaches based on the revenue. The information from the activity-based analysis of my services leads directly into strategy and tactics. I quit performing 99215 exams because most of the companies would not pay for them. A refused claim only increases my costs. The cost of resubmission and documentation is not rewarded with enough revenue to justify its performance. If someone needed a complete evaluation and his or her insurance company reimbursement did not cover my cost, then I would refer the patient to a specialist. The insurance company would gladly pay the specialist more to do the work, the patient would get the necessary evaluation or treatment, and I would not lose money on poorly reimbursed processes.[1]

The primary point to be made with this example is that until the clinic's management could determine the *relative* cost of its different services, it could not react to the pricing problems it believed it faced. The cost differences among the different categories of visits were caused by differences in the activities they required. In addition, until the clinic could document the resource demands and costs for its different products, it would have great difficulty negotiating satisfactory prices.

Assumptions and Accuracy

This example is from the early days of basing costs on analysis of component activities, as opposed to more traditional approaches, which followed costs from department to department. More will be said about this transition later in this book. The physician-manager, who holds an MBA degree, attended a seminar on the activity-based approaches and believed that using it would give him a better understanding of the specific cost of his different products. He was forced to work from general ledger data because the clinic had not been collecting data specifically to support activity-based costing methods. In addition, he did not have a lot of time to devote to this study. Were it not for these constraints, he could have increased the accuracy of the results by modifying the analysis in several ways, based on material covered in Chapter 3.

DIFFERENTIATING COST COMPONENTS   Table 4-3 shows the division of general ledger cost-account balances into fixed and variable categories. These values were established by using historical data from a baseline year. The variable overhead rate was set at $3.99 per patient visit (as used for a single visit at the bottom of Table 4-2) by dividing total variable overhead cost by the number of visits in the year. Realize that this variable overhead rate could also have been found through a cost-behavior analysis by regressing total overhead cost on patient visits and using monthly data. An advantage of the regression approach is that the *goodness*

Table 4-3 **Distribution of Fixed and Variable Costs**

Account	Variable Costs ($)	Fixed Costs ($)
Doctors' Salaries	280,500	
Employees' Salaries	162,264	
Payroll Taxes	30,187	
Supplies	33,161	
Postage	7,644	
Office Expenses		1,332
Building Rent		69,384
Computer		8,010
Supply		14,110
Print		4,315
Rental Equipment		1,415
Depreciation		21,643
Service Expenses		
Accounting		14,545
Computer		4,217
Legal		1,615
Payroll		1,966
Other		14,884
General Expenses		
Malpractice Insurance		16,479
General Insurance		3,034
Maintenance		1,320
Telephone		11,305
Subscriptions		1,363
Other Taxes		713
<u>Nonshared expenses</u>		<u>86,014</u>
Totals	$ 513,756	$276,332
Total cost =		$790,088

of fit would indicate the stability with which overhead rate varied from month to month. It would also indicate if a significant amount of variable overhead was caused by variables other than the number of visits. A poor fit should prompt further effort to find an appropriate causal variable. If regression analysis indicated a fixed cost per period different from that derived from the general ledger analysis shown in Table 4-3, the division of fixed versus variable cost would also need further analysis.

FIXED COST CONSIDERATIONS   Table 4-3 shows that salaries and payroll costs were treated as variable costs. Their dollar-per-hour amounts were applied to the amount of time used for a visit, in order to determine the labor cost of that visit. However, when labor is paid a salary for a period of time, the salary is a fixed cost of that period. As with any fixed cost, the amount per visit depends on the number of visits. This number might be changed in the future through more efficient management of labor time, more time-saving technology, or, if labor is not being used at its capacity, a larger share of the market.

As indicated earlier, the fixed overhead rate was computed at $16.08 per standard 10-minute period of a physician's examination time (as used for a single 10-minute period at the bottom of Table 4-2). If the physician's time was not used to its capacity, this computed figure could be lowered by increasing the number of visits. Relatedly, this example analysis assumed that *all* fixed cost was related to physician time spent in examinations. But if nonphysician fixed-cost resources, such as equipment, are not used to their capacity, even if physician time is, cost per visit could also be lowered by better matching the demand for those resources to their capacities. This can be done in two ways: first, by increasing utilization through increasing patient visits, and second, by decreasing the quantity of fixed cost resources used if demand cannot be increased.

A critical point to be made is that when fixed cost is a material part of total costs and there is unused capacity, the cost per unit of output might be significantly greater than it could be. In this example, if labor costs are recognized as fixed costs to the clinic, Table 4-3 would indicate that fixed cost for the baseline year would be $749,283 of the total cost of $790,088 or 95 percent. Supplies and postage would be the only variable expenses. This would indicate that for this clinic, using fixed-cost resources near their capacity is much more important to the cost per visit than efficient use of the variable-cost resources. It could be that third-party payments are based on services provided by larger practice groups with better utilization of fixed-cost resources. If that is the case, this practice will probably be unable to negotiate higher payments and must increase the efficiency of utilization of its fixed-cost resources. Whether or not this is the case, it certainly should be investigated. There is the unfortunate possibility that further research will show that the clinic is too small to realize economies of scale of larger clinics and cannot become price competitive. This situation emphasizes the value of benchmarking across organizations to check on an organization's relative efficiency.

HISTORICAL VERSUS PROJECTED DATA   The physician-manager stated that his purpose for activity analysis was to see if each type of visit was profitable. Using historical data is appropriate for the purpose of seeing if each visit was profitable in the baseline year, because the cost of each type of visit could be compared to the price received for it. If, however, the purpose is to determine if each visit will remain profitable in the future, historical costs must be adjusted to their future amounts. This requires estimates of future resource price changes and efficiency changes caused by changed technology. Making estimates of these changes is especially difficult when care involves advanced technology that uses expensive fixed-cost resources and when the technology is subject to rapid change. The estimated fixed cost per unit of output then depends on the accuracy of the estimates of the operating life of the resources and the number of visits over which the annual depreciation or lease costs will be spread. Inaccuracies in either of these estimates can cause material inaccuracies in the estimated cost of activities.

OVERHEAD REVISITED The manager understood that from a financial viability standpoint, the clinic's products were the services for which it was paid. The activities needed to complete each billable type of clinic visit were charted based on observation of visits and information from the people involved in the component activities. This analysis was reflected in charts like Figure 4-1. At this point, it was obvious that all the costs necessary to complete a visit were not reflected in the direct costs charted. There were both fixed and variable overhead costs that had to be covered by visit revenue. It is impossible to estimate the full cost of a visit without distributing a portion of the overhead to it. In this example, management used its knowledge of internal cost relationships to determine the basic causes of overhead costs.

Managers decided that variable overhead for a period changed in proportion to changes in the total number of visits. How good this assumption is could be checked by noting the R^2 statistic for a regression of total overhead on the quantity of visits. If the R^2 statistic is high (and the $p<$ statistic is low), it is reasonable that the regression estimate of fixed cost per period is fairly accurate. It will also be fairly accurate as an estimate for a future period if the technology used does not change.

Managers believed that the fixed-cost resources existed to support physicians' work. They, therefore, chose to allocate fixed overhead to each type of visit based on the number of 10-minute physician time blocks used in the visit; however, the fixed overhead does not increase with each 10-minute physician work period. If it did, it would be a variable cost. For instance, part of the fixed cost is an equipment, maintenance contract, a flat fee per year. Within the contract period, additional physician work time will not increase this cost. The same holds true for any fixed cost whose utilization does not exceed the resource's capacity. If, for budgeting purposes, the clinic estimates future fixed cost for a visit using this approach, it will only be accurate if the cost-behavior analysis had a good fit, the array of fixed-cost resources does not change, and the number of visits in the budget period is accurately estimated. If the fixed costs for the period are accurately estimated, the cost per 10-minute period will depend on the number of 10-minute periods in the denominator of the fixed-overhead rate formula:

(total fixed overhead) / (total time blocks) = fixed cost per time block

In short, when fixed costs are a significant portion of total costs, accurate product costing depends on accurate output-volume estimates. Getting these numbers is not difficult when estimating product cost for a past period. However, accurate output-volume estimates for a future period are just that—estimates. Product costing for the future can be no better than those estimates.

This example also illustrates another problem in allocating fixed costs. Lumping all fixed costs into one quantity assumes that all of the different cost objects using the fixed-cost resources will use each component fixed-cost resource in equal amounts. This is rarely the case. Again, using equipment maintenance cost as an example, if one type of visit does not use certain equipment that is used in other types of visits, it should not have the maintenance of that equipment considered part of its cost. These fixed-cost problems cannot be eliminated. They can, however, be reduced by evaluating how the problems affect specific decision processes. Ways to do this will be addressed throughout the remainder of this book.

Case Summary

This rather simple example of cost analysis began with the need for a clinic's management to get accurate measures of the cost of its different prospectively priced products. The clinic suspected that among its products (categories of visits), some were profitable, while others were causing losses. It realized that differences among the costs of its products would be caused by differences in the activities needed to produce and sell them.

- It observed those activities and collected information from the people involved in them.
- The results of this data were organized into an activity flow chart for each product.
- The amount and costs of the resources used in each activity were incorporated into the flow charts.
- The cost of resources whose use was believed to vary with the number of patient visits were taken from the general ledger.
- Average physician, medical assistant, and receptionist time was traced to each product. The remaining variable costs were treated as a variable overhead pool.
- This variable overhead pool was divided by the number of patient visits during the baseline period to create a variable cost per patient visit.
- The remaining costs for the baseline period were assumed to be fixed costs.
- After examining the specific components of the fixed-cost items, the management believed that they were all incurred to support physician activities.

- It, therefore, divided physician time into 10-minute blocks and analyzed the average number of these blocks spent by a physician in producing each type of product.
- Physician costs for the baseline period were analyzed to calculate a physician cost per time block.
- Fixed costs were then assigned to each product based on the standard number of physician time blocks used to produce it.
- For each product, the traceable costs of each activity required were added to the variable overhead cost per visit and the assigned fixed overhead in order to compute the cost of the product.

Having what management considered accurate costs of its different products allowed the clinic to drop products that were creating financial loss; this gave information with which to attempt to negotiate appropriate prices for these products.

Note the assumptions and subjective judgments on which this analysis was based. Inaccuracies in these would, of course, create inaccuracies in the cost estimates. Management assumed that

1. salaries and equipment costs were variable costs.
2. all fixed costs were incurred because physicians spent time with patients, which was proportional to the time spent regardless of the type of patient visit.
3. variable cost not traceable to specific intermediate activities was caused by a visit, and was the same for any type of visit.
4. fixed cost per visit would not vary with the number of patient visits in a period or that the number of patient visits would not vary from period to period.
5. fixed cost resources are being used to their capacities.

All of these assumptions are most likely inaccurate, but the degree of their inaccuracy might be too small to materially affect costs computed. In the following chapters of this part, approaches to analyze the validity of such assumptions will be discussed, as well as the degree possible or appropriate to compensate for them.

DISCUSSION QUESTIONS

1. Why is understanding the relative costs among different products important to financial viability?
2. Explain the advantages of charting the flow of activities and resources into products.
3. Explain how improperly identifying costs as fixed or variable can lead to inappropriate decisions.
4. Explain the value of historical costs when attempting to estimate future costs. Why must they often be adjusted?

KEY POINTS

- Organizations should consider their products to be the service or product for which clients pay.
- Health care delivery organizations have essentially three different products: (1) individually billable services, (2) prospectively priced encounters, and (3) capitated care.
- In the order just stated, each of these products creates more risk for the providers.
- Most health care providers are ill-prepared to manage the insurance risks associated with capitated products.
- Most care-delivery organization outputs are intermediate products combined to produce wellness, which is the final product.
- The cost of a single unit of an intermediate product is materially affected by the level of utilization of the fixed-cost resources used to produce it.
- The cost to produce any product is the sum of the costs of accomplishing the activities needed to complete its production.

PROBLEM

Return to the exercise on page 3-22 in which you categorized the costs of running a dental facility. Based on your best estimates of activities and times involved in a visit that includes x-raying, cleaning teeth, and filling one simple cavity, construct a flowchart, similar to the one in Figure 4-1, of the activities and resources associated with the visit. You need not attach dollar amounts of the resources used.

REFERENCES

[1.]Stuart, T. J. and J. J. Baker. *Activity-Based Costing and Activity-Based Management for Health Care.* (Gaithersburg, MD: Aspen Publishers, 1998).

FORMALIZING THE ANALYSIS OF ACTIVITIES AND COSTS

LEARNING OBJECTIVES

After studying this chapter, students should be able to:

1. Define and explain differences among four general categories of activities.

2. Explain the purpose and basic processes of activity costing.

3. Explain relationships between organization centers and activities.

4. Explain relationships between service and product centers and between external and internal customers.

5. Define and explain the use of cost drivers and the difference between activity drivers and resource drivers.

6. Explain the use of relative value units (RVUs) as resource drivers.

7. Explain the concept of drivers as linkages.

8. Explain why ABC cannot eliminate the fixed cost problem.

9. Explain the steps involved in determining the full cost of a saleable product when taking a top-down ABC analysis approach.

10. Explain the difference between the top-down and bottom-up approaches.

CATEGORIES OF ACTIVITIES

Costing should reflect the fact that resources are consumed by the activities that must occur in order to produce, sell, and distribute a product. These activities can be categorized into four general types according to the breadth of the array of cost objects to which they flow and the ability to trace their cost to units of output.

Organization sustaining activities are those that are necessary to keep the organization functioning. They include executive management, public relations activities, new-product research, financial management, building and grounds maintenance, and personnel administration. These activities support the continued operations of the organization but cannot be traced to specific outputs.

Production sustaining activities include equipment calibration and maintenance, production research, and procedure or protocol design. Many of these activities can be traced to specific outputs but cannot be traced farther to specific units of the output.

Batch activities can be traced to specific production runs of specific outputs but cannot be traced farther to individual units of the output. Batch activity costs per unit of output depends on the volume of output in each production run. Test set-up costs are an example of such batch activities.

Finally, some activities are performed for each unit of output and so can be considered direct costs of each unit. They are referred to as *unit level activities*. Here unit means a single item of production, not a subcenter or department within an organization.

The term *output* is used here rather than *product* because many activities have outputs that are not necessarily billable products. The activity *perform diagnostic radiological test* yields a radiology laboratory output that might be an input to a trauma center activity, which in turn leads to a billable product—an outpatient visit. If the hospital were paid under a prospective ambulatory patient category (APC) system, this would be the case. However, if it were paid under fee for service, the test would itself be a billable product. In both cases, the cost of the test is the cost of performing all the activities needed to complete it.

Activity based costing (ABC) attempts to measure the cost in each activity within each of the four activity categories just discussed. Having done this, an ABC database has a catalog of activity costs that can be aggregated to cost any object that demands those activities. Managers implementing an ABC system have reported that the activity analysis is valuable in itself, because it forces a disciplined look at current procedures. In so doing, it prompts a cross-discipline and cross-departmental analysis of the flow of activities across organization boundaries. This forces the communication that continuous quality improvement efforts have found to be essential to competitive organizationwide performance. This differentiation between outputs and products is not critical to good analysis, but it does help analysts remain focused on the complete flow of activities to products whose sale produces revenue.

DISCUSSION QUESTIONS

1. What is the difference between organization sustaining activities and production sustaining activities? Give examples other than those mentioned that would occur in health care organizations.
2. What is the difference between the sustaining activities and batch activities? Give examples.
3. What is the primary difference between sustaining and batch activities discussed and unit level activities?
4. Why is the process of analyzing the flow of activities within an organization of value in and of itself? Give examples of what managers might learn from such analyses other than acquiring a list of resources used.

ORGANIZATION CENTERS—THE LOCI OF ACTIVITIES

Chapter 1 discusses the concept of specialization underlying the structure of organizations. Experience proves the advantages of grouping like skills and long-term assets using similar technology under the same immediate supervision and control. This creates departmentalization within organizations. A hospital will probably have an executive suite, a personnel department, an intensive care unit, a medical-surgical ward, a surgery department, and so forth. The activities required to meet the organization's objectives are performed within these centers. Specific activity analyses can be done in the centers responsible for the activity needing analysis.

Differences Among Activity Types

The primary difference between the four types of activities previously discussed is the degree to which their outputs can be traced to the different activities using them. Sustaining activities are conducted in departments that support many other centers. They tend to be located in executive management or high-level staff centers within the organization. For instance, the personnel and finance departments perform services for almost all other departments. Their outputs are usually considered to be overhead costs for centers nearer the output of saleable products. For this reason, they are commonly referred to as *service centers* (for Medicare cost-finding they are "general service centers" as discussed in the preceding chapter). The centers whose output is a saleable product have traditionally been called *product centers*. However, under the variety of payment systems that health care organizations face, differentiating service centers from production or product centers is not clean cut. The fact that a clinical laboratory could be considered a product center in one situation and a service center in another has already been discussed. Payment for a hospital discharge under Medicare's prospective payment system is an extreme case. In this situation, the hospital is the only product center. All other centers produce output that flows into the inpatient's care. The hospital is not paid separately for these individual outputs; it is paid one amount for the discharge. This situation is sometimes described by saying that a center can have *external customers* to whom the organization sells its products and *internal customers* (within the organization) to whom service centers transfers their outputs.

Prior to the implementation of prospective payment systems for inpatient discharges and ambulatory care visits, it was logical to call all of the centers that produced billable line items in fee-for-service payment systems *product centers*. ABC systems still keep track of the traditional line items used in a patient's treatment. The costs of providing these items constitute the patient's cost of care. ABC attempts to maximize the accuracy of costing these inputs by carefully identifying and costing each of the activities necessary to deliver each line item. In considering costing an outpatient visit or an inpatient discharge, what had been billable line items under the fee-for-service payment can be thought of as *intermediate products* flowing into the saleable product. The saleable product could be a visit or a discharge. One semantic difference that has evolved with the shift from fee-for-service payment is that the term product center also refers to a center housing the activities producing a countable unit of input to an internal customer. A product center may produce saleable products or intermediate products. Centers like a diagnostic laboratory may be called product centers even if their output is always an intermediate product transferred to other activities. Whether to call a center a service center or a product center becomes less important when analysis focuses on what the center does and follows the flow of these activities from all the centers involved to the outputs that are sold (the organization's products).

Implications for Service Centers

Centers exist in order to gain the advantages of decentralized organization and management of activities by specialists with the appropriate technical skills. A personnel department offers a simple example of accuracy gained by looking inside a service center for various activities provided in different quantities to other activities. Before activity focused analysis, personnel department cost were distributed to other activities using a single, logical basis of allocation. This was often the number of people employed or full time equivalent employees (FTEs). In some cases, closer analysis revealed that most of the department's costs were incurred in two different activities: payroll preparation and personnel action administration. These activities use essentially different sets of personnel and equipment (resources). This meant that they could have separately identifiable costs. Further analysis indicates that payroll preparation costs are caused by the number of payments to workers, regardless of the number of FTEs. Concurrently, personnel action costs are caused by the number of actions processed. Therefore, if personnel department costs are allocated based on FTEs, neither set of costs is allocated by the variable that causes the costs to be incurred. In ABC vernacular, it is said that the cost of the payroll activities is driven by the number of payments made, and the cost of the personnel action activity is driven by the number of personnel actions requested. Therefore, the cost of the two primary activities within the personnel department should be allocated separately. The total cost of running the personnel department does not have a single cause.

The separation of activities is material to the costing process if different users to which their costs are allocated use varying proportions of the activities. Using a single basis for allocation overaverages the costs among the users and fails to capture differences in the *relative* cost of the service center outputs to different users. Indeed, in a hospital, this may be the case in a personnel department. For example, the housekeeping department may have high turnover, which induces large numbers of personnel actions. At the same time, nursing services may be managed well, have a flat organization structure, and therefore have many fewer personnel actions. However, nursing services may also have more people being paid, especially if it supplements the core staff with pool nurses. More accurate allocations would be made by allocating payroll costs by the number of payments and allocating personnel action costs by the number of actions requested. This change isolates the different activities within this service center, finds the variable that drives demand for each, and allocates each activity's costs separately based on that variable.

In the example, nursing services (the cost object) requests personnel actions from the personnel department. The cost of nursing services' use of this service activity is some part of the personnel department's total cost of administering personnel actions. That part is believed to be the proportion of the total number of personnel action requests processed by the personnel department that comes from nursing services. Amounts of this specific activity *administer personnel action requests* can be traced to the cost objects that requested them and the cost of the support activity can be distributed to the objects in proportion to their use of the driver, personnel actions requested.

Cost Drivers

In the vernacular of ABC, the variable or phenomenon that causes a cost to be incurred is referred to as its *driver*. Drivers can be classified into two types: activity drivers and resource drivers.

Activity Drivers

The first steps in performing activity analysis in what has traditionally been considered a service center is to see: (1) if the center performs different activities that use different resources and hence have identifiably different costs, and (2) if discrete units of each activities' output can be traced to specific users. The second step is to determine what causes the center to perform each of these units of activity. These causes are called *activity drivers*. In the personnel department example, the fact that the activity *pay an employee* (a discrete unit of activity) can be traced to nursing services (a user) makes the number of people paid an activity driver.

Resource Drivers

The primary difference between the four types of activities mentioned earlier is the degree to which their output can be traced to the activity using it. A variable that best correlates with the total cost of the support activity can be used as the driver for the variable portion of the overhead cost. The driver is identified using a set of cost behavior analyses. Several drivers that intuitively seem likely to cause the activity are regressed on the activity's total cost over a set of accounting periods. The one whose regression shows the highest R^2 statistic can be chosen as the driver. Though it is true that correlation does not establish causation, using this driver for predicting cost is reasonable as long as the technology applied in the activity does not change. The same driver can be used to allocate the fixed portion of the activity's cost. However, there may be a more rational driver for the fixed portion. In ABC vernacular, these drivers of untraceable costs are often called *resource drivers*. For nursing services (again as the cost object), the variable portion of housekeeping services (an overhead activity) may be allocated by the proportion of hours of housekeeping personnel use in nursing services (a resource driver). Concurrently, the fixed portion may be allocated by floor area (also a resource driver). Note that an activity driver cannot cause changes in fixed costs. Note also that the driver for the variable part of a mixed cost is used much like an activity driver, but it is identified through cost behavior analysis, not by the direct cause-and-effect tracing of the overhead activity. Differentiating activity from resource drivers has to do with how they are isolated. This differentiation is not particularly important to the drivers' application in costing a particular output. The important thing is to visualize the flow of resources and activities that must occur in order to produce the cost object and to identify the factor (or variable called the driver) that best indicates demand for the amount of each activity.

Relative Value Units as Drivers

Relative value units (RVUs) are resource drivers created by assuming a relationship between the use of an untraceable input and variable whose association with a cost object is countable. One approach has been in allocating overhead costs in proportion to the flow of direct costs. In the example given later in this chapter, the overhead cost of doing diagnostic procedures is allocated to different procedures using RVUs as the driver. RVUs are only vaguely related to value; instead, they are related to costs.

RVUs SET AS AN AVERAGE OF DIRECT COSTS A common method of determining the quantity of RVUs used by a specific procedure is to determine the relative amount of costs direct to each procedure. Assume the traceable costs such as supplies, laundry, and so forth for one procedure is $42.65 and for the second of two procedures was $35.73. The average direct cost of the types of procedures performed by the diagnostic imaging internal activity center that performs these procedures is ($42.65 + $35.73)/2 = $39.19. This would be set as the direct cost of a procedure with an RVU = 1. The first procedure would then be assigned an RVU of (42.65/39.19 =) 1.088. The second procedure would be give an RVU value of (35.73/39.19 =) 0.912. The total amount of RVUs for procedures done in a baseline period would be computed, and the total fixed cost of the procedures perform in the period would be obtained from the accounting ledger. The quotient of the total fixed cost divided by the total number of RVUs would produce a *fixed cost per RVU* for the baseline period. This allows RVUs to be used to allocate fixed costs to specific procedures. The total cost per RVU can also be computed if one driver is to be used for both variable and fixed overhead costs. Another example may be helpful.

EXAMPLE

Assume a company is costing different laboratory tests. Using an oversimplified example, assume only four different tests are done and there are only two categories of direct cost: supplies and technician labor. These are measured for each type of test:

Test type	1	2	3	4
Number of test done	500	150	100	230
Direct costs per test				
Supplies	$ 5.00	$ 1.20	$ 7.40	$ 2.00
Labor	10.00	15.00	5.00	20.00
Total direct cost per test	15.00	16.20	12.40	22.00

Therefore, the direct cost of an average type of test is:

$$(15.00 + 16.20 + 12.40 + 22.00) / 4 = \$65.60 / 4 = \$16.40$$

The average cost is assigned a relative value of 1. Therefore, the relative values of the separate tests are:

Test 1 15.00/16.40 = 0.915 RVUs
Test 2 16.20/16.40 = 0.988 RVUs
Test 3 12.40/16.40 = 0.756 RVUs
Test 4 22.00/16.40 = 1.341 RVUs

RVUs are used to allocate total overhead in the laboratory cost pool as follows:

$$\textit{Total RVUs in period} = 500(0.915) + 150(0.988) + 100(0.756) + 230(1.341)$$
$$= 475.5 + 148.2 + 75.6 + 308.4 = 1{,}007.7 \; RVUs$$

If the total overhead costs in the laboratory cost pool were $21,860, then the overhead per RVU would be $21,860/1,007.7 RVUs = $21.70 per RVU. Overhead allocated to each test would be:

Test 1 ($21.70/RVU)(0.915 RVUs) = $19.86
Test 2 ($21.70/RVU)(0.988 RVUs) = $21.44
Test 3 ($21.70/RVU)(0.756 RVUs) = $16.41
Test 4 ($21.70/RVU)(1.341 RVUs) = $29.08

The cost of Test 1 would then total to $15.00 direct cost + $19.86 overhead = $29.10.

Again, this approach assumes that overhead is incurred among test at the same proportions as direct cost. However, capital equipment that creates overhead is often incurred in order to lower direct costs. This means that the proportion of a production department's total overhead caused by a product may actually be the inverse of its relative amount of direct cost. In such cases, significant cost allocation errors can occur when using RVUs based on direct costs to allocate indirect costs.

RVUs SET BY SUBJECTIVE JUDGMENT   A less quantitative way to establish RVUs is available. It uses subjective judgments by those involved in the use of overhead resources to establish the relative use of those resources by different centers or products. As an example, West, Balas, and West[1] describe a situation in which management needed to know the relative amount of dialysis center overhead resources that were used for hemodialysis as opposed to peritoneal dialysis. It simply questioned the dialysis center's clinical personnel and made a studied estimate of the relationship. It found that a hemodialysis treatment required twice as many clinical overhead resources as a peritoneal dialysis. The hemodialysis therefore was given an RVU of 1 and the peritoneal an RVU of 2. Of course, the allocation of overhead costs using this approach to establish RVUs is no more accurate than the estimates of the relative use of resources made by the analysts.

The overhead amount allocated between the two types of treatments was from general overhead, durable equipment, and nursing services costs. The RVU total was computed using two (2) RVUs for each hemodialysis and one (1) RVU for each peritoneal dialysis. Essentially, the RVUs were used as the resource driver for these overhead costs flowing into the two treatments. Doing this assumes that each of these categories of overhead cost is used by the two treatments in the same proportions. This may not be the case.

If this is not the case, a more accurate allocation could be made by constructing a separate set of RVUs for each of these overhead categories or overhead cost centers. In the example, West, Balas, and West subjectively established RVUs for facility costs, administration, medical records, utilities, registered nurses, licensed practical nurses, nursing administrators, and dialysis machine operators. Each RVU was used as the resource driver of overhead costs from its related cost center. They became measures of relative cost.

Implications for Product Centers

Product centers use different amounts of various activities to produce diverse products. Each product demands a set of activities, which in turn, use an array of resources. Because some product-center activities are not traceable to its specific products, resource drivers must be found within production centers as well as for cost flows from an organization's service centers downward to the product center. For instance, the chief pathologist salary is not traceable to specific laboratory tests, so it must be allocated among them using a resource driver such as the standard technician time used. The rationale here is that the chief pathologist's primary activity is supervising technicians; therefore, technician work time drives the pathologist costs.

The overhead pool for a specific activity within a product center, therefore, has two sets of overhead allocations. One is for the organization's service center overhead and the other is for product center overhead. Each separate allocation is in proportion to the driver of the allocated cost. These allocations are added to the cost of direct inputs to compute a total cost of each product center activity. Subsequently, the sum of the overhead and direct costs of the activities used to produce a specific product is the cost of that product.

Drivers as Linkages

Returning again to the personnel department example, confusion is sometimes caused by the intermediary role of a cost driver. For instance, the cost driver *personnel actions* is a link between one of the costs incurred by nursing services and a set of costs within the personnel department. The personnel department must consume resources to complete the activity called *administering a personnel action*. The total amount of this cost that it must incur in a period of time depends on the resources consumed in this activity and the number of times the activity must be performed. Therefore, one of the variables affecting the cost of running the personnel department for a period of time is the number of personnel actions it must process. It can be said that the number of personnel actions to be processed drives the total cost of one of the personnel department's activity centers. From the opposite side of the transaction, one can also say that the number of personnel actions demanded by nursing services is a driver of the cost of nursing services, because it determines how much of the cost of the activity *administer personnel actions* will be allocated to the activity *perform nursing services*. These relationships are illustrated in Figure 5-1.

From either perspective, knowing the cost of administering a single personnel action (an activity) allows one to better understand both the cost of running the personnel department and of providing nursing services. Managing the total cost of the organization is helped by understanding such cost drivers. The cost of the nursing services can be lowered by eliminating unnecessary personnel action requests. In turn, the personnel services cost can be lowered by minimizing the personnel actions it is requested to perform. Notice that a key action to lower the cost

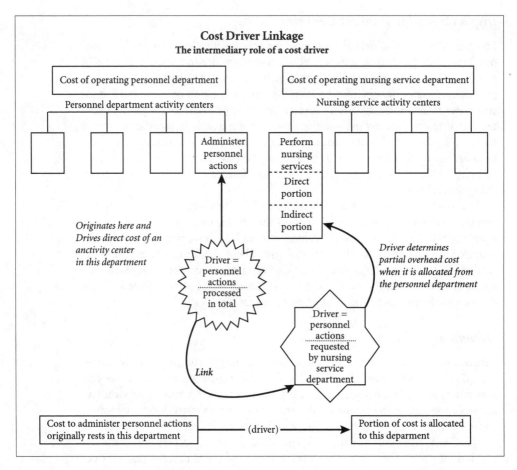

Figure 5-1 **Cost Driver Linkage**

in the personnel department is the reduction of the driver, and this must be done by the centers using the personnel department's services.

Organization Sustaining Activities

Organization sustaining activities are overhead activities conducted at relatively high levels of the organization. The costs of these activities are usually allocated toward production using appropriate resource drivers. Production sustaining activities, such as biomedical engineering actions, might be allocated using resource or activity drivers. For a production run, batch activities are those needed to initiate and terminate the run. They are usually allocated using an activity driver. At the level of a unit of product, these sustaining overhead activity costs are buried in the allocations of activities flowing into the product. This is illustrated in the example at the end of the chapter.

At all levels, activities incorporate direct costs as well as overhead. ABC can analyze costs flows from the level of organization sustaining activities toward the final production activities, or it can analyze the product center activities needed to produce a saleable output and work backward through all the activities and resources that these product center activities demand. Generally, ABC is approached from both directions concurrently. These concepts will be discussed further when considering top-down versus bottom-up analysis.

DISCUSSION QUESTIONS

1. What are the differences between service center and intermediate product centers? What is intermediate about intermediate product centers?
2. What is the advantage of isolating separable activities within a service center? What are the characteristics of separable activities? When is separating activities for costing purposes not useful?
3. What are the characteristics of an activity driver? Why is identifying them important to accurately measuring the cost of a specific output?
4. What is the difference between an activity driver and a resource driver? Which generally leads to more accurate costing? Why?
5. What are some advantages of using RVUs as resource drivers? How can the RVU weights of different overhead activities for different cost objects be determined? Develop some examples for overhead allocations within a hospital or clinic.
6. Why is it appropriate to think of cost drivers as linkages? Give some examples.

COMPREHENSIVE COST ANALYSIS

In choosing among alternative future actions, management must weigh the future revenue change caused by an action relative to future cost changes caused by the action; that is, management must take a marginal view. This means it must look at all the costs incurred by a change in business, not just the production costs. If the question is whether or not to add a product, the marginal administrative and marketing costs are no less charges against the additional sales revenue than are the added production costs. An ABC analysis of this decision would, therefore, require determining the marginal costs of administrative and marketing activities and aggregating those costs into a total cost relevant to the choice between adding the product or not. ABC attempts to provide and track the flow of cost data on all the activities relevant to a choice decision.

Flows to the Cost Objective

As mentioned frequently, the basic focus of ABC is the cost of activities needed to produce a cost object. ABC's attention is on the flow of activities to the cost object. ABC recognizes that the output from one activity may be an input to another. If the cost target is a specific product, that product may need to consume several intermediate products, each of which is itself the output of a set of activities. Analysis of cost objectives therefore demands analysis of the flow of resources to activities and the flow of activities to the cost objective. Charting these flows is discussed in Appendix 5.

The Fixed Cost Problem

This problem is always present when an overhead cost is a fixed cost. For a fixed cost, it is impossible to tell the cost per unit of output unless one knows the total output of the fixed cost resources over the period for which its cost is fixed. The higher the usage, the lower the cost per use becomes. The key points here are that ABC does not solve the fixed-cost problem. However, it does provide help in evaluating how and where fixed cost resources are not used efficiently. This help will be discussed later when the use of cost variances is covered.

DISCUSSION QUESTIONS

1. Why is it important to understand the selling and administration costs of a product as well as its production cost?
2. In what ways and why is the fixed cost problem in product costing not solvable?

EXAMPLE

This will show one branch of a hospital's ABC analysis to estimate the cost of caring for patients in specific DRGs.

Organization and Production Sustaining Costs

The example will follow the flow of institution sustaining activities to the cost of the DRGs in question. To keep the analysis as clear as possible, it is narrowed to the cost of sustaining overhead flows through the diagnostic radiology-imaging center to two DRGs. The approach is the same for all intemediate products contributing to the discharge of any patient under any DRG.

Identifying Cost Targets

Picking the cost targets of primary concern is a necessary first step in an ABC analysis. Targets for initial focus are usually the saleable products of the organization. Their costs are basic to planning and determining profitability. The hospital deals with some third parties that pay fees for services, some that pay for categorized discharges, and others that make capitated payments for care authorized for members of specified populations. DRGs were chosen for this example because payment for discharge under a DRG-like categorization scheme is common. The ABC focus on activity and resource flows enables an ABC system to also accommodate the other two payment forms.

If one starts by analyzing a DRG, one must determine all of the unit-level activities necessary to discharge the patient. Here the unit of output is an inpatient categorized in the DRG in question. The product is the inpatient's discharge. The protocol of care specifies the activities needed. Protocols include the services for which other payers might pay individually under a fee-for-service arrangement. Therefore, to determine the cost of intermediate products flowing into the care of patients in various DRGs, one must cost the items that would be sold in a fee-for-service arrangement. To estimate the cost of providing services under a capitated contract, the provider must also understand the epidemiology of the population the contract serves and the volumes of specific categories (DRGs) of patients the epidemiology indicates. With this additional information and the cost of serving patients in the DRGs involved, the provider can estimate the cost of complying with a capitated contract. Figure 5-2 illustrates.

Institutional Overhead

If a producer is interested in full costs, appropriate shares of the costs of sustaining activities must be determined. This means that these organization and production sustaining activities must be identified as well as the unit-level activities directly involved in the patient's care. The example hospital determined that it performed 15 different organization and production sustaining activities, which it categorized as overhead costs. These are listed along with their cost drivers in Exhibit 5-1. The total cost traced to each overhead activity is divided by the total quantity of the driver used in the hospital during the baseline period to compute an allocation rate. For instance, medical equipment maintenance is allocated by maintenance hours, provision of space is allocated by area of space occupied; and the provision of centralized supplies by the dollar value of supplies used. Note that the focus is on the overhead activities, for which separate cost pools can be established, not the service department in which they are performed. A department within the hospital could contain several activity centers (as in the personnel department example).

Intermediate Activity Centers

Exhibit 5-2 lists the product centers within the hospital and the activities each performs in order to produce its outputs. It also shows the driver for each of the

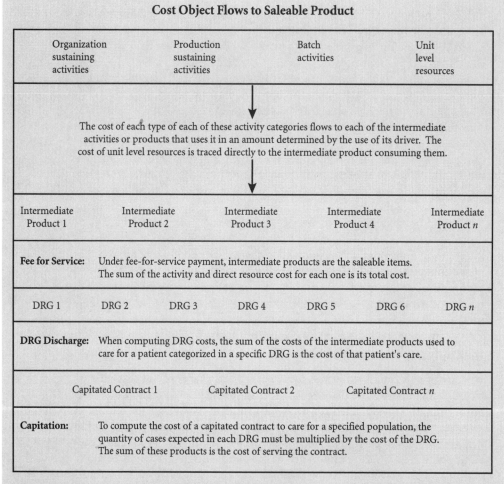

Figure 5-2 **Cost Object Flows to Saleable Product**

center's activities. For instance, to perform a diagnostic imaging test, the hospital must schedule the patient for the procedure, perform the procedure, develop the film, interpret the results, and transport the patient. This hospital has placed all those activities in the same product center and allocated them using an appropriate driver for each activity within the product center.

This is not the only array of centers that could be used. The nursing care, diagnostic imaging, and operating (surgical) centers all transport patients. Some hospitals may choose to create a center that does nothing but coordinate and

Exhibit 5-1   Hospital Overhead Activity Centers and Cost Drivers

Overhead Activity	Cost Driver
1. Supervise employees	Number of employees
2. Perform personnel services	Number of employees
3. Insure equipment	Value of equipment
4. Measure equipment depreciation	Equipment hours used
5. Maintain equipment	Maintenance hours
6. Administer equipment taxes	Value of equipment
7. Provide building space	Space occupied
8. Insure buildings	Space occupied
9. Provide power	Volume occupied
10. Provide central administration*	Number of employees
11. Provide supplies	Value of supplies
12. Maintain medical and billing records	Documents generated
13. Provide food services	Meals served
14. Provide laundry services	Pounds laundered
15. Market hospital services	Patient volume

*Central administration activity costs include the salaries of the president, vice presidents, and other central administrative staff.

accomplish patient transport. Second, all the activities performed in a product center might not be caused by the same driver. For instance, food services (center 4) provides meals and nutritional services. It might be that some patients demand more nutritional planning and education than others. Allocating the total cost of food services simply by the number of special meals, regular meals, and snacks different patients eat disregards that fact. Therefore, the cost of meals could be allocated using volume of meals as the driver and nutritional services allocated using nutrition service RVUs as the driver. Whether or not this should be done depends on the degree to which the types of nutrition services vary among patients. If this variation is significant, the activity *provide meals/nutritional services* should be broken into two activities with separate cost pools and drivers.

Overhead Flow

Figure 5-3 shows the total of hospital overhead costs ($10,892,763) allocated to the intermediate activities by allocating the cost of each hospital overhead activity among the 10 intermediate product centers. Each overhead activity uses its own driver and allocation rate. The resulting overhead cost pools for the activity

Exhibit 5-2 **Production Centers and Their Intermediate Activities and Cost Drivers**

Activity Center	Internal Activities	Cost Driver
1. Admissions	Reservations and scheduling, inpatient registration, billing, insurance verification, admission testing, room/bed/medical assignment	Number of admissions
2. Cardiac Catheterization Laboratory	Schedule, prepare patient, medicate, interpret results, educate patient, perform catheterization, process film	Number of procedures by type
3. ECG Department	Schedule, prepare patient, perform RCG, interpret results	Number of tests
4. Food Services	Plan meals, purchase supplies, prepare food, deliver food, clean and sanitize	Number of meals by type
5. Clinical Laboratory	Obtain specimens, perform tests, report results	Number of tests by type
6. Nursing Services	Transport patients, update medical records, provide patient care, patient education, discharge planning, in-service training	Number of relative value units
7. Pharmacy	Purchase drugs and medical supplies, maintain records, fill medication orders, maintain inventory	Number of orders filled
8. Physical/Occupational Therapy	Schedule patients, perform treatments, educate patients, maintain records	Treatment hours by type of therapy
9. Diagnostic Imaging	Schedule patients, perform procedures, develop film, interpret results, transport patients	Number of procedures by type
10. Surgery	Schedule patients, order supplies maintain supplies, instruments and equipment, provide nursing care, transport patients	Number of hours surgery by surgery suite type

centers in this top-down analysis is shown at the bottom of each activity's square. The sum of the 15 different overhead activity cost allocations to the diagnostic imaging activity formed a product center institutional overhead cost pool of $942,443. Follow the overhead cost flow through the activity *perform diagnostic imaging* on to the three different diagnostic imaging procedures done.

The institutional overhead allocation rates are used again to allocate the 15 overhead activity costs on to diagnostic imaging center's five component

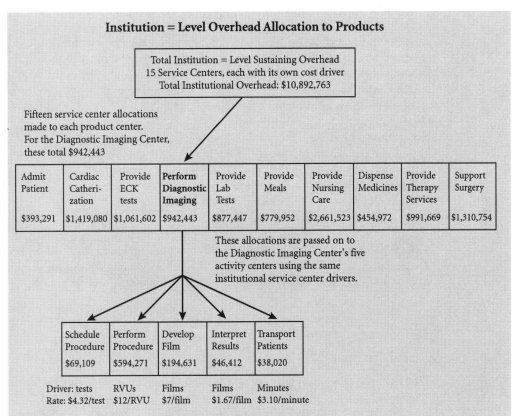

Figure 5-3 **Institution Level Overhead Allocation to Products**

activities. Realize that the allocation to the 10 product centers (departments) was not necessary in order to follow the flow of hospital overhead costs to the intermediate activities. For product costing, the intermediate cost target of interest is the diagnostic imaging center's internal activities, which are needed to produce its various tests, not the center itself. These institution activity results are shown at the bottom of the figure. For instance, the total allocation of institutional overhead to the diagnostic imaging internal activity *develop film* is $194,631.

To allocate the costs of the five imaging center internal activities to specific types of tests, drivers are determined for each of these activities. Analysts determined that scheduling cost are driven by the number of tests scheduled, procedure costs by procedure RVUs, film development costs by the number of films developed, costs of interpreting films by the number of films interpreted, and patient transportation costs by the minutes of transporters' time used. Using the base period data for activity overhead costs and the quantities of each driver used produced the allocation rates shown in the following example. By applying these rates to the quantity of the drivers needed to produce each type of test, hospital overhead was assigned to each type as shown. For each test, the quantity of the driver used in each test was multiplied by the allocation rate per unit of the driver and these were summed.

Using test AAA as an example:

Schedule procedure	1 test × $4.32 per test	= $ 4.32
Perform procedure	1.251 RVUs × $12.00 per RVU	= $15.01
Develop film	1 film × $7.00 per film	= $ 7.00
Interpret film	1 film × $1.67 per film	= $ 1.67
Transport patient	3 minutes × $3.10 per minute	= $ 9.30
Total institution overhead cost of Test AAA		$37.30

Table 5-1 shows how the hospital overhead costs attributable to each DRG were accumulated. An analysis similar to that for diagnostic imaging was done for each of the other nine intermediate product centers and the results were summed.

Table 5-1   **Overhead Cost per DRG**

	DRG 1X1			DRG 1X2		
Activity	Number of Transactions	Rate per Transaction	Overhead Cost	Number of Transactions	Rate per Transaction	Overhead Cost
Admit Patient	1 patient	$43.00	$43.00	1 patient	$43.00	$ 43.00
Perform catherization	2 procedures A	89.41	178.82	1 procedure C	41.21	41.21
Administer ECG test	7 tests	23.00	161.00	4 tests	23.00	92.00
Provide meals	9 special	6.21	55.89	9 regular	3.44	30.96
	6 snacks	2.87	17.22	6 snacks	2.87	17.22
Administer lab tests	4 tests BB	27.00	108.00	3 tests AA	14.00	42.00
Provide nursing care	312 RVUs	4.15	1,294.80	104 RVUs	4.15	431.60
Dispense medications	14 orders	15.67	219.38	6 orders	15.67	94.02
Provide therapy	7 CT hours	7.81	54.67	2 CT hours	7.81	15.62
Perform imaging	2 procedures AAA	37.30	74.60	2 procedures CCC	13.74	27.48
Operate on patient	60 minutes	$14.54	872.40			
Total Hospital Overhead Allocation			$3,079.78			$835.11

Source: Reprinted from J. J. Baker, Activity-Based Costing and Activity-Based Management for Health Care (Gaithersburg, MD: Aspen Publishers, 1998), p. 53.

CONSIDERING MULTIPLE LEVELS OF OVERHEAD

Resource costs are usually traced to activity centers within service departments through the general ledger, then they are allocated to users of the service activities. These can be other service center or product centers. This means that the structure of service departments and their internal activities is important to ABC. Organization and production sustaining activities that are performed in service departments are considered to be at the top of a funnel of activities flowing into cost objects. These cost objects are progressively nearer to the objects whose cost producers want to know. Costing that starts with these overhead activities and allocates accumulations of cost down toward products is referred to as *top-down analysis*.

The analysis in the example is a top-down analysis. It only considered institutional level sustaining costs. There are also resources that are overhead to unit level activities but can be traced (rather than allocated) to each of the 10 product centers. In the diagnostic imaging center, there will be fixed assets and variable cost resources that are dedicated to performing imaging but are not traceable to specific imaging tests. The cost of equipment and management fits this description. The general ledger can assign such costs incurred by the imaging center to it. Some of these center-direct costs can be traced to one or more of the five component activities and should be added to those overhead pools. For instance, some equipment may be used only in performing procedures, other equipment in developing film, and still different equipment in transporting patients. Some center-direct costs cannot be traced to the center's activity pools and must be allocated to them. As an example, the cost of the chief of diagnostic radiology can be traced to the imaging activity (department) pool but must then be allocated among the component activities. This cost is not part of the general supervision considered as hospital overhead. The fact that it is imaging specific should be recognized in the analysis. The chief of radiology's salary can be allocated to the five imaging center activities using the number of employees in the activities as the driver. Costs that are direct to the imaging center and can be traced to specific tests are, of course, charged directly to those tests as unit level costs.

When considering this flow in reverse, from the cost object back through each of the activities necessary to achieve it, one starts by specifying all the activities used directly by the object. Then the activities needed to complete those direct, unit level activities are specified. A producer continues to work backward in this fashion until all the activities needed to produce the target are identified in sequence. This is known as the *bottom-up approach*. In working backward, the producer eventually finds that some activities preceding the activity of interest are overhead activities. At this point, it is necessary to have conducted top-down analyses of these overhead activities so that they can be allocated to the activities that use them. Here top-down and bottom-up approaches merge. The objective is to allocate overhead activity costs in amounts proportional to the amount caused by each user. The best location in which to analyze activities in the flow from sustaining activities to products is the departments in which they occur. It is here that people understand them.

THE SCOPE OF AN ABC ANALYSIS

Management attempting to design an ABC system for its organization may find the scope of the task frightening. The idea of determining every activity necessary to produce each of its products approaches the absurd. Additionally, the accounting analysis required for ABC can become expensive. Obviously, managers must make some trade-offs between the cost of bad decisions made because oferrors in specifying the relative cost of alternative actions and the cost of more accurate measurement from detailed ABC. For example, one tradeoff in ABC-system design is how far to carry the scope. This issue will be discussed more thoroughly in Chapter 9.

KEY POINTS

- Organization activities fall into four categories: organization-sustaining, production-sustaining, batch, and unit activities.
- Activities take place within parts of the organization generally referred to as centers (divisions, departments, sections, etc.).
- Outputs of centers within organizations can flow to external or internal customers.
- Service-center outputs are sustaining activities that serve other centers. They cause indirect costs for other service centers and production centers.
- Production centers produce traceable outputs for sale or inputs to other product centers.
- Outputs of production centers that are inputs to other production centers are called intermediate products.
- Service centers may produce separable outputs that are used by other centers in varying amounts. These separable activities are identified by their use of the same inputs. The cost of these activities is allocated according to the factor that causes them to be done. These factors are called drivers.
- The cost of separable-service center outputs should be allocated separately if doing so would make material changes in the computed cost of centers using the services.
- Activity drivers are specific activities by using centers that cause a service activity to be done. They are countable.
- Resource drivers are factors in using activities that are believed to cause variation in service costs. They are identified by causal logic (often using regression analysis) as oppose to resource tracing.
- Relative value units (RVUs) are ratios of the quantity of an overhead cost (the cost of a set of overhead activities) used by an output. The ratio is relative to the average use among the types of outputs of a center. They can be used as resource drivers for overhead costs.
- Cost drivers link activities and their costs to each other and to outputs.

- Fixed cost per unit of output depends on the quantity of the output. Using ABC cannot change that fact. Therefore, cost per unit of output demands knowing the level of the output.
- Cost analysis that begins with sustaining costs and follows their flow toward the final products is called top-down analysis.
- Cost analysis that starts by isolating all the activities involved in the final production process and works backward through ac-

tivities that must precede these is called bottom-up analysis.
- Activity based costing (ABC) can be conducted by activity within the center performing the each activity. This spreads the costing analysis burden.
- Targeting activities for ABC analysis should begin with those causing the greatest total cost to the organization.

REFERENCES

[1] West, T. D. E. Balas and D. A. West. "Contrasting RSS, RVU and ABC for Managed Care Decision," *Healthcare Financial Management* 50, no. 8 (1996): 54–61.

[2] CPT codes are copyrighted by the American Medical Association.

CHARTING ACTIVITY AND RESOURCE FLOWS

INTRODUCTION

We have discussed the idea that, to reach any objective, produce a product, or make a sale, there must occur a set (or a hierarchy) of activities; think of an inverted pyramid of activities and the resources flowing into them. This pyramid has the output at its pointed base and the inputs to its initial activities across the top. The activities and the resources they use are aggregated as they flow down the pyramid and converge into the demanded output. The inverted pyramid could also be considered as a funnel of activities and resources flowing into the output.

To understand the relationships among the activities necessary to meet output demands, chart (or diagram) the flow. It is possible to attach costs to the resources flowing toward the product and thereby cost the activities at whatever level of activity aggregation (or intermediate product) selected. To say this in a different way, one can cost intermediate products that are made on the way to completing a final output as well as costing the final output. Activity flow charts are, therefore, extremely valuable. Making accurate charts of these flows is a necessary step in costing the outputs. This appendix is an introduction to the charting technique used in Hyperion Business Modeling software. Both Hyperion and Net Prophet are registered trade marks of Hyperion Solutions Corporation. Table 5A-1 and Figures 5A-1 through 5A-3 are used with the company's permission.

BASIC SYMBOLS

Table 5A-1 shows the basic symbols used. At the top of a chart is a set of supply boxes, (the top half of a circle), one for each resource used. As resources are acquired, they flow to inventories (cylinders) or directly to processes (rectangular

Boxes and Their Information

Box Type	Symbol	Data	Examples
Supply		Name Units Capacity $ data, variable Output link (1)	Materials Labor Supplies Energy Outside services
Process		Name Units Entry links (1–10) Capacity Factors $ data, fixed Output link (1)	Labor activities Machine activities Formulations Learning curves Efficiency Cost pools
Demand		Name Units Entry link (1) Volume Factors $ data, variable	Products Services Customers Departments Markets Idle capacity
Route		Name Units Entry links (2–10) Policy Output link (1)	Regular vs. overtime Machine options Labor options Material formula
Inventory		Name Units Entry link (1) Output link (1) Policy Capacity Output link (1)	Supplies Raw materials Finished goods Intermediate products Scrap
Connectors		None	Replace input and output links to avoid crisscrossing lines

boxes). Note that processes are analogous to activities. The output of a process can flow to another process, to an inventory, or if it is a final process, to a demanded output. An output is shown as a demand box (the lower half of a circle). Connectors are like couplers; they connect an outflow to another box without having to draw a line the entire distance from the output box to its destination. Their use will be apparent from examples shown later. Routing boxes also will be discussed later.

Several rules should be noted:

1. Supply boxes have no entry links.
2. Demand and inventory boxes can only have one entry link.
3. Route boxes must have at least 2 entry links and can have a maximum of 10.
4. Process boxes must have at least 1 entry link and can have a maximum of 10. However, they can be chained to allow an unlimited number of entry links to a given process.
5. Demand boxes have no output links; all other boxes have only one output link.
6. Factors, demand volume, route policy, and inventory policy are required data if the associated software for computing costs is going to be used.
7. The units flowing into and out of route and inventory boxes must be the same.

Parameters

Additional information about the flow can be inserted into charts through the use of parameters.

Factors

Process and demand boxes can have factors associated with inflows to them. The factor indicates how many units of the inflow are needed to produce a unit of the outflow.

Capacity

Supply, process, and inventory boxes can be given a capacity to indicate the upper limit of their outflow per planning period.

Volume

Demand boxes can have the volume of demand set by using the volume parameter.

Policy

The method of selecting the extent to which different possible through-put sources are used can be set by assigning a capability policy parameter to the appropriate routing box. The use of an inventory can be controlled by attaching a differential policy to the inventory box. The use of these policies will be demonstrated below.

Unit Factor

Figure 5A-1 is an example of a simple flow of activities and resources involved in the manufacturing in a shop that produces two models of a prosthetic device, Model A and Model B. Inputs consist of two types, wood and labor. Wood is measured by the board foot and labor by hours. There are two input activities, purchasing and marketing. Purchasing activities are measured (driven) by purchase orders (POs) processed. Sales and marketing activity is measured (driven) by sales orders processed. Note that the outflow from these input boxes is terminated by a connector box pointed with the flow. The using activities show connector boxes pointed to the source of a flow. The "W" boxes indicate that wood flows from the

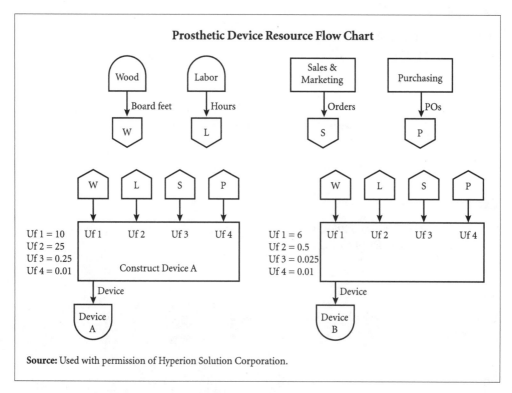

Figure 5A-1   **Prosthetic Device Resource Flow Chart**

wood supply box to both the manufacturing process boxes, as do labor, "L"; sales orders, "S"; and purchase orders, "P." The connector boxes eliminate the need to draw lines from each input box to all the processes that use that input.

Each type of device (demand) has its own charted flows. These are indicated in the process boxes.

Each input used is indicated by a line from the appropriate connector box to the process. Each input line is given a factor; in this case a *unit factor*. For Device A, the factors indicate that one device uses 10 units of wood, which are measured in board feet. It also uses 2.5 hours of labor, 0.25 sales orders (meaning that devices are sold in lots of four), and 0.01 purchase orders (which means that one purchase order covers materials for 100 devices. Note that Device B only uses 6 board feet of wood and a half hour of labor. The unit factor indicates how many units of the input are needed to produce a unit of the output demanded. In this case, demand was stated in terms of devices. It could have been stated in terms of four-device sets, if that is the way they are sold. In that case, for device A, UF-1 would be 40, UF-2 would be 10, UF-3 would be 1, and UF-4 would be 0.04. These would be the amounts of inputs needed to produce a unit of output, a set of four devices.

Constant Factor

Figure 5A-2 indicates that a machine hour of the process "machine parts" used 0.50 hours of machinist's time; this is a unit factor. For an accounting period, the machine lease costs are $30,000; this is a constant factor. The lease cost is paid regardless of the number of parts machined.

Total Factor

A total factor can be used when a standard usage has not been established but historical data on total usage and output is available. The total usage is set as the factor. In Figure 5A-2, during the baseline period of analysis, the shop used 28,161 kWh of electricity; this was a total factor that allowed the software to compute a power cost per part machined. That cost could be used as a rate per part in future budgeting.

Charting Inefficiencies

Figure 5A-3 contains the charting of existing inefficiency or expected wastage. Analysis indicates that it will take 105 test starts to get 100 useful tests; about a 5 percent lossage. The chart therefore indicated that because of this inefficiency, there will need to be 1.05 tests flowing into the efficiency box (treated as a process) in order to get one test completed and flowing into the demand box.

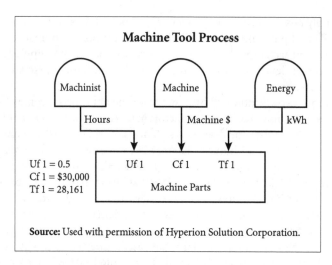

Figure 5A-2 **Machine Tool Process**

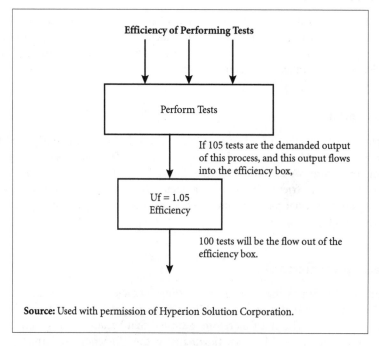

Figure 5A-3 **Efficiency of Performing Tests**

From this example, note the ability of the charting scheme to work backward from output demand to input demand. If the demand box shows that the demand volume is 100 tests, then the preceding efficiency box has a unit function of 1.05. So 105 tests must flow into it to get 100 out. Because the test process box has a supply unit function of 0.1, (105 tests) $\times$ (0.1 liters/test) = 10.5 liters of supplies must flow into the test process. The results of similar backward analysis from output demand are shown for labor and machine hours. This illustrates that software associated with such flow charts can state the total amount of any charted input based on stating the total amounts of all the organization's outputs. It can also show when any capacity constrains would be violated and the amount of the violation.

Summary

This appendix illustrates a method of charting flows of resources and activities in a fashion that lends itself to software programming of the relationships indicated. It is only an introduction to the charting of a generalized analysis system capable of providing extremely valuable projections for planning and sensitivity analysis in support of internal choice decisions.

Exercise

At this point, it would be helpful to express the Process Map shown in Table 4-2 in the form of a flow chart, using the Net Prophet approach just described. A solution is shown in Figure 5A-4.

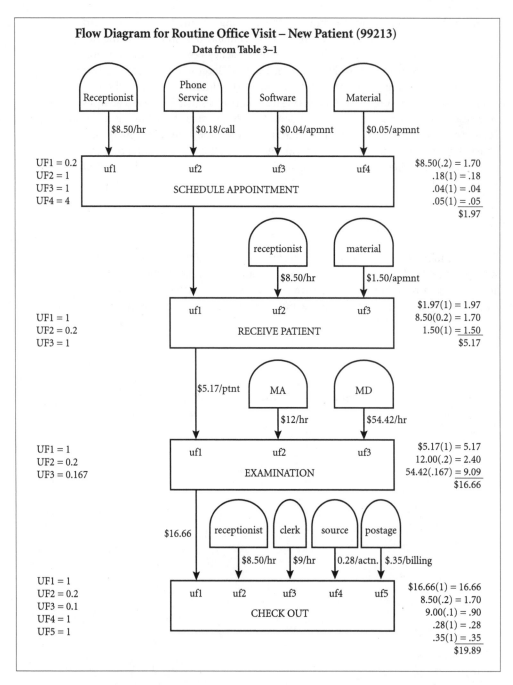

Figure 5A-4   **Flow Diagram for Routine Office Visit–New Patient (99213)**

ANOTHER WAY TO CHART ACTIVITY AND RESOURCE FLOWS

INTRODUCTION

The previous section discussed the idea that to reach any objective, produce a product, or make a sale, a set (or a hierarchy) of activities must occur. If one understands the relationships among the activities necessary to meet output demands, one can then chart (or diagram) the flow. It is possible to attach costs to the resources flowing toward the product and thereby cost the activities at whatever level of activity aggregation (or intermediate product) selected.

Creating a visual representation of the flow in the form of activity flow charts is a necessary step in costing the outputs. It is important to understand that these visual representations can take different forms, and the form they take can be influenced by the ABC software in use. This is because the software takes a particular approach to accumulating and managing the necessary information. It is easier and more efficient to create the activity flow charts in a form that follows the way the software will operate.

The previous appendix to this chapter illustrated the charting technique used by Hyperion Solutions Corporation's Net Prophet II activity-based costing software. The visuals were primarily vertical. For example, an inverted pyramid of activities with the resources flowing into them was described. The example was vertical; that is, the activities and the resources they use were aggregated as they flowed down the pyramid and converged into the demanded output.

This appendix will describe the basic approach of ABC Technologies activity-based costing software, now owned by SAS. ABC Technologies software is used to model, or create, the activity flow charts. Its approach is primarily horizontal rather than vertical. Thus, the resources flow across into the activities, which then flow into the cost objects. This is not a different activity-based methodology; it is merely a different way of accumulating and managing the necessary information and related calculations. This software approach parallels the ABC concepts adopted by Computer Aided Manufacturing International (CAM-I), an industry trade group. CAM-I codified industry standards for activity-based costing.

BASIC APPROACH

The correct level of detail must be chosen for the project's objective. To make this selection, it is necessary to understand the process hierarchy. Then the project moves through four modeling phases as described in this section.

The Process Hierarchy

This approach is built upon a three-part hierarchy of detail: business processes, activities, and tasks. The appropriate level of detail must be selected. Business processes can be, for example, operating processes. A process is composed of a series of activities. An activity is composed of a series of tasks. A process map, built as an initial stage of the project, helps to identify and illustrate what elements are processes versus activities versus tasks.

Modeling Phases

Modeling—and creating the activity flow charts—occurs in four phases as follows.

Phase I: Identify resources, activities, and cost objects
Phase II: Assign resources to activities; assign activities to cost objects; select and assign drivers
Phase III: Enter costs and driver quantities
Phase IV: Calculate costs

All four phases are necessary for an initial project. Only Phases III and IV are required to update an existing model.

BASIC MODULES

Three modules are used for modeling, as illustrated in Figure 5A.1-1. Module 1, "Resources," is at the left of a chart. Module 2, "Activities," is in the middle of the chart, while Module 3, "Cost Object(s)," is at the right of the chart. After resources are accumulated in the Resources module, they flow to the Activities module by means of drivers. Multiple intermediate levels are possible. As the Activity module is completed and activities are thus identified, they flow, with their dollars

Basic Activity-Based Costing Modules

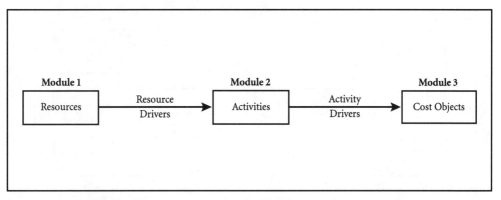

Figure 5A.1-1 **Basic Activity-Based Costing Modules**

traced and/or allocated by means of drivers, to the Cost Object(s) module. (Note that one of the first steps in charting is to select the cost objects.)

Relevant definitions that attach to the various modules are as follows.[1]

Resources: Economic elements that are applied to or used in the performance of activities.

Activities: Work performed within an organization.

Cost Object: Any customer, product, service, contract, project, or other work unit for which a separate cost measurement is desired.

As previously stated, resources flow to activities by means of drivers. These resource drivers are defined as a measure of the quantity of resources consumed by an activity.[2] Figure 5A.1-2 illustrates this concept.

Activities also flow to cost objects by means of drivers. These activity drivers are defined as a measure of the frequency and intensity of the demands placed on activities by cost objects.[3] Figure 5A.1-3 illustrates this concept.

After entering resource costs, resource driver quantities, activity driver quantities, and production quantities, the final step in modeling is to calculate costs. This step is automatically performed upon command by the software.

EXAMPLE

Figure 5A.1-4 provides an extremely simple example of the interaction between and among the three modules.

Activity-Based Costing Resource Driver Example

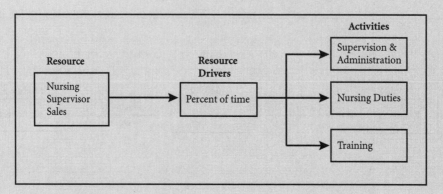

Figure 5A.1-2 **Activity-Based Costing Resource Driver Example**

Activity-Based Costing Activity Driver Example

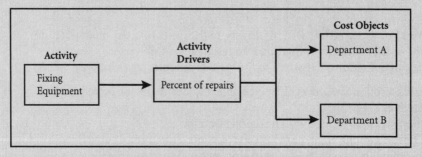

Figure 5A.1-3 **Activity-Based Costing Activity Driver Example**

Activity-Based Costing Model Example

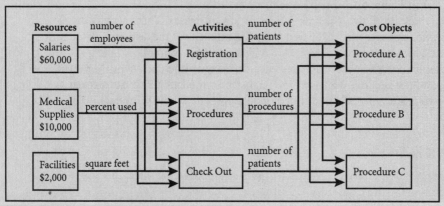

Figure 5A.1-4 **Activity-Based Costing Model Example**

Summary

Many levels of complexity, including multiple levels of intermediate cost pools, are possible. An almost unlimited number of allocation and tracing methods are also possible. Today's advances in computerization has allowed almost unlimited horizons in activity-based costing applications.

References

[1] Adapted from Raffish, N. and P. Turney. *The CAM-I Glossary of Activity-Based Management.* (Arlington, TX: Computer Aided Manufacturing International, 1991).

[2] Ibid.
[3] Ibid.

CHAPTER 6

ORGANIZATION STRUCTURE AND COSTING

Organization emerges whenever there is a shared set of beliefs about the state of affairs to be achieved and that state of affairs requires the efforts of more than a few people. That is, the relationships among people become structures. The behavior patterns or structures derive from a division of labor among the people and a need to coordinate the divided work . . . We can say that organizations are (1) composed of people and groups of people (2) in order to achieve some shared purpose (3) through a division of labor (4) integrated by information-based decision processes (5) continuously through time.[1]

LEARNING OBJECTIVES

After studying this chapter, students should be able to:

1. Define and explain differences among formal organization departments, cost centers, profit centers, service centers, and product centers.

2. Define pseudo profit centers and explain their purposes.

3. Explain the use of transfer prices, various ways of computing them, and the advantages and disadvantages of each.

4. Explain the difference between product center overhead and product overhead.

5. Explain a basic approach to isolating separable sustaining activities in service departments.

6. Explain the steps in following the flow of activities and resources from sustaining activities, through intermediate activities, to fee-for-service, discharge, or capitated products.

INTRODUCTION

Cost analysis is inextricably wrapped in organization structure because creating structure establishes the places within which the activities take place that lead to achieving the shared purposes referred to in the opening quote by Jay Galbraith. Management divides people into groups that use some outputs from other groups and some inputs from outside the organization. Managers' interest in efficiency leads them to want to know the costs of their outputs. Organizations frequently have alternative ways to produce outputs and to acquire the inputs they use in production. They need to know the cost of those alternatives so that the most efficient ones are chosen. How managers visualize the organization's products, the points at which they are completed, and what groups are competent and authorized to make decisions about their specifications and production determines what costs should be measured, how measures are aggregated, how the aggregated costs are used, and to whom costs should be reported.

COMPARING STRUCTURAL UNITS

In order to take advantage of the benefits of labor specialization, an organization would like to join similar skills and technology under common management. The work of cardiological specialists is probably not best supervised and coordinated by accountants, or even by orthopedists. Additionally, when specialized, high-priced, high-tech equipment is used in activities, it is desirable to have individual pieces of such equipment under a single management. This means that management would like to place all the activities using a given piece of such equipment in the same department. Throughout this book, the term *department* is used to refer to a group of people and resources formally differentiated by the organization and having a single individual responsible to the organization for its performance. Departments are usually shown on a formal organization chart. The term *center* is used for both departments and sections of departments. Readers have already seen that a personnel department can produce two distinct outputs, each using distinct personnel and equipment. These sets of resources could be referred to as the *payroll center* and the *personnel actions center*. They are *activity centers* within a service center. Chapter 5, analyzed an activity center that performed diagnostic tests within the diagnostic imaging product center. It is helpful here to establish some definitions to enable distinction between different types of departments, sets of activities, and outputs. Exhibit 6-1 summarizes these definitions.

Cost Centers Versus Profit Centers

All centers within an organization incur costs. The difference between cost and profit centers is that profit centers also create revenue; that is to say, certain sales of the organization may be attributed to a specific center. When both costs and revenue can be attributed to a center, it is a profit center. When hospitals are paid for individual laboratory test, radiological treatments, therapy sessions, surgical procedures, and the like, the centers that house the final activities producing these outputs can be considered profit centers. As mentioned earlier, the specific outputs for which a health care delivery organization is paid depend on the method of payment. Some payments may be for specific interventions, such as performing a diagnostic test. Other payers may pay a specified amount for a patient's discharge, regardless of the array or quantity interventions used in the patient's care. What an organization's products are depends on how they

Exhibit 6-1 **Structural Units**

Department	A unit shown on the formal organization chart of an organization.
ABC Cost Center	A unit within an organization to which costs can be traced or allocated but revenue cannot.
Profit Center	A unit within an organization to which both costs and revenue can be traced.
Pseudo Profit Center	A unit within an organization to which costs can be traced but revenue must be attributed through the use of transfer prices.
General Service Center	A unit in an organization whose output is not sold to external customers but produces organization- and production-sustaining activities for other units of the organization.
Product Center	A unit of the organization that produces a countable products that can be traced as a direct input to a subsequent product as opposed to flowing to an overhead pool, or a center that produces a product that is sold.
Intermediate Product Center	A center that produces a product that is a direct input to a subsequent product (a special case of a product center).
Activity Center	A center within a service or a product center where an activity is performed whose cost can be separated from other activities and traced or allocated to a subsequent overhead center or product. Activity centers are the locations at which costs are incurred.

are paid. This complicates the differentiation of cost and profit centers. Addressing management's desire to know how much specific departments and activities are contributing to the organization's profit (and hence financial viability) will be discussed later.

Service Centers

Cost accounting literature commonly differentiates between service departments and product (or production) departments. The terminology is a bit confusing because every department produces something. The traditional differentiation was that service departments serve other departments in the organization, whereas product departments produce discreet outputs for sale, which meant that they could also be called profit centers.

However, as management thinks of the flow of resources to a saleable output, this definition is inadequate. Departments that only perform services for other departments are referred to as service departments or service centers; they are frequently called overhead departments. This book will refer to them as departments when the emphasis is on their place in the formal structure of the organization; they will be referred to as centers when the emphasis is on the flow of resources to a saleable product. What separates service centers from other centers is that their outputs are institutional- or production-sustaining activities. These usually must be allocated to their users by using resource drivers, but this is not always the case. For instance, in the examples thus far, the cost of insuring equipment (a sustaining activity) was treated as being driven by the value of equipment insured. This meant that the cost of insurance was allocated to other centers in proportion to the value of the equipment they controlled (a resource driver). However, within the personnel department, the cost of administering personnel actions (another sustaining activity) was treated as if driven by the number of personnel action a using center requested. This is an activity driver.

Using activity drivers to allocate service center costs is somewhat like tracing unit costs. The driver can be traced to the using center; in fact, it comes from the using center. The number of personnel action request from any given center can be counted. However, the costs of one unit of the activity are not directly traceable to it. For instance, to get the cost of administering a personnel action, the total cost of operating that activity center within the personnel service center was divided by the number of actions it administered during a baseline period. This average cost per action was multiplied by the number of action requests from a user to allocate an appropriate amount of this service cost to that user.

The costs of service activities become part of the overhead costs of intermediate products. Notice that the costs of the hospital overhead activities in the example in Chapter 5 were allocated to the overhead cost pools of the 10 product centers as an intermediate step in allocating them to activities performed within those 10 centers. That example described the subsequent flow of those 15 overhead costs to the 5 specific activity centers within the diagnostic imaging center. Four of these activity center overhead cost pools were further allocated to specific imaging procedures (intermediate products) using activity drivers. The fifth cost pool, transporting patients, used the time patients spent in transport as a resource driver.

Product Centers

Costing the output of product centers is viewed somewhat differently. Traditionally, product centers were considered departments that finalized production of a saleable item. However, when the product is a patient discharge under a DRG-based prospective payment systems, the whole organization is the product center. In this case, according to the traditional definition, there are no internal product centers. However, producers can expand the definition of a product center to one that produces a countable product that can be traced to a saleable product, as opposed to being traced to the overhead pool of another product center. Products traced to subsequent product centers are called *intermediate products;* the centers that produce these products can be called *intermediate product centers*. Considering clinical laboratories illustrates this idea. A clinical laboratory is a product center. It can act as a reference laboratory and produce test results as products sold to users outside the organization (external customers). It can also act as in intermediate product center, producing test results for organization clinics (internal customers). In either case, its products are distinct, countable outputs of a set of activities internal to the laboratory—and these outputs can be traced as inputs to external and/or internal customers. Chapter 5 described how hospital overhead was allocated to specific diagnostic imaging tests and how the overhead cost of these tests was traced to specific DRGs, which were the products sold.

Allocations of sustaining overhead costs are not the only overhead costs that occur within a product center. Product center costs include four categories:

1. Allocations of organization- and production-sustaining overhead
2. Overhead costs that are traceable (as opposed to allocated) to the product center but are not further traceable to specific products—product center overhead
3. Overhead costs that are traceable to producing a specific product but not traceable further on to specific units of the product—product overhead
4. Cost that are direct to each specific unit of a product

The first three categories are indirect to the production of a unit of product. They flow into the overhead cost pool of the activity center producing the specific product being costed. An example is the overhead costs flowing through the diagnostic imaging center to produce *procedure AAA*. The example in Chapter 5 showed only the flow of hospital sustaining overhead.

■ It first flows to the five activities within the diagnostic imaging product center.
■ Then these shares of hospital overhead flow further on to the overhead pools of specific products, using the appropriate driver for each of the five activities.
■ A complete analysis of the flow of costs of overhead activities to products would also have to include *product center overhead*. This would include such activities as providing chief radiologist services and scheduling within the center.
■ A complete overhead analysis of the cost of a unit of a specific product would also need to include product overhead. This would include the cost of such resources as a piece of equipment that was used only for the specific type of product.

The example at the end of this chapter will illustrate how these resource categories and their costs can be applied to a unit of a product costs. The nomenclature used in discussing structure and cost flows was summarized in Exhibit 6-1.

DISCUSSION QUESTIONS

1. What characteristics are required of department within an organization in order to consider it a *profit center?* How does it differ from a cost center?
2. We can contend that all centers of activity within an organization have an output. What then differentiates a product center from a service center?
3. What are the characteristics of an intermediate product? How does it differ from an internal service? Give examples of intermediate products and internal services in a primary care clinic.
4. How does product center overhead differ from product overhead?

TRANSFER PRICES AND PSEUDO PROFIT CENTERS

Earlier we discussed the ability to divide a care delivery organization into profit centers if groups of patients with identifiable revenues (paid by fee for service, discharge, or per-diem) used the same resources in the same production center and none of these resources needed to be shared with other patients. To do this requires a large organization with enough patients in that set to use the center's fixed cost resources efficiently. Here *efficiently* means near capacity. For instance, a coronary care center could be a profit center if its volume of patients were large enough to warrant its own ward and laboratories. This enables all costs related to coronary patients to be traced or allocated to the coronary care center.

For smaller organizations, there is an alternative accounting tool to allow centers providing intermediate care products to be treated as profit centers. When low utilization of the fixed costs assets necessary to produce intermediate products within a potential profit center would create inefficiency, the center can "buy" intermediate products from the centers within the organization that produce these intermediate products. For instance, the coronary care center can buy bed-days from the hospital's medical-surgery ward and tests from its clinical laboratory. Keep in mind, however, that the reason to have profit centers is to get a better understanding of the financial performance of different parts of the organization. Using the laboratory as an example, if the tests it performs are "sold" to the direct patient care centers, the laboratory can be treated as a profit center, as it was under fee-for-service payment. However, problems arise in setting the transfer (or internal) prices. The higher the transfer price, the better the performance of the supplying center appears, at the expense of the users of its products. A great deal of research and writing has been done about appropriate ways to set transfer prices.[2] Some alternative are:

- the actual cost of transferred production
- the marginal cost of the transferred product
- the market price of the transferred product
- the standard cost of the transferred product

It is important to realize that the amount of a single transfer price has no direct impact on the reported profitability of the organization as a whole. The revenue to the seller is canceled by also being the cost to the user. Transfer prices are used to enable treating internal centers as profit centers. How transfer prices are set should therefore depend on how management wants to use centers' profit information. This information is often used to understand the relative contribution of different sectors of the organization to the organization's overall performance. It is also used as a basis for determining performance-based motivational actions, such as awarding bonuses. As with any choice decision, the uses and appropriate attributes of transfer prices should be determined before the manner of computing them is set.

1. If the transfer price is to reflect the financial contribution to the organization of the center *selling* its product internally, it should represent the price that the seller could get if it sold the product outside the organization, its *market price*. By using this transfer price, the selling center's revenue figure indicates the revenues it would have earned if the organization had sold the product rather than using it internally. From the seller's perspective, using the *production cost* (either actual or standard) would be unfair because the seller would get no credit for profit made by the organization through the seller's effort.

2. If the marginal cost of production is used, the transfer price is less than actual cost and the selling center's apparent profits are lowered to a level unacceptable to the sellers, especially if middle management bonuses are based to a significant degree on department profits or surpluses.

3. If the transfer price is to reflect the financial contribution to the organization of the profit center *buying* the product internally, it should represent the cost that the organization should suffer to produce it, its *standard cost*. (The classic definition of standard cost is the per-unit cost of an output under good (or best) performance.) It would not be fair to the buying center to be charged for inefficiencies of the selling center by using the actual cost of production. It would also not be fair to the buying center for all profit derived from the product to be awarded to the producing center by charging the market price. The contribution to the quality of the final product has much to do with the revenue it will earn and is significantly affected by the work of the buying department.

This limited analysis of alternative transfer prices illustrates that a single number cannot support decision purposes relevant to both the seller and the buyer—however, there is no reason that it should. For management decision purposes, there is no reason that profit center profits should sum to the organization profit. The organization profit is determined by financial accounting practices. Transfer pricing is used to produce center-specific information for internal decisions. The objective should be to produce the most meaningful information relevant to decisions about each center. This is probably done by using market price as the output price for the center producing/selling the intermediate product and standard cost for the input price of the center using/buying the intermediate product. The authors contend that ABC can produce the most accurate *standard full costs* for intermediate products and services transferred among internal centers. Probably the best source of the *market prices* for the intermediate products is research conducted by the organization's purchasing department. This research should not incur additional costs, because the purchasing department should track outsource prices as part of a continuing, "make-or-buy" decision process. If standard costs and market prices for the internally transferred items are kept in a database, computing center-specific profit information for management evaluation can be rather easily done through spreadsheet programming.

DISCUSSION QUESTIONS

1. What is a pseudo profit center?
2. Why are transfer prices sometimes established for intermediate products?
3. What problems arise when trying to set transfer prices that will meet the objectives of transfer pricing?
4. Why do the authors contend that the sum of the management accounting profits across all profit centers need not equal the total profit of the organization?

USES OF CENTER-SPECIFIC COST INFORMATION

Up to this point, several different groupings of personnel and other resources have been called centers. Divisions within the formal organization structure are generally referred to as departments. However, there could be several hierarchical levels of these centers such as subsidiary, division, department, section, and work group. The organization is generally considered as a hierarchical structure of departments that is documented on an organization chart. Management is concerned about two basic aspects of departments' performance: (1) Are they efficient? and (2) Are they contributing to financial viability? Of course the more efficient any department is, the more likely it is contributing to viability. Efficiency is usually measured by comparing costs to some benchmark. If a department can be treated as a profit center, its periodic profit or contribution should answer the second question. This question, however, is more difficult for service centers and intermediate product centers.

Service Centers

Costs that flow direct to service centers are traced to each center through the general ledger. The costs a service center caused by using the outputs of other service centers can be added through service activity cost allocation, like those overviewed in Chapter 5. Department costs (as opposed to the separable costs of activities within a service department) are generally used to measure the efficiency of service departments. To do this, there must also be some measurement of output and some reference levels of appropriate cost given the department's service output. ABC contributes to the ability to make comparisons of cost and output by specifying the activities that the department must accomplish. In the previous personnel services example, these activities are paying employees and processing personnel actions. At the end of an accounting period, the average cost of doing these can be computed. This is done best if each activity uses an identifiable and exclusive set of resources, so that each activity cost per unit of its driver can be computed. The benchmark for comparison could be management's standard cost per unit. Other sources of benchmarks are historic costs per unit from similar organizations. These are often available from trade associations or in summarized data furnished by consulting firms.

ISOLATING SEPARABLE SERVICE ACTIVITIES   In a previous example, an analysis of a personnel department discovered that the department conducted two separable activities. These activities were used in different amount by other activities and each used resources that were not shared with the other (thus they are separable). This is what is meant by *separable activities*. Identifying separable activities requires that analysts examine the work of service departments shown in the formal organization chart to see if separable activities exist within them. This demands observing the work done and talking with those who do the work. Analysts often begin by having service department personnel describe what they do and list the outputs resulting from their activities. The next step is to observe how these internal outputs are combined to produce outputs used by internal customers. This process can be reversed by asking the service department personnel what their department does for its internal customers. It is often helpful to then go to those internal customers and inquire as to what the service center does for them and what they want the center to do for them. It is quite possible that money is being wasted in service outputs that at one time were useful but that technology or other changes in the user's activities have made unnecessary. When a service department's outputs are identified, an analysis can be made within the service department to identify the activities that must be accomplished to produce those outputs. When analysts understand the outputs and the activities each demands, they can determine if some of the activities are separable.

The process of asking the service department personnel what their department does for its internal customers will often reveal nonvalue-added tasks and activities. One researcher observed a medical records department where significant nonvalue-added tasks were a source of daily irritation. Actually, two separate significant nonvalue-added tasks were occurring. One was in the activity of completing charts and the other was in the activity of transcribing medical records. In the case of completing charts, the medical records personnel responsible for this activity were having to "chase down" doctors to get signatures to complete the charts. Obviously, this was not part of their official job description, but it was consuming significant amounts of time; up to an estimated one-half of an FTE. In the case of transcribing medical records, the medical records personnel responsible for this activity were finding large portions of the dictation illegible. They were forced to contact the responsible doctor and get the illegible information interpreted. This is known in manufacturing as "re-work." In this case, it took time amounting to more than one entire FTE just to "re-work" the faulty transcription information. When the matter was investigated by management, only 5 percent of the doctors on staff were responsible for an estimated 90 percent of the faulty information. Needless to say, this nonvalue-added time as revealed by ABC analysis was promptly corrected.

Information from internal customers confirms what service department activities are needed. Information from observations within the service department reveals if some of its outputs are separable and should have their costs allocated using different drivers. As shown in Chapter 5, knowing the cost of specific service activities used to different extents by various users increases the accuracy of estimating the cost of different products. As in the personnel department example, not dividing these activities and allocating their costs separately causes the cost of each to be inaccurately distributed among the users of the center's outputs.

Product Centers

Chapter 5 illustrated how institutional and production sustaining activities performed in service centers are allocated to the production activities performed in product centers. However, products also demand resources that:

- can be traced to their product center but not to specific products; these are called *product center overhead.*
- can be traced to specific products but not to units of the products; these are called *product overhead.*
- *direct costs* or unit level resources that can be traced to each unit of each product made.

Product center overhead, such as the salary of the center's manager, is a component of the product center's total overhead pool. If some elements of cost in this pool have identifiable drivers, these overhead costs are allocated to activity centers similar to the way hospital overhead was handled in the Chapter 5 example. Product overhead is allocated to units of the product it supports using an appropriate driver. For instance, the cost of a piece of equipment used only in cardiac surgery could be allocated using time of use as the driver. Direct costs are, of course, charged directly to each unit of product. The following product center application of cost information illustrates these procedures.

DISCUSSION QUESTIONS

1. What is the purpose of setting benchmarks for the cost of specific activities? What are the sources of appropriate benchmarks?
2. What is the source of direct cost data for specific centers? What requirements does getting this data put on the general accounting system?
3. What is the role of output measures in benchmarking and efficiency measurement?
4. Why is finding rational drivers essential to establishing accurate cost information for any center within an organization?

Example

Implications of the interaction of structure and costs can be shown by examining the ABC analysis of an actual radiology department.

A Product Center Example: Diagnostic Radiology

The organization to be considered is a hospital that does not sell radiological procedures to outside users but produces them as intermediate products contributing to the discharge of its patients. The purposes of cost analysis is to cost the procedures and gain an understanding of the structure of resource usage among them. The hospital performs an array of imaging procedures that use a common set of shared overhead activities. These procedures are performed in a radiology department in order to optimize coordination of specialized skills and equipment. Their costing is done within the department, an intermediate product center. The department uses the following institution sustaining overhead activities:

1. Provide building space and depreciation
2. Provide labor benefits
3. Provide administration, teaching, and other overhead

This last category can be thought of as a remainder pool.

The radiology department also has product center overhead activities, whose costs are traceable to it but allocated to its component activity centers.

1. Transport patients
2. Receive patients
3. File films and documentation
4. Manage the department

These overhead activity costs, along with direct costs, flow into five different component activities whose outputs are (1) radiological diagnostics,

(2) ultrasound tests, (3) nuclear medicine procedures, (4) CT tests, and (5) radiation therapy.

Radiological activities and the *radiology department* are synonymous with reference to cost. Similarly, the *component activities* and *procedure types* become synonymous. Costs of the activity *perform ultrasound tests* are costs of the diagnostic radiology center. The radiology department's indirect costs are allocated among component activities cost pools using a cost basis appropriate for each indirect cost category. *Perform ultrasound test* would also be a component activity. ABC gains accuracy in the estimates of indirect costs of specific products by not lumping the cost of the different product center overhead activities into a single overhead pool and then allocating that pool among its component activities using only one driver. As with the personnel department example discussed previously, any one driver chosen may not be appropriate for one or more of the component overhead activities, hence reducing the accuracy of the allocations.

Table 6-1 shows how radiology product center overhead activities (*transporting patients, receiving patients, filing,* and *managing radiology processes*) have been allocated to the five radiology component activities or procedures. Realize that a cost behavior analyses had to be done for each of these overhead activity in order to find the most appropriate driver to use in its allocation. The results were that transporter costs were allocated to component activities using the volume of procedures done. Reception and management costs were allocated using direct-cost amounts, and the driver of filing costs was determined to be the number of films processed. The bottom portion of Table 6-1 shows the three drivers, the number of units of each driver used in each of the five production activities, and the total units of each driver used during the baseline period.

The data show that the total transporter activity costs for the product center was $550,000. The total number of radiological procedures was 500,000. Based on this historical data, the cost of transporting per unit of driver was:

$$\$550,000/500,000 \ procedures = \$1.10 \ per \ procedure$$

Because there were 120,000 ultrasound tests done, transporter costs allocated to these tests (#558) were:

$$\$1.10(120,000) = \$132,000$$

This approach was also used to allocate the cost of the other four product center overhead activities among the five procedures. The total of these radiology product center overhead allocations to the ultrasound tests (#558) was $195,375.

Table 6-1 **Product Center Overhead Allocations to Its Internal Activity Centers**

Activity	Cost	Driver	#557 Diagnostic Radiology	#558 Ultrasound	#559 Nuclear Medicine	#560 CT Scan	#561 Radiation Therapy	Total
Transport patients	$550,000	A	$110,000	$132,000	$ 88,000	$154,000	$ 66,000	$550,000
Receive Patients	360,000	B	60,000	36,000	72,000	108,000	84,000	360,000
File	117,000	C	90,000	3,375	13,500	4,500	5,625	117,000
Manage Production	140,000	B	40,000	24,000	48,000	72,000	56,000	240,000
Totals	$1,267,000		$300,000	$195,375	221,500	$338,500	$221,625	$1,267,000
Allocation Drivers								
A.	Volumes		100,000	120,000	80,000	140,000	60,000	500,000
B.	Direct Costs		$1,000,000	$600,000	$1,200,000	$1,800,000	$1,400,000	$6,000,000
C.	Number of Files		400,000	15,000	60,000	20,000	25,000	520,000

Table 6-2 Summary for Diagnostic Radiology Testing Activity Center Costs (#557)

Account Number	Cost Description	Amount ($)	Dir.Labor Vrble. ($)	Indirect Vrble. ($)	Labor Fixed ($)	Other ($)	Supplies ($)	Eqpmnt. ($)	Total Vrble. ($)	Total Fixed ($)
Activity Center Direct Costs										
4010	Direct Labor, Variable	500,000	500,000						500,000	
4020	Indirect Labor, Variable	100,000		100,000					100,000	
4030	Indirect Labor, Fixed	100,000			100,000					100,000
4210	Office Supplies	25,000					25,000		25,000	
4310	Film & Med/Surg Supplies	90,000					90,000		90,000	
4320	Diagnostic Expenses	35,000					35,000		35,000	
4700	Equipment Service Contract	50,000						50,000		50,000
4740	Equipment, Rental	10,000						10,000		10,000
4900	Misc., Travel, Library	10,000				10,000				10,000
5100	Depreciation	80,000						80,000		80,000
	Total	1,000,000	500,000	100,000	100,000	10,000	150,000	140,000	750,000	250,000
Diagnostic Imaging Product Center Overhead Allocations										
	Transport Patients	110,000		110,000					110,000	
	Receive Patients	60,000			60,000					60,000
	File	90,000		90,000					90,000	
	Manage the Product Center	40,000			40,000					40,000
	Total	300,000		200,000	100,000				200,000	100,000
Institutional Overhead Allocations										
	Depreciation, Building	75,000								75,000
	Benefits	125,000	62,500	37,500	25,000				100,000	25,000
	Administration	250,000							202,500	47,500
	Provide Space	150,000								150,000
	Remainder Overhead Pool	100,000								100,000
	Total	700,000	62,500	37,500	25,000				302,500	397,500
Total Expenses		$2,000,000	$562,500	$337,500	$225,000	$10,000	$150,000	$140,000	$1,252,500	$747,500

Table 6-2 (#557) shows how institutional overhead, product center overhead, and direct product costs for the activity center *diagnostic radiology* (#557) were aggregated to compute a cost per test. In this analysis, direct costs include both product overhead and product direct costs. Realize that to find the totals of each direct cost (the first cost category in the table), each line cost must be flagged in the ledger of accounts by an account number for the diagnostic radiology activity within the radiology product center. After direct cost, the component activity's totals for product center overhead categories are taken from Table 6-1. Lastly, diagnostic radiology's allocation of institutional sustaining overhead cost are shown. These institutional costs and their drivers were previously analyzed using a top-down approach similar to that done in Chapter 5. The remaining columns of Table 6-2 simply break the total of cost category figures into component costs of interest to managers, such as labor versus nonlabor and fixed versus variable. Decisions based on marginal analyses (to be discussed in Chapter 13) need these further breakdowns.

From Table 6-2, the total cost of performing diagnostic tests in the baseline period was $2,000,000. The number of tests performed was 100,000. The average cost per test of the intermediate product *diagnostic radiology test* was therefore $20. Analyses similar to the one shown in Table 6-2 were also done for the other four categories of radiological tests. Note that this activity approach takes into consideration that different radiological tests use different amounts of institutional services, direct to product center costs and direct to individual product costs. It is this consideration that produces adequately accurate estimates of the costs of separate products.

So far, this example has computed the average cost of diagnostic test as opposed to other radiology center product categories. However, the center does 18 different diagnostic tests. Analysis of costs within the center could be done in greater detail if costing was done to the level of each different type of diagnostic test. An analysis like that shown in Table 6-2 could be done for each of the 18 different tests. To do this, the general ledger would have to separate accounts for each direct cost item for the individual tests. It would have to measure the quantity of the product center drivers that applies to each different test as well as the institutional overhead drivers that apply to each test. If it did this, it would have analyses such as the one in Table 6-2 for each type of output produced in the each of the radiology department's five internal product centers. The benefit is that it would have costs per product for each of the department's products rather than simply an average cost for each of the radiology department's internal product centers. This would involve more measurement, bookkeeping, and computer time. Managers must decide if the more accurate product costs is worth the additional accounting costs.

In this particular case, a more detailed analysis was done and showed that radiology tests ranged from $16.34 to $20.46 per test with an average of $19.30. Managers must decide that different patients using different sets of these tests would cause their radiology costs to vary enough to make a material difference in their cost to care. For instance, one category of patient might use three tests whose costs are $16.34, $19.73, and $18.09, totalling $54.16. Another category might use tests costing $20.40, $19.39, and $18.91, totalling $58.70. The difference would be $4.54. For any patients using three radiology tests, the maximum difference in radiology test costs could be $(20.46)3 - (16.34)3 = 12.36. For such tests the cost could range from 15 percent below to be 6 percent above the average cost. Management felt that failure to do the more detailed costing, at least for a trial period, could result in materially undercosting some patients. This, in turn, could lead to materially underpricing some patient categories, especially if this variation in radiology test cost was compounded by similar variations in other intermediate product costs.

Note that this cost analysis of diagnostic radiology procedures is built on the organizational structure of the hospital. This is especially evident in Table 6-2. Here, categorization of costs follows the structural location of cost pools: the direct to diagnostic radiology costs, imaging center overhead cost pools, and institutional overhead pools. Analysis at these levels is necessary to estimate the full cost of each diagnostic test. Intuitively, this approach takes into considerations many more influences on differences in costs among various products than are considered when all the costs placed in a production center's cost pool are allocated among its products using a single basis, such as volume of procedures, as is frequently done.

Example Summary

This example of ABC application raises some questions about the categorization of direct and overhead costs. In Table 6-2, the *Direct Costs* title in the first section of the table refers to costs that are direct to the #557 cost pool, not necessarily direct to a single test. The first entry, *Direct Labor, Variable*, is direct to tests and therefore is traced by the time used for each type of test. The next two items measure the variable and fixed portions of labor that are direct to the diagnostic radiology cost pool but indirect to specific tests. Again, realize that stating these costs involves separating labor cost traced to the pool into the portion that is further traceable to specific tests and that which is not.

Another assumption should be noted. The last four items under *Direct Costs* assume that equipment-related cost for the diagnostic radiology tests are not also used by the other four categories of radiology department outputs. If they were, these costs would constitute radiology product center overhead, not costs direct to the #557 cost pool. These observations illustrate that in order to properly classify costs, analysts must understand the processes and utilization of resources used at the product centers. This information is best gained by talking with people and observing at the points of production.

DIRECT VERSUS INDIRECT COSTS

The main criticism of costing methods not based on activity analysis is their inadequate method of allocating indirect costs, in particular their overaveraging of these costs. ABC overcomes a large problem by breaking overhead costs into separate pools for different activities and allocating them separately to the users of those specific activities. In ABC, a direct cost is a cost that is traced directly to a cost target. For example, supplies issued for a particular procedure and the operating room nurse time devoted to that procedure are *direct costs* of that procedure (activity). In ABC, an *indirect* (or *overhead*) *cost* is a cost that must be allocated because it cannot be directly traced to the activity being costed. For example, the cost of supervision of nursing services might be allocated to a surgical procedure on the basis of direct nursing hours used in the procedure. Whereas direct cost is traceable, indirect costs are not. Attempting to compensate for this structural difference among different types of costs is a primary reason for using ABC. Because indirect costs cannot be traced (or the cost of doing the tracing is prohibitive), they are *allocated*. A specific allocation is based on a driver of the cost being allocated. In the example, the cost of nursing supervision is thought to be driven by direct nursing hours.

FIXED VERSUS VARIABLE COSTS

When indirect costs are a mixture of fixed and variable resources, cost behavior analysis might be able to separate the fixed cost amount from the variable cost rate per a specific driver. (Recall that variable costs change *in total* in proportion to changes of a cost driver, while fixed costs do not change in total despite changes in a cost driver.) The appropriateness of any probable driver can be measured by the goodness of fit revealed by cost behavior regression. Because *fixed costs* are cost elements of an activity that do not vary with changes in the volume of the driver, ABC cannot overcome the basic problem in allocating fixed cost. That is, the amount of cost associated with a unit of the driver will depend of how many units of the driver exist in the period over which the cost is fixed. To allocate a fixed costs, management must assume a volume over which it will be spread. This is frequently done before the fact in order to provide decision support information. If the assumed volume is not the actual volume that occurs, estimates of the cost per unit of activity will be inaccurate. Methods to understand the degree to which this phenomenon might affect cost information are discussed in Chapter 11.

COST FLOWS TO HEALTH CARE PRODUCTS

Chapter 4 describes three basic categories of health care products that are based on what is paid for by those who purchase health care. Another look at the costing implications of selling products in these different categories may be helpful now that product costs have been explained in more detail. When payment is by fee for service, the center that completes the making of each billable item can be credited with the revenue received from it. That product center can be treated as a profit center.

It was mentioned earlier that, with increasing amounts of health care revenue coming through prospectively set fees for categories of patient discharges, per-diem payments, and capitated paying systems, fewer profit centers exist within health care organizations. Under these payment schemes, revenue can be traced to the hospital but it is not further traceable to the specific departments producing the components of patients care. However, producers like to break organizations into profit centers in order to get part-by-part measures of financial performance. They like to know if the company is making or losing money in particular sections of the organization or in particular organization activities. To the extent that sets of revenues can be attributed to specific sectors within the organization and the cost of running those sectors can be isolated, producers can consider them profit centers. The ability to do this depends primarily on the services for which they are paid, the volume of patient under each payment scheme, and their ability to construct meaningful transfer prices.

Major Diagnostic Categories

To illustrate, assume that an organization is paid under a prospective payment system using DRGs to categorize patients and that it is paid a set amount for treating each patient depending on the patient's DRG. Also assume that a specified set of DRGs uses fixed cost resources that are not used to treat patients outside this set. There are, of course, additional variable costs consumed by these patients and therefore assignable to them as a group. All the revenues for these patients can be associated with that set of costs. In addition, these revenues are associated with no other costs except institution level overhead. An internal center managing the care of these patients could be considered a profit center. Under what conditions might this be the case? Extremely large hospitals might be large enough to warrant a unit with all the necessary services to care for those patients. No fixed costs would be shared with other patients; all the costs (aside from institutional overhead) required to earn the revenue from these patients would be direct to this center. The center would, by definition, be a profit center. For this to happen, the patient volume would have to be great enough to support a ward, diagnostic laboratories, a surgical suite, therapeutic units, and so forth of sufficient size to be efficient when serving only these patients. Some large health care delivery organizations have divided themselves by *service lines* according to major diagnostic categories (MDCs). MDCs are a good example of a criterion for forming profit centers, because they are broad categories of similar patient types and include a specific set of DRGs. These DRGs tend to use similar types of personnel and other fixed cost resources. When these resources are put into a separate production center, that center meets the criteria for a profit center, even under DRG based prospective payment. Another advantage of using MDCs is that, in the

Exhibit 6-2 **Major Diagnostic Categories**

	Diseases and disorders of the:
MDC1	Nervous system
MDC2	Eye
MDC3	Ear, nose, mouth, and throat
MDC4	Respiratory system
MDC5	Circulatory system
MDC6	Digestive system
MDC7	Hepitobiliary system and pancreas
MDC8	Musculoskeletal system and connective tissue
MDC9	Skin, subcutaneous tissue, and breast
MDC10	Endocrine, nutritional, and metabolic
MDC11	Kidney and urinary track
MDC12	Male reproductive system
MDC13	Female reproductive system
MDC14	Pregnancy, childbirth, and puerperium
MDC15	Newborns and other neonates with conditions originating in the perinatal period
MDC16	Blood and blood-forming organs and immunological disorders
MDC17	Myeloproliferative and poorly and differentiated neoplasms
MDC18	Infections and parasitic diseases (systemic and unspecified sites)
MDC19	Mental diseases and disorders
MDC20	Alcohol/drug use and alcohol/drug-induced organic mental disorders
MDC21	Injuries, poisonings, and toxic effect of drugs
MDC22	Burns
MDC23	Factors influencing health status and other contacts with health services

United States, they are standard designations with standard definitions. A list of MDCs is shown in Exhibit 6-2. How DRGs might be used to define a service line is depicted in Exhibit 6-3.

Capitation

Remember, a requirement for a profit center is that specific revenues must be traceable to it. Under capitation, a predetermined payment is made to the pro-

Exhibit 6-3   **Products of a Cardiac Service Line (a product center)**

Cardiac Pacemaker Services

DRG 115	Permanent cardiac pacemaker with acute myocardial infarction, heart failure, and shock
DRG 116	Other permanent cardiac pacemaker implant
DRG 117	Cardiac pacemaker revision except device replacement
DRG 118	Cardiac pacemaker device replacement

Cardiac Disorders

DRG 121	Circulatory disorders with acute myocardial infarction and cardiovascular complications, discharged alive
DRG 122	Circulatory disorders with acute myocardial infarction without cardiovascular complications, discharged alive
DRG 123	Circulatory disorders with acute myocardial infarction, expired
DRG 124	Circulatory disorders except acute myocardial infarction with cardiac catherization and complex diagnosis
DGR 125	Circulatory disorders except acute myocardial infarction with cardiac catherization and complex diagnosis
DRG 126	Acute and subacute endocarditis
DRG 127	Heart failure and shock

Chest Pain

DRG 140	Chest pain
DRG 143	Chest pain

viding organization regardless of resources used. Revenue is not attributable to specific centers within the provider organization. The revenue is associated with populations of clients, not specific patient episodes. However, the profitability of a given capitated contract can be estimated if the costs of the each episode of care for people in the capitated population can be totaled. The cost of any one of these episodes is the total of the costs of the activities needed for the care delivered. Even though capitated payment prevents organizations from being able to fully understand the financial performance of its internal units, ABC allows it to understand the performance of specific capitated agreements because it enables understanding the costs incurred in serving these agreements. ABC can estimate the cost of caring for specific categories of patients. Estimates of the number of patients in each category that will need to be cared for can be made from the epidemiology of the population being capitated. Summing the products of the estimated cost of a patient in each category by the number of patients expected in that category provides an estimate of the cost of delivering care under the contract.

Other Organizing Schemes

Recently, a chief financial officer (CFO) reported that their hospital had updated their organization structure to be based on five service lines: medical, surgical, women's and children's care, mental health, and rehabilitation. Columbia\HCA has organized around eight somewhat heterogeneous product lines: cancer, cardiology, diabetes, behavioral health, worker's compensation, and emergency care. Continuing care retirement communities sometimes choose to consider four service lines divided by their level of care: skilled nursing facilities, nursing facilities, assisted living units, and independent living units. This division could be further divided by patient groups who are subsidized as opposed to private-pay patients, because this dichotomy affects tracing revenues to each of the two subgroups. In any of these approaches to organization, the ABC can be done in much the same way it is described in this chapter. Separable sustaining activities can be identified. Production center and product overhead activities can also be identified and costs assigned to them for the service, product center, and direct costs they use. These can than be distributes among the units of product outputs by the product centers along with unit direct costs. This process produces information on the costs of all the centers along the flow of resources to the organization's products as well as unit costs for the products.

DISCUSSION QUESTIONS

1. Why does executive management want to divide the organization into profit centers?
2. How does the manner of payment for health care affect the organization's ability to divide itself into profit centers?
3. What conditions allow an organization to form profit centers when they might otherwise be illogical?
4. What constraints are put on the ability to gain the advantages of having profit centers when payment is by:

    a. Fee for service
    b. Per diem rates
    c. Prospectively set prices for discharges
    d. Capitated contract

KEY POINTS

- Organizations are given a structure of work groups and managers in order to apply specialized expertise and technology efficiently.
- In order for a center to be evaluated as a *profit center*, it must have traceable revenues as well as costs.
- Cost centers have only identifiable costs. Service centers and intermediate product centers are cost centers.
- Transfer pricing allows cost centers to be treated as profit centers. Such centers are called pseudo profit centers.
- When transfer prices are used to create pseudo profit centers, prices that increase selling center profits decrease the buying center profits.
- The sameness of resources used to treat conditions within each major diagnostic category (MDC) make structuring care delivery by MDCs potentially helpful. However, the profit centers would need to be quite large to use fixed assets efficiently.

Capitation payment systems are not facilitated by any specific structure. Having all clients under the same contract cared for by the same center would help cost the contract. This would, however, require extremely large centers in order to use fixed assets efficiently.

EXERCISE

Your receiving department accepts, inspects, and distributes within your hospital all shipments from all vendors. Some of these shipments go to central supply and are re-distributed by central supply to the end-users. Others go directly to the end-user. You currently allocate the cost of receiving shipments to the activities receiving them according to number of shipments they receive. You suspect that this may overaverage the allocations of the cost of operating the receiving department among the departments it serves. How would you go about investigating your concern?
Required:

- List the activities that you suspect are necessary in operating a receiving department.
- List the individuals you would talk with in order to confirm your prior beliefs and identify more component activities within the broad activity of receiving shipments.
- List questions you would ask them.
- List the types of documentation that could help identify activities within the department, their relationships, and their approximate costs.
- Lists steps you would take to determine if some of these activities, or groups of them, should be treated separable activities for costing purposes.

REFERENCES

[1] Galbraith, Jay R. *Organization Design* (Reading, MA: Addison-Wesley Publishing Company, 1977. p. 3).

[2] Thomas, Arthur L. *A Behavioral Analysis of Joint-Cost Allocation and Transfer Pricing.* (Manchester, UK: University Press, 1977).

CHAPTER 7

AGGREGATING ACTIVITY COSTS

After studying this chapter, students should be able to:

1. Estimate the cost of sustaining service activities caused by outputs of other centers within the organization.

2. Explain how batch-level activities can be analyzed and their costs attached to products.

3. Explain how product center overhead, direct-to-unit costs, and intermediate product are aggregated in order to compute unit costs.

4. Explain the difference between top-down and bottom-up analysis and the appropriate use of each.

INTRODUCTION

We have considered four categories of activities that cause costs within organizations, (1) organization sustaining, (2) production sustaining, (3) batch, and (4) unit, listing them from the top down. That is, the first concerns services that are centrally produced and support other activities throughout the organization and the last includes the final activities needed to produce a specific unit of a specific product. The primary care clinic example in Chapter 4 demonstrated a general approach to a rather simple analysis of the overhead and direct cost of a specific product—a primary care outpatient visit. An example in Chapter 5 showed how institutional sustaining overhead costs can be followed through intermediate product centers to the cost of salable products. The example in Chapter 6 showed the allocation of production center overhead to specific production activities within the center. These are costs that are direct to the production center but indirect to the production of specific categories of outputs.

As illustrated in earlier chapters, the costs of organization sustaining overhead activities flows to a given product through the other services and production activities needed to make the product. The same is true of production sustaining activities except that they support the production activities directly. Performing personnel administration would be considered an organization sustaining activity while maintaining production equipment would be considered a production sustaining activity. Returning to the example in Chapter 5, Exhibit 5-1 shows the cost of the organization sustaining activity *provide personnel services* is allocated using the driver *number of employees*. This overhead cost is allocated to all other activities because they each have employees. The production sustaining activity *maintain medical equipment* is allocated only to centers that have medical equipment. In that example, part of the allocation of the cost of personnel services activities is allocated to the intermediate product activity *develop film*, which is done in the diagnostic imaging center. The allocation is based on the number of employees involved in developing film. Other parts of the cost of personnel services are allocated to other activities in the organization in proportion to the number of employees involved in each of those activities.

Product Center Overhead

In addition to organization level sustaining overhead just described, centers cause costs that can be traced to them (as opposed to needing to be allocated) but cannot be traced further to any of their specific products. In the Chapter 5 example, the salary of the chief radiologist cannot be traced to a specific test or type of test. The salary can, however, be traced to the center. Another such example is the lease costs for equipment used only in diagnostic imaging but is common to several of its five component activities. These direct-to-center costs are allocated to the different internal activities using an appropriate driver for each cost. The chief radiologist's cost may use as its driver the number of personnel in the activity; lease costs of common-use equipment could use hours of use as the driver. Note that equipment used by only one of the component activities would be a direct cost of that activity. The Chapter 5 example does not include these allocations of intermediate center direct costs that must be allocated to separable activities performed within each center. That example deals only with the allocation of institutional sustaining activities.

All of the direct-to-center overhead can be lumped into one overhead pool. However, if different categories of the direct-to-center costs can be allocated more precisely by using separate drivers, the overhead pool can be allocated more accurately. Different degrees of detail with which cost flows can be analyzed exist. As product center overhead is broken into a greater number of distinct pools with distinct drivers, costing results should become more accurate. Intuitively, the more detail, the more accurate the costing result. However, increased detail in flow analysis also creates increased accounting costs. A balance between accounting cost and the value of the resulting information should be sought. A key reality is that there is no one right way to analyze the flows. The examples in the remainder of the book will illustrate approaches that, though similar in basics, are somewhat different in detail. The costing objective is to get adequately accurate cost data. This is cost data whose value in support of management decisions is greater than the cost of measuring and reporting it.

Figure 5-3, the accompanying analysis of the cost of a specific test, and Table 5-1 indicate that a certain amount of the organization's cost of providing personnel services is buried in the cost of the diagnostic procedures (AAA and CCC) and flows through these procedures to the cost of a DRG discharge. Other portions of the personnel services costs will flow to the DRG through other intermediate activities, such as *nursing care, therapy services*, and *laboratory tests*. The costs of sustaining activities flow to intermediate products by allocating them to activities that use them. The costs in those activities flow through their outputs to succeeding activities for which they are inputs. Eventually these flows are merged in the costs of the final activities needed to create the cost object of interest. Table 5-1 shows this process for two DRGs. The final inputs to each DRG are those identified in an analysis of activities needed to produce the discharge of a patient in the designated DRG.

DISCUSSION QUESTIONS

1. What are the differences between institution level sustaining activities and direct to product center overhead costs?
2. How is each of these categories of cost allocated to the next intermediate activity as costs flow toward a specific cost target?
3. How are activity overhead cost pools used in following costs to a specific cost target? Why are they necessary? Give several examples.

EXAMPLE HOME HEALTH CARE

An example of product center activity analysis may be helpful at this point. A multiservice home health care system is interested in determining how much it costs to deliver its different services. It is part of a larger health care system that owns hospitals, outpatient facilities, and medical office facilities as well as the home care system. The home care system is currently organized into centers for each of seven different product lines. These are:

Standard home care   Infusion therapy services
Pulmonary home services   Wound care
Mental health home services   Diabetes education
Maternity home services

Each product line has its own management team, personnel, and equipment that support an array of products. For instance, the *standard home care center* produces:

Skilled nursing visits   Speech therapy visits
Aide visits   Medical social visits
Physical therapy visits   Dietician visits
Occupational therapy visits

To support the activities needed to perform these visits, sustaining activities occur at both the corporate level and the standard home care system level. The first step in allocating the part of corporate overhead activities to the standard home care activities was to determine which corporate activities were caused by the standard home care center. A way to do this is to ask what activities needed to sustain the standard home care activities are produced at the corporate office? Corporate activity analysis was based on both corporate personnel's knowledge of their work and the standard home care center management team's knowledge of its support from the corporate headquarters.

- First, analysts simply asked corporate staff personnel to list the services performed at that level for the health system's component divisions. This list was shown to the standard home care management for confirmation or correction.
- Analysts then identified the listed activities that used the same resources and did not share resources with other activities. These sets of activities were, therefore, separable activities.
- Next, analysts asked those involved in these separable corporate overhead activities to identify things that prompted them to perform the activities. These things were potential drivers of the costs incurred by the activities.
- Finally, to find the most predictive driver, analysts ran regression analyses of these potential drivers on the cost of the activities, using historical data. For each separable activity, the potential driver that produced the highest R^2 statistic was used as its driver in allocating the corporate overhead activity's costs to the product centers.

The following activities and drivers were identified:

Activity	Driver
Perform marketing services	Sales dollars
Perform financial accounting services	Financial transactions
Collect accounts receivable	Quantity of billings
Negotiate purchase contracts	Contracts negotiated
Furnish space	Square feet furnished
Pay employees	Payments made
Perform general corporate administration	Number of employees

These costs are allocated among all of the parent organization's product line centers and on to product centers within the product lines. The *general corporate administration* activity cost pool took on the function of a *remainder* overhead pool. Activities whose costs could not be separated from the other activities or whose costs were not material were put in that pool.

There are also sustaining activities at the standard home care center. The costs of these activities are direct to that center but indirect to the seven types of visits (products) it produces. The process for identifying these activities was similar to that used at the corporate-activity level. The analysis results were:

Activity	Driver
General administration	Number of employees
Scheduling	Number of visits
Supply management	Dollar value of supplies used
Common equipment repair	Maintenance orders
Common equipment rental	Time used

The cost of overhead activities performed at the corporate and the standard home care center levels are allocated to separate cost pools for each of the seven standard home care products. The driver for allocating the total of costs in each of the seven product center overhead cost pools to specific visits is the number of visits produced by each center. The total overhead cost in each product center pool was divided by the number of visits, and the result was the cost per visit. The number of visits was used as the driver of overhead cost at the unit level because management did not believe that different visits of the same type caused materially different amounts of overhead. If analysis of overhead costs had indicated that some overhead was caused by the length of a visit while some was caused simply by the having a visit, two overhead pools would be created. One would be allocated at an amount per visit, as just described. The other pool would be allocated to a visit in proportion to the length of the visit.

Example Summary

To summarize, overhead costs can be caused by activities at the institution (or corporate) level and at intermediate centers. A cost analysis should try to find a driver that causes each separable set of overhead activities. That driver is then used to allocate the cost of its associated activity as far toward the final cost target as it can. At some point, the cost of any given overhead activity may have to be assigned to the overhead pool of a product center or a product and allocated as part of the more aggregated overhead costs to individual units of the product.

Look at an example using activities and centers discussed previously. The sustaining center *personnel services* contains a separable activity *pay personnel*. The cost of this activity is allocated to other activities using the driver *number of people paid*. This overhead cost is allocated through the *diagnostic imaging center* on to the *develop film* activity. At that point, the cost of paying its personnel is put into the *develop film* activity's overhead pool.

Concurrently, the costs of the diagnostic imaging centers administrative personnel, which are direct to the diagnostic center, are allocated among its subcenters using the number of people employed as the driver. Once allocations of all the institutional and product center overhead costs are added to a component activity's overhead pool, the total pool is allocated to the subcenter's products. In the case of the *develop film* activity, the overhead allocations were added to the direct costs of developing film to establish the total cost of the *develop film* activity. The total cost of this center (or activity) was assigned to specific diagnostic tests using the number of films involved as the driver. Figure 7-1 illustrates this process.

The overhead allocations and direct cost of each test were summed to find each test's cost. The cost of each test then becomes a direct cost of the treatment of a patient.

DISCUSSION QUESTIONS

1. How can separable corporate overhead activities be identified?
2. How can drivers of separable activities be identified?
3. Why must caution be used when allocating fixed costs using a driver identified by typical cost-driver analysis?

BATCH-LEVEL OVERHEAD ACTIVITIES

The flow of resources into some production activities is not a continuous stream. The same products may not be produced at a set rate. They may be produced in batches of various quantities. These batches may involve costs of activities necessary to get ready for a run of production of a specific product or to terminate the run. These are called *batch activities* and their costs are called *batch costs*. Batch costs tend to be nearly the same, regardless of the size of the production run. Like fixed costs, the batch cost per unit of output of a production run depends on the number of units in the run.

In manufacturing, it is not uncommon for a production activity to get an order for a certain number of a specified product. When this happens, the production center pulls the technical drawings and production instructions,

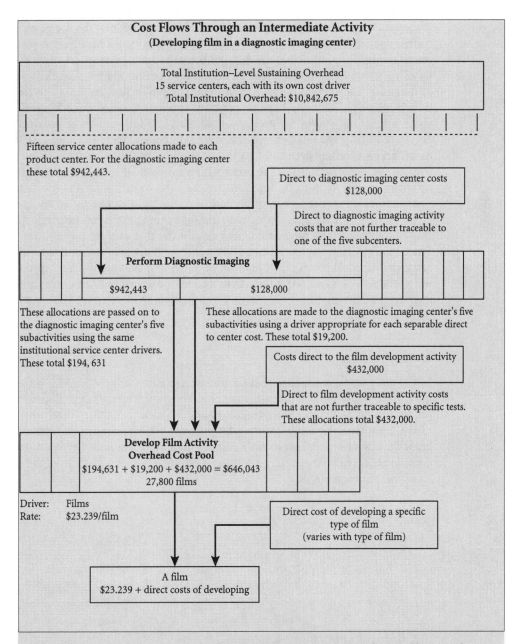

Figure 7-1   **Cost Flows Through an Intermediate Activity** [Developing film in a diagnostic imaging center]

withdraws the needed materials from the warehouses, schedules the use of machines, configures them to produce the specified product, schedules the personnel needed for production, and then performs the direct production activities. Usually preparatory activities need be done only once no matter what the size of the order. The order is referred to as a *job*. The production center is referred to as a *job shop*. The cost of the preparatory activities is called a *batch cost* or *set-up cost*. At the end of the production, usually an additional set of activities necessary to clear the job from the shop in readiness for the next set up exists. Acute health care has been referred to as the ultimate job shop. This reflects the fact that each patient is a job order with a quantity of one. Therefore, set-up costs for interventions for a patient are the costs of caring for that patient. The entire batch cost for a run of a single unit of output can be traced to that unit and so is a direct cost of that unit. However, some intermediate products may be the output of a production run of quantities that vary from run to run. The laboratory example at the end of this chapter illustrates an occurrence of batch costs in health care. Cost analysis of batch cost is done similarly to the way sustaining costs are identified. Analysts must observe production runs and identify the one-time activities needed to enable individual runs. They must then measure the costs of those activities.

UNIT COSTS

ABC defines unit costs as costs that are traceable to a unit of product. This is the same as the definition of a direct-to-unit cost. These costs do not need allocation procedures. In fact, allocation procedures are fall-back procedures used when costs are not traceable to the cost target of interest. When management wants to know the cost of a given target, ABC analyzes the immediate activities that must occur to obtain it. When the target is a single unit of a product, the costs of these activities are unit costs.

EXAMPLE

The following example of the application of ABC to costing clinical laboratory tests (though overly simplistic) should help clarify the ideas just presented.

A Clinical Laboratory Example

In applying ABC to this laboratory, the first task is to identify all of the activities required to perform the tests. The laboratory is responsible for performing four tests: P, Q, R, and S.

Each test requires:
1. Processing and delivery of supplies and materials by the hospital supply department.
2. Maintaining test equipment, done by the hospital biomedical engineering department.
3. Providing tools and equipment, done by laboratory management.
4. Setting up tools and equipment for a test batch. These tools are provided by the laboratory.
5. Performing the test, done by laboratory technicians.
6. Documenting and distributing the test results to the appropriate parties, done by laboratory clerks.

After identifying the activities, the amounts of resources required to carry out each activity must be determined. Costs outside the laboratory (sustaining activities) were $46,284, incurred by the hospital to provide and maintain equipment. This corporate overhead was allocated using maintenance technician hours consumed as the driver. The cost to process and distribute supplies is driven by the dollar amount of supplies used. For the laboratory, this amounted to $8,510.

Within the laboratory, $154,750 was spent in setup activities, $147,000 was traced to internal clerical support activities, and $30,856 to furnishing tools and equipment. An appropriate amount of cost from each of these activities is part of the full cost of each test. Determining the amount of each of these costs to be allocated to each type of test is discussed here.

Supply Processing and Distribution

Supply processing and distribution (P&D) is a production sustaining activity whose resource driver is believed to be the *dollar value of the supplies furnished*. This resource driver was determined through an analysis of the supply P&D activity combined with cost behavior analysis to judge the goodness of fit of potential drivers. The rate was computed at $0.005 per dollar of supplies used. Supply P&D was allocated to each test using this rate and the standard direct supply cost for the test. Realize that the supply costs for each test type were measures by counting the cost of direct supplies used to perform each test.

Test	Supply cost/test	$\times$	$ per $ of supplies	$=$	Supply P&D cost per test
P	$5.00		$0.005		$0.0250/test
Q	$3.20		$0.005		$0.0160/test
R	$12.50		$0.005		$0.0625/test
S	$2.00		$0.005		$0.0100/test

Maintenance

In this example, maintenance is performed by a hospital-level service department. It can be considered a production-sustaining activity and is allocated using the resource driver *machine hours* (mach. hrs). Therefore, the cost of the maintenance department (which could be thought of as the cost of maintenance activities) is allocated using machine hours. In the baseline period, $46,284 of maintenance were used to support 77,140 machine hours for a rate of $0.60 per machine hour.

Test	Mach. hrs	×	$ per mach. hr	=	Maintenance cost per test
P	0.220		$0.60		$0.1320/test
Q	0.050		$0.60		$0.0300/test
R	0.600		$0.60		$0.3600/test
S	0.828		$0.60		$0.4968/test

Calculating Laboratory Test Setup Costs

Observation of setup procedures indicates that the cost of this overhead activity varies significantly across the four different setups, because the setups use varying amounts of each input. Table 7-1 shows the computation of the setup cost for each test. Wages of setup technicians are available from payroll data. The technician time to do each setup can be measured by observation of the work, and a standard can be determined. The number of setups for each type of test during the baseline period can simply be counted. A standard cost for the setup for each type of test can be set by dividing the total of costs to each type of setup by the number of those setups performed. In simple cases such as this example, it can also be had by tracing the direct costs of doing a single setup. When, for each type of test, the total set-up cost for a period is divided by the average number of tests performed, an average setup cost per test results. Realize that this procedure has put all the costs traceable to setting up for each type of test into a cost pool for that setup. It then divides the total pool cost by the number of tests performed to arrive at a cost per test of the setup activity. Note that this process uses historic data to establish *standard* setup costs, which are *batch* costs allocated using the activity driver *setups done*. A set-up cost is thereby computed for each type of test.

This computation was possible because costs flowing to each type of setup were separable and the average number of tests resulting from each type of setup could be measured.

There are two assumptions buried in this specific example. First, the standard setup cost is the result of the total number of setup activities and

Table 7-1 **Calculating Laboratory Test Set-up Costs**

Test Type	P	Q	R	S
a. Setup labor time (hrs)	0.05	0.08	0.12	0.15
b. Wage rate ($/hr)	30	30	30	30
c. Labor cost per setup (a × b)	$1.50	$2.40	$3.60	$4.50
d. Supply cost ($)	10,000	8,000	12,000	18,000
e. Setups	5,000	6,000	16,000	2,500
f. Supply cost per setup (d / e)	$2.000	$1.333	$0.750	$7.200
g. Set-up tool cost ($)	$3,000	$2000	$4,000	$ 7,000
h. Setups	5,000	6,000	16,000	2,500
i. Tool cost per setup (g / h)	$0.600	$0.333	$0.250	$2.800
j. Total cost per setup (c+f+I)	$4.100	$4.066	$4.600	$14.500
k. Total tests	100,000	60,000	80,000	5,000
l. Setups	5,000	6,000	16,000	2,500
m. Average tests per setup (k / l)	20	10	5	2
n. Average set-up cost per test (j / m)	$0.2050	$0.4066	$0.9200	$7.2500

their costs in a given historic period. This is referred to as the baseline period. Analysis of data from a different period could give different results. If management believes that conditions in the future may change from those of the baseline period, it should adjust the computed cost per setup before using it as an input to decisions about the future. Second, if the ratio of the number of setups done to the total number test produced changes, the cost per test will change. For instance, if there is an emergency request for a test "P" and it must be produced by itself rather than in a batch of 20, the setup cost for that particular test will be ($4.100/setup)/(1test/setup) = $4.100/test, not $0.205. This is an example of how knowing the cost of intermediate activities and products creates flexibility in costing targets in different situations.

Tools and Equipment

For the baseline period the total tools and equipment (T&E) cost for the laboratory was $30,858. This information comes from depreciation schedules for laboratory T&E. Specific T&E cost were not traced to specific tests. It appears that the same T&E resources are used in all tests. Therefore, this amount is a joint cost allocated at the unit level. It is believed that these costs are driven by the amount of machine time used in the laboratory. Therefore, the dollar amount is allocated to specific tests using the resource driver, machine hours (mach. hrs) demanded by each test.

The amount per test is:

$30,858 / 77,140 total mach. hrs = $0.40 per mach. hr

T&E cost per test:

Test	Mach. hrs	×	$ per mach. hr	=	$ per test
P	0.220		0.40		0.0880
Q	0.050		0.40		0.0200
R	0.600		0.40		0.2400
S	0.828		0.40		0.3312

The approach to determining the overhead cost attributable to a unit of product follows a consistent pattern. A logical cause for changes in cost per period caused by producing the product is hypothesize from knowledge of the production process. It can be tested through regression analysis using historical data. If it shows strong predictive power, it is used as the cost driver for the overhead resource in question. In this case, it is machine hours. The regression analysis also shows the cost per unit of driver; in this case, $0.40 per machine hour. Finally, this rate is used to allocate the indirect cost-to-cost objects. In this example, using ABC, the cost object is an intermediate product rather than a final product. However, even if the fit indicated by the regression analysis is good, one must remember that if a large part of T&E cost are fixed, the amount per test is only accurate if the total amount of machine hours does not vary materially in the future. This is because the fit only applies to the variable portion. The fixed portion of a cost per unit of output will always depend on the quantity of the output during the period in which fixed costs are fixed.

Clerical Support

Observation of clerical activity demanded by the various tests indicated that there was no material difference in the cost of this activity among the tests. It was therefore appropriate to divide the total cost of clerical activity resources by the number of tests done in a period to compute a clerical cost per test: $147,000/ 245,000 tests = $0.600 per test. Clerical support can therefore be treated like a unit-level activity using the activity driver *number of tests performed.* Realize that if clerks are salaried, as with any fixed cost, this clerical support cost per test is only accurate in the future if the total number of tests does not change. ABC does not alter this fact. Where fixed costs are a material part of indirect costs, ABC cannot produce an accurate cost figure without knowing the volume of production.

Remaining Costs

The remaining costs involved in producing each test are the unit-direct costs for the test. These are measured by observing the direct resources consumed by each test. One of these is the material used to perform the test. The cost per test is simply the number of units of each material used times its cost per unit. As discussed earlier, whether labor is a fixed or unit (variable) cost depends on the way it is acquired and paid. In this particular organization, laboratory technician work is done almost entirely by technicians in a labor pool. These technicians work in a flexible scheduling system in which they work only when they are needed and are paid only when they work. This allows the laboratory labor cost to be treated as a direct cost. In this example, the rate is $30.00 per hour or $0.50 per minute. The labor cost for each test is, therefore, the number of minutes taken to do the test multiplied by $0.50.

Table 7-2 shows the cost of each type of test computed using the ABC approach. This table aggregates the cost of the component activities needed to produce them. The flow of these costs is then shown in Figure 7-2.

Table 7-2 **Average Cost per Test (in dollars)**

Resources	P	Q	R	S
Direct material	5.0000	3.2000	12.5000	2.0000
Direct labor	1.5000	3.0000	1.2000	3.0000
Department overhead activities				
Clerical support	0.6000	0.6000	0.6000	0.6000
Setup	0.2050	0.4067	0.9200	7.2500
Tools and equipment	0.0880	0.0200	0.2400	0.3312
Corporate allocated overhead				
Maintenance	0.1320	0.0300	0.3600	0.4968
Supply P&D	0.0250	0.0160	0.0625	0.0100
Total Cost	$7.5500	$7.2727	$15.8825	$13.6880

DISCUSSION QUESTIONS

1. What are the primary differences between a job shop and other approaches to production?
2. Why is the job shop concept applicable in health care delivery?
3. What sorts of activities cause batch costs? Give some examples.

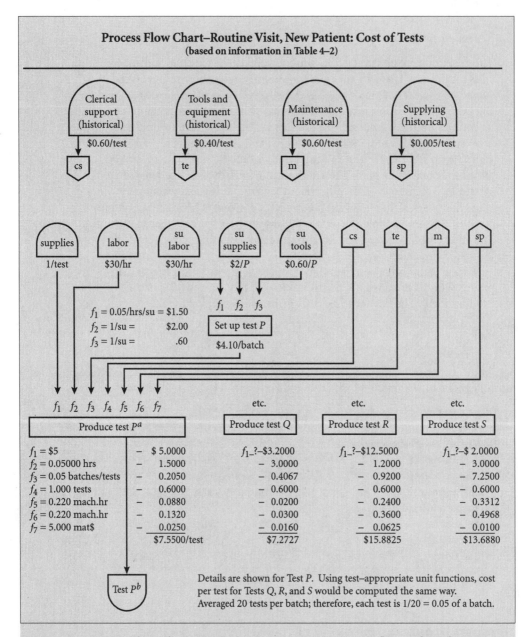

Figure 7-2   Process Flow Chart–Routine Visit, New Patient: Cost of Tests (based on information in Table 4-2)

4. In the examples given, how is overhead caused by the batch activities identified, measured, and allocated to the output of the center suffering the batch costs?

5. What information in addition to the cost of a batch activity is needed to allocate batch costs to output?

BOTTOM-UP AND TOP-DOWN ANALYSIS

No matter what the cost object might be, activity analysis involves both bottom-up and top-down analysis. When the primary interest is in a specific final or intermediate product, it is logical to start with an analysis of the activities and resources needed in the final production phase and work backward through all the activities needed to create these. Eventually, and perhaps rather early on, analysts will find that overhead activities are necessary to support certain intermediate activities. At that point, it becomes necessary to find allocation procedures that are as accurate as efficient accounting procedures can produce. This will involve studying overhead activities to see which ones are separable; that is, which ones use separate sets of resources and are used by different cost targets in different proportions. This involves a top-down investigation. When analysts attempt to create a general activity based costing system, it may be more direct to start with sustaining overhead activities managed at the top of the organization hierarchy and work downward through intermediate products to the final, saleable product. Figure 7-3 and Figure 7-4 illustrate the two approaches.

While working in either direction, analysts will find activities that support specific sets of production activities. The example here was set-up activities for runs of clinical tests. These batch costs cannot only occur in producing intermediate products, such as clinical laboratory tests or diagnostic imaging, they can also occur on sustaining activities such as the payroll function. In paying employees, much of the total effort may be calling up software and entering data. These are set-up activities. Once they are done, running the computations, printing checks, and mailing the checks or making automatic deposits may be relatively inexpensive.

DISCUSSION QUESTIONS

1. Why does activity analysis of a specific cost target require both bottom-up and top-down analysis?

2. Pick an output of a health care product center. What are the sources of the information that must be available in order to do a bottom-up cost analysis? A top-down cost analysis?

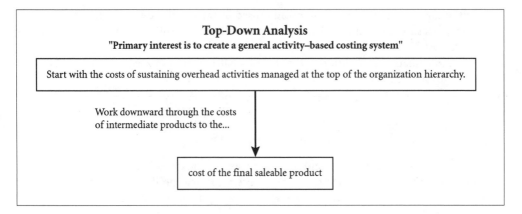

Figure 7-3 **Top-Down Analysis**

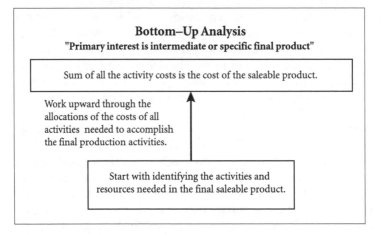

Figure 7-4 **Bottom-Up Analysis**

A REFLECTION

When following the cost of activities through intermediate products to saleable products or other cost targets, it may appear that the approach depends on playing with words. For instance, one could say that the diagnostic imaging center produces ultrasound tests—a product. One can also say that the imaging center performs ultrasound test—an activity. One can even say that the location of the production of ultrasound tests, along with its fixed resources, is a cost center or an intermediate product center or an intermediate activity center. Any of these perspectives is correct. Activity based approaches tend to use activities as the subject of analysis because the activities necessary to produce an output generate its cost. More important, with reference to understanding differences in costs of various outputs, is to understand the degree to which different outputs use varying amounts of different activities as well as direct resources. In fact, as was just implied, the outputs of prior activities frequently are the traceable cost inputs to a later activity.

EXAMPLE

This example explains how one hospital used ABC to analyze operating room costs incurred to perform a specific surgical procedure. In this chapter the example is used to illustrate the aggregation of activity and resource costs along the flow to the given cost target—an orthroscopic knee surgery.

The hospital is a not-for-profit community hospital that serves a three-county area and operates a clinic 30 miles away. The hospital began to use an activity based accounting system in 1996. The ABC system was set up parallel to the financial accounting general ledger system, although data from that system is used. Kaplan and Cooper suggest this separation, especially in early phases of ABC application.[1] A distinct advantage is that the accounting information system in place does not have to be disturbed. ABC was implemented department by department. Concurrent analysis of separated departments prompted a primarily bottom-up approach. Prior to developing an ABC system sustaining overhead was allocated using a single driver for each overhead category. The ABC system was planned to enable reports that could show managers:

- What resources flow to specific procedures in what quantities and at what costs. (This extends to showing the relative cost of different protocols for the same procedure.)
- The utilization of fixed cost resources and a measure of unused capacity.
- The gross margin for each procedure, when revenue can be directly attributed to surgical procedures.
- The gross margin for the production center, when revenue can at least be traced to the production center.

Within the surgery center, this required analysis of the differences among its various surgical procedures. Any operating room (OR) procedure incorporates the direct labor, direct supplies, and any specialty equipment used in the procedure. It also includes the procedure's share of OR overhead and of institutional overhead. Inputs to the procedure were broken into eight activities. These activities with their drivers and allocation rates are (shown in dollars):

1. Acuity-3 surgery: An activity costed per minute   9.27 per minute
2. IV set-up: An activity allocated by occurrence   2.52 per occurrence
3. Surgical preparation: An activity allocated by occurrence   15.08 per occurrence
4. Arthroscope: An OR resource allocated by usage   18.41 per use

5. Video equipment: An OR resource allocated by usage — 3.40 per use

6. Tourniquet equipment: An OR resource allocated by usage — 0.01 per use

7. General closure: An activity allocated by RVU — 0.42 per RVU

8. Phase II recovery: An activity allocated per minute — 2.35 per minute

To arrive at the cost of the five activities, an analysis was necessary for each one.

Figure 7-5 shows the aggregating of these activity costs as the activities flow from sustaining actions to the arthroscopic knee operation. Analysis of this flows to as acuity-3 surgical procedure are discussed in Chapter 8. These acuity-3 costs total $9.27 per minute of OR-suite time use. This rate per minute is carried forward as the cost of one element in the knee arthroscopy's total resource use. Similar analyses were done for the other two activities involved in the surgery: surgical preparation and IV setup.

Of the inputs required to complete a knee arthroscopy, the cost of the three resources (arthrosope, video equipment, and tourniquet equipment) were determined by finding the annual amount spent for each of them and dividing that amount by the number of procedures that are to be done during the period of interest. An illustration of direct charge for specialty equipment is given in Table 7-3. This table shows the asset's acquired value and the annual depreciation cost for each of the five components of the arthroscope. The annual usage for the past 2 years is also shown, then the annualized usage for the current year is estimated. The financial column shows the calculated current year's cost per arthroscopy. This figure is found by dividing the annual depreciation by the current year's usage figure: $930.60/274 = $3.40. A similar analysis is done for the video equipment and for the tourniquet equipment. Note that the cost per procedure depends on the number of procedures performed in the period, because the resources have a large component of fixed costs.

Errors in estimates of the volume of the workload will, therefore, cause errors in the estimate of the cost per procedure. ABC cannot correct these errors. Because of this fact, volume estimates need careful scrutiny and cost per procedure should receive analysis of its sensitivity to volume changes.

Analyses were also done for the follow-on activities: closure and recovery. Figure 7-5 shows these flows and the costs of each activity and resource required. The demand box indicates the estimated full cost of doing the surgery associated with DRG 222. This is an output of the surgery center. It is also an intermediate activity in the discharge of a DRG 222 patient.

Example | **155**

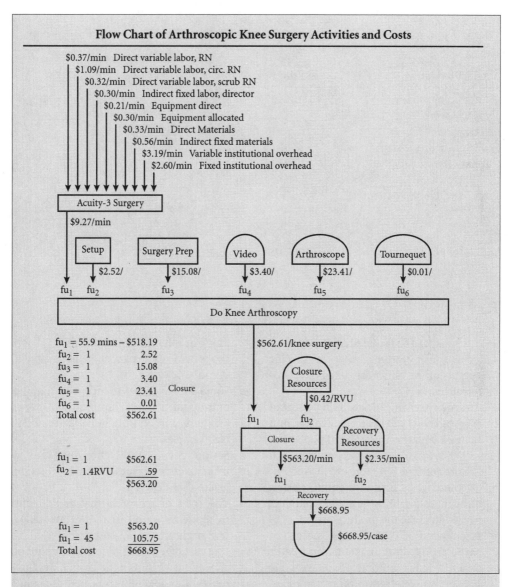

Figure 7-5   Flow Chart of Arthroscopic Knee Surgery Activities and Costs

Table 7-3   **Capital Equipment Charge Operating Room Arthroscope**

Asset Description	Acquired Value ($)	Annual Value ($)	Forecast Usage	Cost per Use
Arthroscopy camera (fully depreciated)	9,761.20	0.00	274	
Telescope and lenses	6,361.36	636.12		
Duckbill upbiter & basket punch	1,531.25	153.12		
Forceps 3.4mm backbiter Arthrotek	905.45	90.60		
Isometric ligament positioner	507.06	50.76		
		$930.60	274	$3.3964

KEY POINTS

- Costs that can be traced to an activity center but not traced further to specific outputs of the center are called direct-to-center costs.
- An activity center can have a single pool of overhead costs and use a single driver, or it can have an array of overhead pools each with its own driver. The second approach is more accurate but more expensive.
- Overhead costs flow to a product's cost through allocations to the activities needed to make the product.
- Batch overhead costs are costs needed to have a production run that makes a batch of a particular output. These costs are usually the same regardless of the quantity of the batch.
- Batch costs per unit of output, therefore, depend on the size of the batch.
- A job shop is a production center that produces outputs to fill specific orders for specific quantities of specific products.

- Many health care organizations act as job shops with each patient being a single-output job.
- Some inputs to a patient's care may be outputs of a production batch. Laboratory tests and pharmaceuticals are possible examples.
- Set-up costs for production runs are the most common types of batch costs in health care delivery.
- The costs of resources that are directly traceable to a unit of output are called unit or direct-to-unit costs.
- The cost of a unit of output is the sum of allocations of sustaining costs, direct-to-center costs, and unit costs of all of the activities needed to produce the output.
- The analysis of these activities and their costs can be done by starting with the output and analyzing backwards through all of the activities needed to produce it. This is bottom-up analysis. It can also be

done by starting with sustaining activities and analyzing down through the increas-

ing array of activities to achieve the output. This is top-down analysis.

REFERENCES

[1] Kaplan, R.S. and R. Cooper, 1998. *Cost and Effect: Using Integrated Cost Systems to Drive Profitability and Performance.* (Boston: Harvard Business School Press, 1998), pp. 18–21.

CHAPTER 8

DETERMINING ACTIVITY STRUCTURES AND COST DRIVERS

INTRODUCTION

To this point, we have discussed how sustaining, intermediate center, batch, and unit costs should be assigned to successive production centers and eventually to units of output. The assignment logic is based on the fact that costs of creating an output are caused by the activities needed to produce the output. These include the costs of both direct and indirect resources used in those activities. The costs of direct resources for a cost target are rather easily computed, because, by definition, these resources can be traced to the target.

Indirect (overhead) costs, however, create significant costing problems. Indirect costs are caused by activities whose outputs are not traceable to specific users. An example used is the sustaining costs of running a personnel department. This collection of costs cannot be traced to various users of the personnel department's efforts. However, different segments of these costs might be separated and assigned to the specific activities that use them. In so doing, the accuracy of costs computed for the using activities may be greatly increased.

This is possible if:

- The overhead activities can be divided into separate sets with distinct costs, and these activities can be traced to the specific cost targets that use them. Such a set is called a *separable activity*. In the personnel department example, activities were divided into those involved in paying personnel and those needed to process personnel actions.
- The cost of each separable activity can be measured and is independent of the cost of other activities.
- Demand for each cost target's use of a separable activity may be caused by a specific activity by the target, which is called the *activity driver*. This was illustrated by realizing that the total cost of paying personnel was driven by the number of people paid and the cost of processing personnel actions was driven by the number of actions requested.

When these requirements for using an activity driver cannot be found, a *resource driver* is determined. A resource driver is a variable that can logically be considered to cause changes in an overhead input in question. A previous example is the realization that total maintenance costs might be caused by the number of hours of maintenance labor used by a cost target.

How the array of activities performed in a department can be divided into separable activities and how the cost of each of these activities can be separately estimated has not yet been discussed, nor has much been mentioned about how drivers can be identified. This chapter will consider these topics.

ISOLATING SEPARABLE ACTIVITIES

Earlier it was pointed out that using one variable, usually called an *allocation basis*, to distribute the cost of an overhead department or an overhead activity within a production department tends to overaverage the cost of its outputs. In the personnel department example, it was noted that various users of personnel department services used different services in different amounts. To accurately determine how much of the personnel department's cost is caused by each user, this fact should be considered. Analyzing the causes of an overhead department's costs requires that its separable activities be identified. The first step is to identify what the department does, then the analyst must determine which sets of these overhead activities can be considered separable activities. Several sources of help exist in doing this.

Documents

An array of documents exists within most organization that can give the analyst a head start on understanding the structure of activities within parts of the organization that handle overhead functions. Reviewing these documents before working with the people performing overhead activities increases the speed with which an analyst can isolate separable activities and their resource use. One caution should be mentioned. If these documents are not kept up to date, they are of little help and can even slow the analysis process by creating bad guidance. It pays to check the currency of the organization's work documentation before spending too much time with it.

ORGANIZATION CHARTS   Organization charts help the analyst to see where activities are conducted and can provide a list of departments and their managers. This allows the analyst to relate resources used by specific activities to cost information in the general ledger and to know whom to contact to coordinate further analysis.

JOB DESCRIPTIONS   Within any department, a list of activities performed can be created by examining the job descriptions of its personnel. The descriptions will also indicate who is involved in different aspects of each of the department's outputs. This information also helps in understanding the personnel resources used in activities supporting various outputs.

PROCEDURE MANUALS   Departments frequently have procedure manuals that describe how various outputs are to be produced. These manuals obviously define the activities carried out within the department. They also give insight to the nonpersonnel resources used in each activity.

Interactions

After reviewing documentation related to activity structuring, the analyst can get more detailed insight by observing the work of the department and discussing the work with those doing it. This can involve three approaches: (1) observation, (2) interviews, and (3) group discussions.

OBSERVATION   The analyst may become what is referred to as a *complete observer*.[1] The complete observer is removed from the activities and is not noticed by those involved in them. This situation is difficult to achieve. Workers will usually realize they are being observed. This may, of itself, change their behavior. For this reason, it is important that workers understand the purpose of the analysis is to track the flow of resources in order to understand who uses what components of their work. Convincing workers of this usually demands the cooperation of executive management and their immediate supervisors, as well as the union steward if one exists. This type of problem in implementing ABC will be discussed more thoroughly in Chapter 9.

Finding separable activities starts with the list of activities discovered in the document review. The object of observing work within a department is to detect groups of these activities that produce specific outputs used in different amounts by the different customers. For such a set to be a separable activity, it must also use a set of resources that are primarily dedicated to it. In the personnel department example, the analyst found that payroll activities and personnel actions were handled by different people using various equipment, software programs, and supplies. The costs of these two activities could, therefore, be separated. Concurrently, some departments within the hospital had a large number of people on the payroll but a stable workforce with a flat personnel structure while other departments had a small workforce with high turnover and frequent disciplinary and promotion actions. This meant that the two separable personnel department activities should be allocated separately, because they have different costs and various customers used different amounts of activity.

There are two potential problems with the observational approach to activity analysis. The first is the possibility that the results will have limits to their validity, especially when the analyst is not previously familiar with the activities of a department. The greatest threat to validity is that all the activities relevant to the cost of an output may not be included. The second problem relates to the reliability of the findings. Different observers may see the spectrum of activities in various ways and appraise the costs of their inputs differently. The reliability problem can be lessened by repeated observations using different analysts and by testing for interrater reliability, but this is often more time consuming and expensive than its results warrant.

INTERVIEWS   The most common way to improve the results of observation alone is to interview individuals with expertise on the activities being analyzed. Efficient analysis of production activities usually involves gaining a fundamental understanding of activities through document review and as unobtrusive observations as can be made. This beginning should be improved by interviews. Because the purpose of the interviews is to understand the activities in a specific department of an organization, the techniques used need not be aimed at gaining generalizable, industry-wide truths. Therefore, interviews need not be highly structured, though some questions are common to most situations.

The following is a series of lead-in questions that can help identify activities performed, their outputs, the users of the outputs, and the degree to which they use common inputs.

- What are the outputs of this department (or overhead activity)?
- Who uses them?
- What are the outputs of your work?
- Who uses them?
- What resources do you use?
- How much of each resource do you use to produce each of your outputs?
- Are some resources used to support several different outputs?

- What proportion of these joint-use resources is used by each output it supports?

The first four of these questions assist in determining what activities produce outputs for external customers and which support the internal products. This information can then be used to specify the flows of activities. The last three questions help identify the specific resources used. This information helps to determine which external outputs use separable resources and can therefore be costed separately. Answers to these two questions identify what are called separable activities within an overhead department or function.

Fontana and Frey suggest some general rules to follow in this kind of interviewing.[2]

- Never let another person interrupt the interview, answer for the respondent, or give his or her opinion on the question.
- Never suggest an answer or agree or disagree with an answer.
- Do not give the respondent any idea of your personal views on the questions.
- Never attempt to improve the answer by adding to it, deleting portions of it, or making word changes.

When interviewing several people about the same activities, ask the basic questions in exactly the same way to each interviewee. After this is done, the analyst can ask more question in order to delve deeper or clarify prior answers. Great effort should be made to ensure that the data collected is solely the opinion of the interviewee.

GROUP DISCUSSIONS   It is possible that the information gleaned from interviews will vary somewhat among interviewees. The analysts must evaluate these differences based on their understanding of differences in the backgrounds and perceptions of those interviewed. Some of the uncertainties caused by differences among interviewees can be eliminated by group discussions. In group activity analysis, as with individual interviews, the participants must be well informed about the activities in question. This means the group should be composed of people involved in the activities. The analyst must assure that the group realizes the purpose of the discussion is to understand the activities performed, their flow, and the resources they use, and is not intended to establish responsibility or performance standards. This is especially true if the group is composed of both workers and supervisors.

If the department being analyzed is large and involves many activities, the information available from individual interviews is probably needed. For smaller departments with fewer activities, a group discussion may serve the purposes of both individual and group interactions. It is important that the group have representatives with knowledge of each of its activity areas, outputs, and customers.

At the same time, as single discussion group should be limited to between 6 and 10 people.[3] Smaller groups may lack the expertise and knowledge coverage needed while larger groups may not allow individual members to adequately pursue ideas. This means that in a department with complex activities, several groups may be needed.

The benefits of a group discussion rest in the ability of members to mutually stimulate thought and produce more comprehensive analyses than might come from a set of individual interviews. It also enables the creation of consensus among personnel as to outputs, customers, activity flows, and resources needed. The questions proposed to the group will be essentially the same as those used in individual interviews, except modified for responses by several people.

The analyst acting as moderator of a group attempting to describe and understand the activities of its organization should take two moderator roles as described by Krueger.[4]

1. *Seeker of wisdom.* The moderator assumes that the members have the insight and understanding needed and will share it if they are asked the right questions.
2. *Referee.* Provide balance within the group when there are opposing points of view.

Generally, group interviews done to analyze activity structures are rather unstructured. The idea is to get respondents to stimulate each other in order to maximize the comprehensiveness of the data gathered. The rules for individual interviews are appropriate if modified slightly to apply to groups. Additionally, the analysis must work to assure that all members of the group participate and that no members are allowed to dominate the flow or intimidate other.

A Comment

After separable activities have been identified, it is often quite informative to go to the internal customer using the activities' outputs and ask why the outputs are needed and how they are used.

It is not uncommon to find that the output is not used or is not used as its producer thought it would be. When the output is information, analysts often find that its need no longer exists or that somewhat different information in another format would be more useful. One of the benefits of activity based costing is the efficiency produced by this sort of cross-boundary communication done as part of its analysis. Eliminating such unnecessary support activities obviously increases efficiency. Eliminating unnecessary information from reports increases their usability.

DISCUSSION QUESTIONS

1. What are separable overhead activities? Why are they of interest?
2. What documents can help gain early understanding of specific activities within an organization. How?
3. What guidelines should be followed when interviewing workers or leading group discussions in order to gain understanding of the structure of activities?
4. What are the advantages of observation over interviewing and vice versa?
5. If you were attempting to understand the activities performed in your biomedical engineering department, how would you proceed? What questions would you ask?

Isolating Drivers

The cost of any cost object (or cost target) is the sum of the costs of a series of preceding activities, the resources used in those activities, and the resources used in the activity that produces the cost object in question. To understand this flow, one must know what activities precede the final activity and what additional resources are needed in the final activity.

Activity Drivers

In any overhead department or function, one establishes separable activities as just described. The next question is: "What causes these activities to be done?" This factor is the activity's driver. It is the link between the activity in question and the cost of the objects for which it is an input. In our personnel department example, paying personnel is a separable activity. An individual instance of this activity is required when an individual must be paid. Therefore, the requirement to pay individuals is the driver; it is an activity driver. It is used to link a part of the personnel department's costs to users of that activity. In determining the cost of running nursing services, one of the input activities is the cost of paying its personnel. This is established by multiplying the cost of the activity *pay a person* by the number of people paid in the nursing services. An activity driver is identified by determining what instigates the activity. In the case of the activity *administer personnel actions*, the question was: "What makes the personnel department do this?" The answer was: "A request from a department within the organization."

In determining the cost of an activity, the cost of other resources used in the activity itself must be added to the cost of previous, necessary activities. These fall into two categories: (1) direct costs and (2) allocated overhead. Detecting the direct cost can be done by examining the activity's procedure documentation, observation, and interaction with the producers to establish how much of what specific resources are used. If the general ledger has direct resource accounts for each separable activity, a historical measure can be made by dividing the total of these expense accounts by the number of times the activity was performed in a baseline period. Because management accounting information is to be used in making decisions about the future, such historic figures may be of limited value to decision makers. Adjusting them to be of more use in management decisions will be discussed in Chapter 11.

Resource Drivers

When a separable overhead activity is conducted in response to a countable activity of the service's user, the relationship between the overhead activity and what causes it to be done is easy to establish. In fact, once these separable overhead activities are defined, they are treated like direct costs. This is because activity drivers allow them to be linked to their cost object much like the general ledger links direct costs to the place where they are used. Detecting the drivers of other overhead resources presents more of a problem. For these types of overhead, no one-to-one relationship between a unit of the overhead activity and an activity by its user exists.

These other overhead costs are those for which tracing to specific users is either virtually impossible or too expensive to be worthwhile. Examples are building maintenance, executive management, housekeeping, and production scheduling. For these costs, analysts examine factors that could rationally drive the amount of the overhead cost for a period. For example, it is rational that the cost of housekeeping is driven by the square footage of the area that must be cleaned. Cost objects would then be charged the proportion of housekeeping costs that is their proportion of the total area that must be kept. Executive management can be considered caused by the number of people who must be managed; the number of middle managers in the organization or perhaps the total cost of resources that must be managed. Any of these variables are potential drivers of executive management costs. Selection from a logical array of drivers is usually done by running a regression analysis of historic data on each potential driver and seeing which has the highest correlation with the cost category being analyzed, as measured by the R^2 statistic. Obviously, isolating resource drivers is considered more subjective than establishing activity drivers.

Accuracy in measuring the use of resource drivers can be increased by stratifying users. For instance, analysts may realize that some areas of the facility demand more housekeeping effort than do others. They could then classify work centers by the relative amount of housekeeping effort needed. Perhaps there would be three categories:

Category A uses less than the average amount of effort. It is given a weight of 0.7.

Category B uses the average amount of effort. It is given a weight of 1.0.
Category C uses a larger amount of effort. It is given a weight of 1.5.

The driver for allocating housekeeping costs would be changed from simple square foot proportions to proportions of the weighted square footage. This adjustment compensates for the fact that all areas do not incur the same housekeeping cost per unit of floor area. The value of this adjustment can be checked by regressing housekeeping costs on the new weighted area measures and seeing if the R^2 statistic is significantly improved.

Such adjustments will be discussed in detail when relative value units (RVUs) are explained later in this chapter.

Analysis of Resource Use

After identifying separable overhead activities and their activity drivers, managers identify other overhead activities that are not driven by activity drivers. For these, one establishes resource drivers, as just discussed. After doing this, it is necessary to measure how many resources are used for each unit of the driver and the cost of these resources. Management can begin collecting this information as separable activities are identified. One of the factors that allows management to aggregate a set of activities into a single separable activity is that they use a set of resources that can be separated from those used by other activities. In personnel department example, a distinct set of people, supplies, and equipment was used by activities needed to pay employees while another set was used in processing personnel actions. After determining such differences, the specific amounts of the specific resources used must be measured.

OBSERVATION AND INTERVIEWS   In an optimal situation, these resources are traceable to the different separable activities. Usually, however, some of the resources used by each separable activity will be shared.

This problem can often be overcome by a subjective analysis of the relative amounts of the resources that are used by each activity. One way of doing this is to use a resource driver to assign the shared resource. In the personnel department, management may find that some pieces of office equipment or certain personnel are used on both separable activities. The use of these personnel may be in proportion to the number of transactions of either type; a transaction being defined as a person paid or a personnel action processed. In this case, the resource driver for allocating the cost of these workers would be the number of transactions. Alternatively, the relative use of shared office equipment may be quite simply determined by asking the workers what percentage of time the equipment is used to support each activity.

RELATIVE VALUE UNITS   Another approach to determining a driver for machine usage would do to establish office machine relative value units (RVUs) similar to the way RVUs were established in Chapter 5 to allocate laboratory fixed costs. Interviews or observation might show that these machines are used 0.12 hours in preparing the payroll entry for an individual and 0.50 hours in processing a personnel action. The time used by the average activity is:

$$(0.12 + 0.50)/2 = 0.31 \text{ hours}$$

The RVU for each activity is:

$$Payroll\ activity\ 0.12/0.31 = 0.387$$
$$Personnel\ action\ 0.50/0.31 = 1.613$$

If the total cost of using these machines for a period of time is $25,000 and the total number of RVUs used in that period is 180,000, cost per RVU would be:

$$\$25,000/180,00\ RVUs = \$0.139\ per\ RVU$$

The cost of shared office equipment would be allocated to the activities at a rate of $0.139 per RVU. The RVUs charged to the payroll activity would be 0.387 times the number of its transactions. The amount charged to the personnel actions activity would be 1.613 times the number of its transactions.

ENGINEERING WORK STUDY   In order to understand the amount of direct resources needed to complete an activity, the resources used can simply be counted. Often documentation of the procedures used in the activity lists the supplies and equipment that are needed. This counting is complicated somewhat when labor is an input. For current purposes, treat direct labor as a variable cost. Situations in which it should be considered a fixed cost will be discussed later. The amount of labor needed to complete an activity will depend on the skill and experience of the workers, the amount and type of capital they work with, and their level of effort.

The use of time studies of human work has existed for a long time, undergone much research, and now has extensive literature. Simple activities, such as making a bed, are rather easily measured. In fact, if a charge nurse were asked to state a standard time for making a bed, he could probably come within a few seconds of a standard established using rigorous engineering techniques. However, for fairly complex activities or tasks within activities, determining an expected amount of time to complete a task should be done by a specialist trained in work measurement.

The usual approach is to make repetitive measurements of the time used for the task and compute an average of those times. Because this can rarely be done unobtrusively, workers may well slow their pace in order to reduce the speed at which they will be expected to work. The average time is therefore adjusted by a performance rating. For instance, if a task the analyst believes the observed workers are operating 15 percent slower than would be done at a normal pace, the performance-rating factor would be − 0.15. If the average task time were 20 minutes, the normal time (NT) for the task would be set at:

$$20 - 0.15(20) = 17 \ minutes$$

The standard time (ST) for use in predicting productivity or future costs is the normal time plus an allowance. These allowances account for appropriate time spent in washrooms, on coffee breaks, and for other appropriate personal or administrative reasons. The allowance factor is the percentage of total work time that is allowed for these other activities. The formula for standard time is:

$$ST = NT \ (1 + allowance)$$

The reason time studies of human inputs should be done by people experienced in such work is that establishing sound performance ratings, and to some extent allowance factors, takes experience. Accurate judgments about these factors must be made if the standard times established are to reflect efficient work habits yet be fair to the workers. Unachievable work standards do not promote efficiency; they tend to promote low morale and lack of proper attention to tasks. Excessive time pressure has proved to increase the risk of errors in clinical settings. This, in turn, can cause both rework and litigation costs.

A MACROLEVEL TIME STUDY   In order to gauge labor's effect on specific activities, time studies can also be done at a macro level. In the face of forthcoming prospective payment, a mid-western home health agency thought it should better understand the cost of treating different types of patients. It divided its home visits into categories dependent on the type of patient visited. Because the major cost of a visit is the professional time spent to complete it, the agency conducted a time study of visits to patients in each category. The first step was to identify the categories of patients whose visits would be costed separately. Chronic conditions with high frequency visits and high probability of hospital admission were picked for initial study. A study of chronic obstructive pulmonary disease (COPD) patients will be used as an example of these macro studies.

The second step was to interview registered nurses (RNs) specially trained and experienced in home visits to these types of patients. The purpose of the interviews was to create a comprehensive list of the activities and resources used in their visits. Analysis of the information from these interviews indicated that activities could be divided into three groups: (1) activities before the visit, (2) activities during the visit, and (3) activities after the visit. Analysis of interviews across the different types of patients showed that that the activities before and after a visit did not differ greatly among the types of patients. Figure 8-1 illustrates the data sheet used to record the times of components within these three groups of activities for COPD patient visits. The left-hand column shows the components of these groups. In the right-hand column, the RN/respiratory

RN-Respiratory Therapist—Patient Visit Sheet

Your Name _____ Today's Date _____

Patient's Name _____ ID # _____

Before Visit   **No. of Minutes**

    Review patient's previous problem   _____

    Telephone contact to schedule visit   _____

    Gather or replenish supplies   _____

    Check voice mail reports on patient from other nurses   _____

    Travel–related activities   _____

During Visit

    Introductory activities   _____

    Obtain paperwork/consent signatures   _____

    Assessment/observation of immediate conditions   _____

    Do assessment–systems by systems checklist   _____

    Focused pulmonary assessment

        Pulse oximetry   _____

        Check O_2 when relevant   _____

        Check other respiratory equipment   _____

        Assess use of nocturnal therapies   _____

    Perform clinical care as necessary   _____

    Draw lab work and complete requisitions   _____

    Initiate charting in the home during visit   _____

    Check medications supplies; review medications box   _____

    Supervise care and cleaning of equipment   _____

    Telephone calls from the home for clinical purposes

        Physician   _____

        DME supplier   _____

        Home health agency   _____

        Members of family (as needed)   _____

    Patient education   _____

    Care of caregiver   _____

    Other _____   _____

After Visit

    Travel–related activities from visit   _____

    Log–in time spent   _____

    Charting, if needed   _____

    Return follow–up telephone calls

        Physician   _____

        DME   _____

        Members of family (not reached while in the home)   _____

        Other case management calls reference this patient   _____

    Drop off specimens at the lab, when necessary   _____

    Total Minutes (carried forward to the summary sheet) _____

Source: Reprinted from J.J. Baker, Activity-Based Costing and Activity-Based Management for Health Care p. 230 (Reading, MA: Aspen Publishers, 1998)

Figure 8-1   **RN-Respiratory Therapist—Patient Visit Sheet**

therapist records the time spent in each component activity. Additionally, each visiting nurse completes a daily time sheet for activities performed for each patient subsequent to those directly related to visits. Figure 8-2 illustrates the form used to record activities performed after visits are completed. A daily time sheet is also prepared for activities not related to specific patients. This sheet is illustrated in Figure 8-3. Finally, a daily summary sheet for each nurse is prepared, as illustrated by Figure 8-4.

The data from these sheets comes from what can be called *participant observers*. The extent to which these observers have a personal interest in the information gained from them can bias that information. Because the sum of times consumed by daily activities cannot exceed the total work time for each day, the summary sheet data acts as at least a partial control on the effect of bias. It prevents individual task times from being generally inflated. Some control of this sort should be used when there is a strong motivation for measurement bias to occur. This bias could also be controlled by the analyst applying performance factors to the task times. However, when the analyst is not a direct observer of the activities, this control becomes highly subjective and fraught with low reliability.

Knowing the wage rates of the visiting nurses combined with this labor resource use information allows computation of the cost of the activities involved each type of visit. Realize that each category of visit is treated as a separable activity.

DISCUSSION QUESTIONS

1. What is the difference between an activity driver and a resource driver?
2. What is the similarity between separable overhead activities and direct costs?
3. What is the relationship between the general ledger and costing overhead?
4. How do analysts go about picking the best resource driver from among logical alternatives?
5. What are stratified cost objects with reference to resource drivers? Why are they used? How are they used?
6. When is it appropriate to use RVUs as resource drivers?
7. What are the basic steps in doing and using a labor time study? Why are they done? What are their potential weaknesses?
8. How do macrolevel time studies relate to separable activity analysis?

EXAMPLE

Understanding the separation of activities and isolating of drivers may be helped by returning to the knee arthroscopy example discussed at the end of Chapter 7. Figure 8-5 is a duplication of Figure 7-5.

Subsequent Visit-Related Activities

Your Name _____   Today's Date _____

Telephone: Case Management Calls re: Patient Clinical Care   **Today's total time**

Patient's Name _____   _____

Patient's Name _____   _____

Patient's Name _____   _____

Patient's Name _____   _____

Patient's Name _____   _____   _____

Telephone: Physician Calls

Patient's Name _____   _____

Patient's Name _____   _____

Patient's Name _____   _____

Patient's Name _____   _____

Patient's Name _____   _____   _____

Telephone: Patient or Care Giver

Telephone: Insurance-Reimbursement-Recertification

Patient's Name _____   _____

Patient's Name _____   _____

Patient's Name _____   _____

Patient's Name _____   _____

Patient's Name _____   _____   _____

Telephone: Other Visit Related

(Describe) _____

_____

_____   _____

Complete Forms in the Patients' Records

Submit Daily Visit Reports   _____

Hospital visits when patients are hospitalized

Patient's Name _____   _____

Patient's Name _____   _____

Patient's Name _____   _____   _____

      Total Minutes (carried forward to the summary sheet)   _____

Source: Reprinted from J.J. Baker, Activity-Based Costing and Activity-Based Management for Health Care p. 227.

Figure 8-2   **Subsequent Visit-Related Activities**

Nonvisit-Related Activities

Your Name _____	Today's Date _____

Consultations on Specialty Care	Time in Minutes
_____	_____
_____	_____
_____	_____
_____	_____
_____	_____
_____	_____
_____	_____
_____	_____
_____	_____
_____	_____

All Other Nonspecific Visit-Related Activities

Boarding patients	_____
Completing day sheets	_____
Inservice programs for staff members, reference specialty care	_____
Quality improvement meetings	_____
Staff meetings	_____
Marketing with specialists	_____
Professional growth responsibilities	_____
Other (describe) _____	_____
_____	_____
_____	_____
_____	_____
Total Other	_____
Personal (describe) _____	_____
_____	_____
_____	_____
Total Personal	_____
Total Minutes (carry forward to the summary sheet)	_____

Source: Reprinted from J.J. Baker, Activity-Based Costing and Activity-Based Management for Health Care p. 228.

Figure 8-3 **Nonvisit-Related Activities**

Daily Time Summary Sheet

Your Name _____ Today's Date _____

Begin Time _____ End Time _____ Total Time _____

Visit Summary (Totals from RN Respiratory Therapist visit sheets)	Today's time (minutes)
Patient's Name	

Visit: _____ suppl. sheet # _____   _____

Visit: _____ suppl. sheet # _____   _____

Visit: _____ suppl. sheet # _____   _____

Visit: _____ suppl. sheet # _____   _____

Visit: _____ suppl. sheet # _____   _____

Visit: _____ suppl. sheet # _____   _____

Visit: _____ suppl. sheet # _____   _____

Visit: _____ suppl. sheet # _____   _____

Visit: _____ suppl. sheet # _____   _____

Visit: _____ suppl. sheet # _____   _____

Total Minutes of All Visits Above: _____

Summary of Subsequent Vist-Related Activities: _____

Summary of Nonvisit-Related Activities   _____

Total Minutes   _____

Note: Total minutes should equal total time at top of this sheet

Source: Reprinted from J.J. Baker, Activity-Based Costing and Activity-Based Management for Health Care p. 227.

Figure 8-4 **Daily Time Summary Sheet**

This hospital simplified its costing of specific types of surgeries by categorizing surgical procedures according to the types of resources they consumed and used the duration of the operation as the driver resources per minute. The result was a limited set of procedure categories with the same cost per minute. The different categories were called *acuity levels*. Performing an acuity-3 surgery involves the 10 inputs listed at the top of the figure. The driver of costs associated with this general surgery category is the time over which it is performed. The analysts, therefore, chose to cost its inputs per minute. For some inputs, such as labor, this is a natural thing to do because they are paid by time employed.

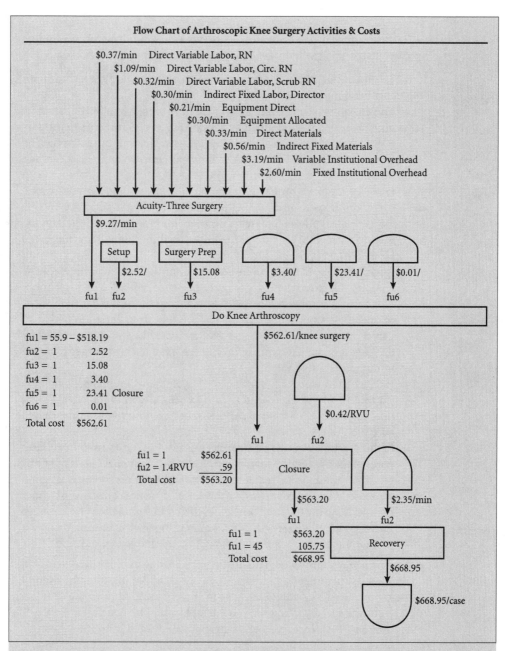

Figure 8-5   **Flow Chart of Arthroscopic Knee Surgery Activities and Costs**

For others, time had to be treated as a resource driver and the cost per minute computed from general ledger data. Examine these inputs individually.

- The three categories of nurses used in the surgery are charged at their cost per minute.

- The director's salary, a fixed cost, could have been driven by the total cost of all surgeries. It would then be allocated to level-3 surgeries in proportion to their proportion of total surgery costs. This amount could then be divided by the total time spent in those surgeries to arrive at a cost per minute.

- Direct equipment probable is equipment that is used only in level-3 surgeries. Its cost can be stated per minute by dividing its total cost by total minutes of level-3 activity. Because this is a fixed cost, the rate per minute is accurate only if the total time used for level-3 surgeries is the same from period to period.

- Allocated equipment is equipment used for a variety of activities. The allocation is driven by time of use. It is also a fixed cost per period; therefore, its cost per minute will also not be accurate if the total minutes of operating room utilization are not constant from period to period.

- Direct materials for level-3 surgeries are stated as a cost per minute by dividing the total direct material costs charged to those surgeries by the minutes used to do them.

- Indirect fixed materials, like allocated equipment, are materials that are charged to the surgical center (as opposed to level-3 surgeries). Their total coast is divided by total surgical suite time to arrive at a time-driven allocation rate.

- In this organization, all institutional overhead is allocated to the overhead pools of the operating departments. A cost behavior analysis was done by regressing the allocations to the surgery center on the time surgical suites were used. The result provided the variable institutional overhead per minute. Dividing the fixed portion of this cost by total time of suite usage furnished a fixed overhead cost per minute. Again, this is accurate only if the amount of time use does not vary from period to period.

Reviewing these procedures for costing a defined level of surgical procedure shows that various approaches can be taken. For instance, the overhead pool was allocated to each type of surgery based only on the time taken by the surgery. There was no attempt to allocate equipment-related institutional costs by equipment value or labor-related institutional cost by labor time. This increased detail may have improved the differentiation of level-3 surgeries from those at other levels. The analyst evidently decided that the decision support value of the more detailed analysis was not worth its additional cost.

Having determined the cost per minute of surgical level-3 operations as one input to the knee arthroscopy, similar analyses were done for the separable activities and other resources necessary in this procedure. These are the IV setup, surgery preparation, and the arthrosope, video, and tourniquet equipment. Summing these costs and assuming the average surgery takes 55.9 minutes gives an average cost of $562.61.

Follow-on activities needed to complete the surgical episode were analyzed similarly. These are reflected in the costing of the closure and recovery activities.

ADDITIONAL COMMENTS

The accuracy of subjective or qualitative information development techniques discussed in this chapter is sometimes questioned. The legitimacy of such results from appropriately conducted research is well documented in decision science literature.[5]

The knee orthroscopy example indicates that the costs of separable activities can be analyzed separately, although the analysis cannot be completed until all the preceding activities used by the activity in question have been analyzed. The reason that, in that example, institutional overhead was allocate to level-3 surgeries using the total of institutional overhead costs is probably because separable institutional overhead activities with specific drivers had not yet been analyzed. Despite this limitation, the level-3 surgery, IV setup, surgery preparation, and knee orthroscopy could be analyzed concurrently by the people involved in each of these activities. The ability to do this means that the total time needed to complete activity based costing of an array of high cost or frequently employed activities is not as great as it would be if the component analyses had to be done one at a time.

KEY POINTS

- The cost of an overhead activity consists of direct and indirect components. The output of an overhead activity is an input to another activity.
- Clusters of overhead activities that use resources not shared with other activities and whose output can be traced to its user are called separable activities.
- Separable activities can be treated similarly to the treatment of direct costs and allocated using an activity driver.

- Overhead activities that are not separable are allocated based on a logical resource driver. The quality of a resource driver can usually be measured through regression analysis.
- Analyzing the structure of activities should usually start with review of organization charts, job descriptions, and procedure manuals.
- Interviews and group discussions with involved workers about activities are used

to increase understanding of activity structures.

- The need for the activities engaged in by a department or overhead function should be confirmed by its customers.
- The quantity of nonlabor resources used by an activity can be measured by observation, interviews, and tracing ledger accounts.
- RVUs can be used as resource drivers when different cost objects use different amounts of a nontraceable overhead resource.

- Measuring labor usage can be done by interviews and time studies.
- Labor time studies can be made through timing of specific actions by uninvolved observers. For complex activities, these should be trained specialists.
- Macro time studies can be made by averaging self-measurement of activities or groups of activities by an array of workers in those activities.

EXERCISES

PROBLEM 1

Your organization provides day care for employees' children less than 7 years of age. The day care center cares for about 200 children distributed rather equally across the 7-year spectrum. You would like to know what this costs per child in order to establish cost-sharing rates for the employees. You suspect that children fall into different categories and that the categories have different costs.

List the actions you would take to:

1. Specify how children should be categorized.
2. Determine what activities are demanded by each category.
3. Discover if the activities are separable.
4. Conclude the cost of the activities.

PROBLEM 2

Review the section of this chapter entitled "A Macrolevel Time Study" on page 169, along with the accompanying four figures illustrating time sheet information. The text states: "Knowing the wage rates of the visiting nurses combined with this information on the use of labor allows computation of the

cost of the activities involved in each type of visit. Realize that each category of visit is treated as a separable activity."

Required:

1. Arrange the categories of visits into separable activities.
2. Using blank copies of the forms, make some assumptions as to minutes spent. Fill out the forms using your assumptions.
3. Compute the cost of the activities involved in each type of visit.

Assume the wage rate of the visiting nurses is $24 per hour before fringe benefits and $30 per hour including fringe benefits. (Fringe benefits include such items as payroll taxes and health insurance.)

PROBLEM 3

An ambulatory surgery center (ASC) is a distinct facility that provides exclusively outpatient surgical services. Excellent ASC, located in Midtown, Any State, tracks its volume by the number of surgeries. It regards its surgeries as being of three types; that is, either high, medium, or low complexity. As the ASC business manager, you define complexity as length of time in the ASC operating room, measured in 15-minute segments. You would like to know what it costs per type of activity as a first step in establishing internally generated RVUs for Excellent ASC. You suspect that the activities fall into different categories and that the categories have different costs.

You have gathered the following information. A typical procedure involves preparation of the patient in one area of the floor plan, and performance of the surgical procedure in one of the operating rooms. Patient recovery takes place in a separate recovery area within the floor plan. The floor plan also includes a waiting room, a check-in or registration area, and a check-out area, along with two administrative offices, a filing area, and a locked supply room.

List the actions you would take to:

1. Specify how the business of the ASC should be categorized.

2. Determine what activities are demanded by each category.
3. Conclude if the activities are separable.

As business manager, you have also gathered the following statistical and financial data about the ASC operations. There are four operating rooms and 12 preparation/recovery beds. The preparation/recovery staffing includes two RNs and two technicians. There is typically one RN in each operating room plus one RN floater. The business manager makes $60,000 annually and the secretary/receptionist makes $20,000 annually. The RNs make $24 per hour without fringe benefits and $30 including fringe benefits. The technicians make $15 per hour without fringe benefits and $20 per hour including fringe benefits.

4. Make the necessary assumptions and compute the direct cost of the activities you have identified.

REFERENCES

[1] Adler, P. A. and P. Adler. "Observational Techniques" in *Handbook of Qualitative Research*, N. K. Denzin and Y. S. Lincoln, eds. (Thousand Oaks, CA: Sage Publications, 1994), p. 337.
[2] Fontana, A. and J. H. Frey. "Interviewing: The Art of Science" in *Handbook of Qualitative Research*, N. K. Denzin and Y. S. Lincoln, eds. (Thousand Oaks, CA: Sage Publications, 1994), p. 364.
[3] Morgan, D. L. *Focus Groups as Qualitative Research* (Thousand Oaks, CA: Sage Publications, 1998), pp. 43–44.

[4] Krueger, R. A. *Focus Groups: A Practical Guide to Applied Research* (Thousand Oaks, CA: Sage Publications, 1994), p. 105.
[5] Guftason, D. H., D. Fryback and J. Rose. "An Evaluation of Multiple Severity Indices Created by Different Index Development Strategies," *Medical Care* 6, no. 7 (1983): 674; and Alemi, F. "The Value of Introspection in Modeling Decisions Under Time Pressure, Dissertation," *Abstracts International* (1983): 83.

CHAPTER 9

PLANNING, DESIGNING, AND IMPLEMENTING AN **ABC** SYSTEM

LEARNING OBJECTIVES

After studying this chapter, students should be able to:

1. Discuss management's motivation and priorities when planning an ABC system design.
2. Explain management criteria and project decision making when designing plans for the system.
3. Discuss the elements of designing the ABC system and its implementation.
4. Explain the stages of implementation.
5. Define multiple cost systems.
6. Describe system implementation with ABC upgrades.
7. Explain the difference between direct costs and indirect costs.

INTRODUCTION

Management accounting can make excellent use of an activity-based costing (ABC) system, and such a system provides a wealth of information for the health care manager. Because installation of an ABC system requires both capital expenditures and staff-time expenditures, it is important to provide careful planning and knowledgeable project supervision. In this chapter, we describe a set of system planning and implementation steps that are the keys to a successful project.

PLANNING AN ABC SYSTEM DESIGN

Planning the ABC system design is the first step in the project and it is essential to get management to communicate their motivations and their priorities. Only then should the actual project criteria be set and decision making proceed.

Determining Management Motivation

To be successful, an ABC project requires managerial support. Many good projects have never achieved their full potential because of internal opposition. One way to anticipate areas of opposition is to determine the project motivations of managers. How do they feel about it? Why would they support the project?

The organizational motivation worksheet shown in Exhibit 9-1 is a useful tool to reveal these primary motivations. Of the four motivations shown on the worksheet, two are reactive (maximize profitability and control resource consumption) and two are proactive (maximize productivity and obtain information for decision making).

Determining Management Priorities

Managers are more likely to support an ABC project if they have had input into the project planning process. Because an ABC system should be chosen to fit primary priorities of the organization, one way to gain useful input and support at the same time is to ask the managers to rank their priorities for the capabilities of an "ideal" ABC system. Each manager involved in planning would fill out his or her own list. The worksheet shown in Exhibit 9-2 provides the format to rank a list of priorities.

Applying Management's Criteria to the Project

Human nature dictates that managers are more likely to be in favor of the ABC system proposal if it supports their own management style. In other words, a detail-oriented manager will be interested in the nuts and bolts of the system, while a top line-oriented manager will be more interested in the outcomes produced by the system. It is important to provide the correct information about the project in order to satisfy each type of manager.

After reviewing management's criteria, the project manager will first conduct a general search for suitable systems. When suitable vendors are located, the

Exhibit 9-1   **An Organizational Motivation Worksheet**

For each item listed, indicate your degree of interest by marking a number from 1 to 5 beside it, with 5 indicating the highest degree of interest.

Project Motivations	High 5	4	3	2	Low 1
Maximize profitability					
Maximize productivity					
Control resource consumption					
Obtain information for decision making					

Exhibit 9-2 **An Organizational Priority Worksheet: Choosing from Costing Alternatives**

For each item listed, indicate your degree of interest by marking a number from 1 to 5 beside it, with 5 indicating the highest degree of interest.

Project Priorities	High 5	4	3	2	Low 1
Product/service pricing					
Cost-reduction efforts					
Process improvement					
Quality improvement					
Performance measures					
Resource management					
Underutilized capacity					
Capital investment					
Strategic assessment					
Analysis of organizational-risk levels					
Time line					
Integration					

project manager will then issue a request for proposals, or RFP. It is important to insist upon sufficient detail in the RFPs so that a good understanding of system capabilities can be obtained. It is also important to insist that the RFP responses be as uniform as possible, so that adequate comparisons can be made among and between vendors.

The ABC system will incur costs for hardware, software, and training. There will also be costs incurred for internal staff time and for outside consultant's fees. All costs to be charged by the vendor should be revealed at the time of proposal. (For example, it is common for the cost of training to be understated in initial proposals.) All expenses that will be borne internally, such as staff time, should also be computed and included in the system cost. Exhibit 9-3 provides a starting format for recording and tracking RFP information received. After initial RFP responses are received and reviewed, the top two or three vendors are invited to make a second, more detailed, proposal. The second round generally includes additional demonstrations of system capabilities plus and greater detail about inputs and outputs. The checklist example in Exhibit 9-3 would then be expanded into detailed listings of individual cost components for each vendor's proposal.

Exhibit 9-3   **Project Cost Component Checklist**

Project Costs Include:

Software cost	
Hardware cost	
Staff time incurred	
Consultants' fees	
Training costs	

Decision Making

In most cases, the vendors' proposals will not be directly comparable. Management can also expect that every item desired will not be achievable, mainly because some will not be available while others will be too expensive. So how can an appropriate decision be made? The elements involved in decision making can be quantified in a two-step process: (1) the benefits of an ABC system are assessed and (2) the trade-offs are assessed.

Exhibit 9-4 provides a format for two checklists. In the first checklist, the benefits received from the ABC system are compared to the project cost. Trade-offs are also summarized for decision-making purposes. Trade-off detail is contained in the second checklist within Exhibit 9-4 with common trade-offs already listed. The project team should be fully aware of the give and take involved in this type of system decision, and the checklists assist in this process.

Exhibit 9-4   **Project Decision and Trade-Off Checklists**

Project Decisions Affect:

Benefits Received from Performing ABC	
Project cost	
Trade-offs	
Project Trade-Offs Include:	
Flexibility/adaptability	
Responsibility accounting	
Profit centers	
Time-frame requirements	
Alternative special-purpose budgets	
No change to basic accounting system (if so desired)	
Constraints	

EXERCISE

Two final proposals have been received. Both are priced at $100,000 but the components are different. What are the strengths and weaknesses of each proposal?

Proposal 1 costs are quoted as:

Software cost	$ 10,000
Hardware cost	$ 25,000
Estimated staff time required	$ 5,000
Consultants' fees	$ 40,000
Training costs–external	$ 20,000
Total	$100,000

Proposal 2 costs are quoted as:

Software cost	[included in hardware quote]
Hardware cost	$ 60,000
Estimated staff time required	$ 20,000
Consultants' fees	$ 10,000
Training costs–external	$ 5,000
Training costs–internal	$ 5,000
Total	$100,000

DESIGNING THE ABC SYSTEM AND ITS OPERATION

Designing the ABC system, its operation, and its implementation involves multiple elements as discussed in this section.

Determining Stages of Implementation

The stages of implementation affect both capital expenditure and staffing hours. Some organizations commit to a series of contracts that match implementation stages. This approach may spread the capital expenditure over more than 1 fiscal year. Other organizations commit to the entire expenditure in a single contract. Obviously, the timing of stages directly affects the number of hours required for internal staffing.

Determining Responsibility Structure

It is important to formally document both internal and external responsibility for the system. Just as there is a charge-master coordinator, there must be an ABC system coordinator. Figure 9-1 sets out a responsibility matrix. Each is discussed.

Figure 9-1   **Internal/External System Responsibility Matrix**

Responsible Party	Implementation	Maintenance
Internal		
External (vendor)		
Internal	Documentation	System Updates
External (vendor)		

IMPLEMENTATION RESPONSIBILITY   Each step of implementation should be set out. The vendor's external responsibility should be designated, and all steps not covered by the vendor's contract then become internal responsibility. Some organizations outsource part of the tasks not covered by the vendor's contract. In this case, the responsibility matrix would show two separate vendors, each accountable for certain areas.

DOCUMENTATION RESPONSIBILITY   Each step of required documentation should also be designated. The vendor's external responsibility should be noted. Be aware that some vendors will provide off-the-shelf manuals only. These manuals will not contain any customized adjustments to the company's system. The internal responsibility is to document every item that the vendor does not cover.

MAINTENANCE RESPONSIBILITY   Some maintenance is routinely covered in the contractual obligations of the external vendor. There will remain, however, additional tasks that internal personnel will have to complete. The lines of distinction between internal and external is especially important in the case of maintenance.

SYSTEM UPDATE RESPONSIBILITY   The system is not yielding full benefits to the organization unless it is updated. Furthermore, the updates should occur on a set schedule. The vendor may be contractually obligated to provide computerized updates. However, this is often a gray area that should be addressed in the initial contract. The internal responsibility will generally include providing updates of statistical and service delivery information.

Determining Actual Detail of System Structure

Chapter 8 discusses determining activity structures and cost drivers. Review the introduction. Remember that costs of direct resources are rather easily determined because, by definition, these resources can be traced. Likewise, Chapter 8 points out that activities need to be distinguished from one another (thus, "separable activities"), and drivers need to be determined for each type of activity.

Now, to determine system detail, the actual method by which resources will be traced, allocated, and thus divided in the new system must be perfectly clear. This method should be documented before the work of implementation begins. This step is essential because the segmenting of the activities and the selection of drivers will determine all outputs of the ABC system. One must clearly understand how this system detail will work. If one loses control of this piece, one will lose control of the project.

DETERMINING INPUTS   Determining inputs is not a task to be left entirely to the vendor. It is a system for the company and should be customized to the greatest extent possible. Inputs should be consistent with outputs that are useful to the company. Input information should also be readily available somewhere in the organization. (This point is sometimes ignored by the vendor.) Issues to consider include relationship to the financial accounting system, specific relationship to the general ledger, and measures or statistics desired.

DETERMINING OUTPUTS   The preceding section on the actual detail of the system structure noted the actual method should be documented before implementation because segmenting of the activities and the selection of drivers would determine all outputs of the ABC. The system outputs should match management's priorities and desires to the greatest extent possible.

The degree to which the system matches management's expectations is determined by the type of system selected, as previously discussed. Management has to understand that the choice of system determines what that system can or cannot do for the company.

EXAMPLE

The following example illustrates a performance measure (operating margin) and the detail necessary to compute it. If computation of operating margins is a desired part of the ABC project, then the definition, computation, and assigning of costs are all important inputs and the margin computation is an important output.

Some organizations measure performance by the operating margin generated. The operating margin is generally expressed as a percentage and is determined as follows:

(operating revenue − operating costs) × *100 / operating revenue*

COMPUTATION OF OPERATING COST   This computation is dependent upon the definition of cost. The amount and type of operating cost assigned to a cost center will obviously affect this measure of performance. How will the proposed ABC system assign operating costs to cost centers?

ABC SYSTEM'S METHOD FOR ASSIGNING COST   The ABC system's method for tracing direct cost and assigning indirect cost will directly affect the operating-cost portion of the margin computation. If the operating margin is a performance measure, then the method becomes of intense interest. Figure 9-2 illustrates one way in which an operating margin can be reported. The company can expect lobbying from department managers who feel they can influence these computations. Management should be prepared with arguments about how the system works on an objective and impartial basis.

Determining Report Structure

Another planning aspect of system implementation is determining report structures. Many internal reports are generated in various formats and for various purposes. The report is the final product that the manager sees and hopefully uses. It is best to not plan report structure in a vacuum; instead, get feedback from the managerial users.

Determining System Update Schedule

Although the report structures are a joint project, determining system update schedules is a function that should be controlled by the "owner" of the ABC project. The system updates are necessary and important because they require funding and manpower that has to come from someone's budget. The update schedule planning must therefore also consider whose budget will be funding these updates.

Scope of ABC Analysis

As mentioned in Chapter 5, management attempting to undertake an ABC system for its organization may find the scope of the task daunting. However, the purpose of ABC is not to determine every activity that is necessary to produce each of the organization's products. So how far does management carry the scope? If the overall project is too large to tackle at once, consider implementing by stages, as discussed in the next section. Implementation with multiple-cost systems readily allows scope of analysis in the ABC system to be adopted at whatever level management desires. Finally, the incremental implementation ap-

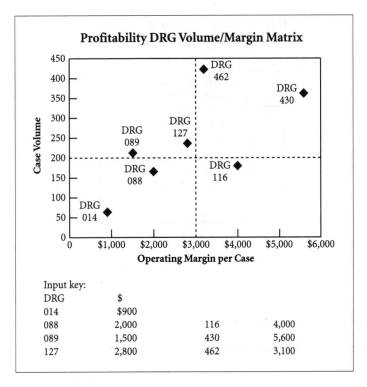

Profitability DRG Volume/Margin Matrix

Input key:

DRG	$		
014	$900		
088	2,000	116	4,000
089	1,500	430	5,600
127	2,800	462	3,100

Figure 9-2   **Profitability DRG Volume/Margin Matrix**

proach (discussed toward the end of the chapter) is ideal for controlling the scope of ABC analysis.

Also, management must review overall overhead allocations in terms of scope. (Ideally, this step should occur in planning, but in reality, it often occurs during implementation when the true size of the project becomes visible.) Overhead allocations are usually in layers or levels. These include production center overhead (within the center itself) and sustaining overhead (within the hospital itself). In a health system of more than one hospital, home office or corporate office administrative overhead cost also exist and in the health system, there may also be regional office administrative overhead. Figure 9-3 illustrates this point. Management must consider how deep into the layers the analysis needs to go, especially in the initial implementation. At a minimum, it should probably cover the hospital, although even that scope can be implemented incrementally. But why does the analysis, at first anyway, cover the regional office and the corporate office? The following exercise will illuminate the purpose of the ABC analysis.

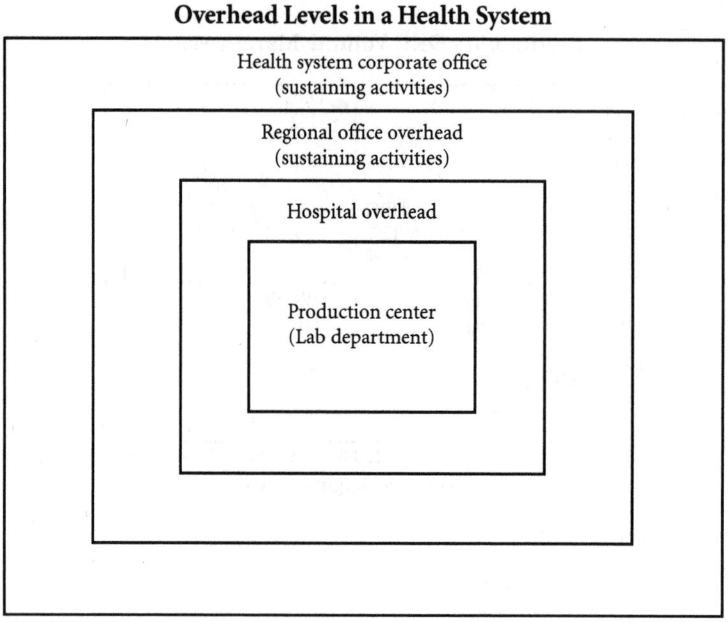

Overhead Levels in a Health System

Health system corporate office
(sustaining activities)

Regional office overhead
(sustaining activities)

Hospital overhead

Production center
(Lab department)

Figure 9-3 **Overhead Levels in a Health System**

IMPLEMENTATION BY STAGES

The actual implementation of an ABC system can be segmented into stages. A discussion of the stages is contained in this section.

Setting Up Project Management

PROJECT TEAM The internal project manager needs three things: (1) the authority to operate; (2) office space dedicated to the project; (3) and his or her time allotted to the project. The designated team should be selected to represent information technology team members along with primary users of the system and the resulting information. The training manager should also be a member of the project team.

The internal project manager sets (and enforces) milestones from the vendor, identifies acceptable performance, and controls performance and delivery time lines with penalties. Hopefully, these milestones and penalties have been made a part of the initial contractual arrangements.

REPORTING AND DOCUMENTATION The project manager supervises inputs and records driver descriptions. The manager tracks required documentation delivered as part of the project and reviews it for adequacy. (Note that supporting work papers should also be delivered and retained.) The project manager also issues status reports to management within the organization and, overall, communicates and coordinates information about the system.

Implementing Pilot Projects

Attentive organized management is the key to pilot project implementation. Certain elements such as timing and testing are necessary no matter what area is selected for the pilot.

TIME LINE   The manager is responsible for the time line, and it requires constant vigilance to stay on schedule. Staffing is a constant problem, because the temptation is to pull staff off the pilot project to cover other management emergencies.

TEST RESULTS   The pilot project's inputs, outputs, and reports should be tested. A periodic status report (a monthly report, for example) is the best way to stay on schedule with testing pilot results.

ADJUST METHODS   It will be necessary to adjust methods in the pilot. Adjustments are necessary because that is the purpose of the pilot—to discover flaws and correct them in a smaller operation that is easier to control and evaluate.

Training

Managers and staff involved with the ABC system all require training, and the program must be consistent and thorough. Different levels of training are required for staff and for managers, depending upon their level of involvement. An overview is sufficient for certain individuals, while comprehensive training will be required for others.

Implementing the System

After the pilot program has been completed, some organizations believe in immediately implementing the system across the company. Other organizations choose to implement it in a planned sequence instead of all at once. An example of a planned sequence might be department by department.

The system-wide implementation should be timed to occur shortly after the pilot project has been completed and evaluated. The timing of the implementation must be considered in relation to the organization's annual cycle. For example, it is not good practice to interfere with the closeout stages just before the end of the year. Training should continue on a regular schedule.

Performing System Evaluations

The system should be evaluated at least quarterly for the first year after implementation, semiannually for the second year, and at least annually thereafter. The ABC system should still be evaluated, even if evaluations of other systems within the organization are not a standard procedure. The evaluation process is important for two reasons: First, it makes management accountable for the project, and second, it allows successes of the system to be recognized.

Maintaining Project Structure

The manager who is responsible for the ABC system must work to maintain both staffing levels and supervisory structure for the project. It is not acceptable for accountability to remain, while staffing disappears because new supervisors do not understand the value of the project nor the benefits it provides to the organization. The manager must take positive steps to never let this situation occur.

ENCOURAGE COMMUNICATION The wise manager will encourage communication about implementation of the system. He or she will accept and consider suggestions and will encourage communication across organizational barriers.

PLANS FOR ONGOING SYSTEM IMPROVEMENT Maintaining the structure also means planning for ongoing system improvement. This means the current and future budgets need to contain a designated amount for improvements to the system.

IMPLEMENTATION WITH MULTIPLE COST SYSTEMS

The general propensity to have multiple cost systems has been discussed by Kaplan.[1] He believes that diverse uses of cost information may well require more than one cost system. He, therefore, proposes three cost system usage categories. The first system merely values inventory and meets the requirements of outside reporting. It is the most simplistic from a costing standpoint. The second system allows the control of cost at a responsibility center level, thus providing swift feedback to operational personnel. The third and highest level system is a product cost system; it can support strategic management decisions.

Two years later, Kaplan expanded on his position concerning multiple cost systems.[2] He now states that present technology is not yet capable of what he termed *cost-system design*, which could instead be called *cost-system evolution*. His cost-system evolution and its effect on the three uses of cost information (as just discussed) are summarized as:

Stage 1. Poor data quality—is inadequate to meet any of the three needs.

Stage 2. Focus on external reporting—tailored to meet financial reporting needs, provides inaccurate product costs for (strategic support) and limited feedback for (operational control).

Stage 3. Innovation: managerial relevance—provides operational control information with emphasis on direct measures for operating performance.

Stage 4. Integrated cost systems—provides expanded activity-based cost system to support financial reporting as well as product cost for (strategic support) and provides feedback and input interface on budgeting and current operations to support operational control system.

IMPLEMENTATION WITH ABC UPGRADES

We agree with Kaplan's proposition that multiple cost systems are necessary due to diverse uses of cost information and that present technology is not yet capable of meeting all cost needs in one system—especially for health care purposes. In many cases, another system running parallel to the existing system will answer health care cost accounting needs.

Management might consider a cost system running parallel to the existing system, which will increase its ABC precision as additional information is added to it. One can term the increasingly sophisticated parallel system as an *ABC upgrade implementation*, as it has a rolling implementation capability.

One can expand upon Kaplan's four stages by perceiving each stage as a range of capability, moving from low through moderate to high capability within the assigned stage. Thus, in Kaplan's four-stage cost-system design, his Stage 3 defined as "innovation: managerial relevance", includes developing activity based cost systems to provide (product costs for strategic support) and developing operational performance measurement system to support (operational control). Instead, one can propose an initial parallel cost system that begins at the low end of Stage 3 and moves "upward" through the moderate range and on into the higher ranges of Stage 3 as its components are upgraded; thus an ABC upgrade implementation.

The benefits of this approach answer the challenge of creating and implementing an ABC-oriented system that can meet the cost-benefit test, can initially be put into place in a reasonable time frame, and whose ABC capability can be sequentially improved upon in a rolling implementation subsequent to initial installation, all without disturbing the existing system, which functions primarily for financial reporting purposes.

An ABC Incremental Implementation Approach

To illustrate a low-range ABC incremental implementation approach we turn to an emergency department (ED) example. This example is adapted from an article authored by Holmes and Schroeder[3] that illustrated ABC *estimation* of unit costs for ED services. As an ABC *estimation*, the example does not meet Kaplan's Stage 3 definition, but is within his lower Stage 2. This example provides the potential for an ABC system to be developed beyond the estimation stage as illustrated. (Using the proposal, if it developed out of the estimation stage, it could develop to a low-range Stage 3.) This potential shall be noted as we work through the example.

Full Costs Are Not Relevant

Holmes and Schroeder argue that full costs for individual services provided (called *fully loaded costs* by some managers) have little bearing on profitability or management in health care today.[4] The prevalence of substantial contractual allowances negates the use of full costs for charge setting—and many of the indirect costs present in full cost amounts have been arbitrarily allocated to the individual services. Instead, for many decisions a case is made for the relevance of incremental costs; the cost of an additional unit of service or the avoidable cost if one unit less is provided. Holmes and Schroeder propose that better management decisions will result by accepting what they term *feasible imperfect information* (e.g., containing some estimates) on incremental activity-based costs rather than using traditional full-cost data.[5]

Their proposition is supported by Christiansen and Sharp, who look at the problem from the standpoint of responsibility accounting.[6] These two advocate reporting on the basis of a manager's controllable costs (e.g., subject to the manager's decision) rather than incorporating the manager's noncontrollable costs (e.g., outside existing decision-making powers). Their argument additionally supports the philosophy of the incremental activity-based costs presented in this example.

Incremental ABC Estimates

The incremental activity-based cost estimates are discovered in a series of eight steps, as follows.

> Step 1. Identification of all relevant costs.
>
> Step 2. Clustering into groups for counting and costing such as ambulatory patient groups (APG) or physicians' current procedural terminology (CPT) groups. These services create similar demands for ED functions.
>
> Step 3. Identifying and counting the activities or cost drivers for each service group. Such activities or drivers are the characteristics of the service that trigger the performance of an ED function.

Step 4. Applying the activity measures or cost drivers that allow determination of internal (production center) direct expense and internal (production center) indirect expense.

Step 5. Accounting for external costs allows determination of external (nondepartmental) indirect expense.

Step 6. Sorting of costs in support of ED functions, discarding those that are not relevant or not affected by volume or availability of services.

Step 7. Estimating the costliness of each ED function, permitting quantification of the relationship between costs and the triggering characteristics.

Step 8. Aggregating the "functional costliness" (individual activity costs) for all ED functions of a service to determine the incremental cost of one unit.

Upon completing the eight steps, a rough unit incremental cost has been calculated. Tables illustrating the calculations just described and accompanying comments follow.

Example

STEP 1. IDENTIFICATION OF ALL RELEVANT COSTS   In this example, costs are categorized into three types: direct, production center, and external. Direct costs can be captured directly (in ABC terminology, they are traced). To summarize, the incremental ABC-estimates approach starts with the basic cost center treatment that is traditional to Medicare cost reporting. That is, departmental costs have been charged directly to the center while external costs have been allocated to the department from other departments or cost centers. Direct costs that can be identified and traced are isolated, labeled as direct, and subtracted from the production center costs. Management now has three types of cost: (1) *direct or traced production center cost;* (2) the remaining cost that originated in the production center, designated as *indirect or allocated production center cost* and (3) the *external allocated costs* that occur outside the production center and originate within other cost centers.

Table 9-1 illustrates costs that have been charged directly to the emergency department. Their total is labeled "gross departmental costs" on Table 9-1. As explained, the direct costs that can be identified and traced are isolated and as such labeled "direct" on Table 9-1. The remaining costs are designated as indirect production center costs; they are labeled "indirect" on Table 9-1.

Table 9-1 **Departmental Costs Recorded in the Emergency Department (ED) Production Center**

Cost Center Line Item	Gross Center Costs	Less Direct Cost	Equals Indirect Cost
Labor-clinician	$ 93,532	$46,778	$46,754
Labor-nursing	89,359		89,359
Labor-technician	15,944		15,944
Labor-admin/clerk	5,422		5,422
Medical supplies	280,610	226,747	53,863
Subtotal	$484,867	$273,525	$211,342
Medical equipment	34,632		34,632
Total	$519,499	$273,525	$245,974

The total production center direct cost is carried forward from Table 9-1 and now set out in Table 9-2. They are then divided into costs for specific services in the remaining columns of the report.

STEP 2: CLUSTERING AND COUNTING OF SERVICES A classification system must be chosen to sort the ED services. *Common procedural terminology* (CPT) codes would be a routine choice. APCs (ambulatory payment classifications) might also be a choice. In this example, DRGs have been chosen and two particular DRGs (236 and 486) utilized. DRG 236 represents fractures of the hip and pelvis, while DRG 486 represents other operating room procedures for multiple significant trauma. Because an actual report would show all the relevant DRGs—not just two—a final column on Table 9-2 is labeled "other DRGs follow." The same concept carries through to the other tables in this example.

STEP 3: IDENTIFYING ACTIVITY MEASURES OR COST DRIVERS The cost-driver statistics are set out in Table 9-3. As other examples in this book have demonstrated, cost drivers may be measured, may reflect protocols or clinical pathways, or may reflect published norms. Choices are affected by the degree of accuracy desired.

STEP 4: APPLYING THE ACTIVITY MEASURES OR COST DRIVERS The cost drivers in Table 9-3 are now used to allocate indirect center costs to cost objects. In this case the cost objects are the DRGs. Table 9-4 illustrates the end result whereby specific cost drivers have been used for each cost type.

Table 9-2 ED Direct Costs (Traced Costs) by Service

Center Line Item	Total Direct Cost	DRG 236 Fractures Hip & Pelvis	DRG 486 Other OR Procedures for Multiple Significant Trauma	Other DRGs Follow
Labor-clinician	$ 46,778	$ 5,844	$10,808	xx
Labor-nursing	—	—	—	—
Labor-technician	—	—	—	—
Labor-admin/clerk	—	—	—	—
Medical supplies	226,747	9,069	20,270	xx
Subtotal	$273,525	$14,913	$ 31,078	xx
Medical equipment	—	—	—	—
Total	$273,525	$14,913	$ 31,078	xx

Note: — indicates that there are no entries.
xx indicates that part of total departmental direct cost has been assigned to other DRGs.

Table 9-3 Cost Drivers and Allocation Bases Used to Assign Costs to Services

Center Line Item	Cost Driver	Total Allocation Basis	DRG 236	DRG 486
Pathway minutes-clinician	Pathway-CL	122.8	2.7	2.5
Pathway minutes-nurse	Pathway-NS	52,194	897	715
Pathway minutes-technician	Pathway-TCH	5,191	68	72
Protocol minutes- administrative/clerk	Protocol-AD	1,722	31	30
Operating room minutes	ORmins	16,595	483	430
Nursing acuity hours	NAcuity	3,285	76	46
DRG weights (from CMS database information)	DRG Weights	144.4	2.8	2.4
Radiology films	Radfilms	553	7	7
Pharmaceuticals by standard weighted amount	Wtd procs	30	10	9
Standard electrocardiographs	EKGs	126	3	1
Laboratory tests by standard relative value	RVUs	1,486	51	39
Standard respiratory therapies	RTs	36	1	0
Anticipated units of blood	BUs	212.5	6	5.2
Standard immunizations (tetanus)	Shots	11	0	0

Table 9-4 **ED Indirect Costs (Allocated Costs) by Service**

Center Line Item	Indirect Cost	% Variable	Cost Driver	DRG 236	DRG 486
Labor-clinician	$46,754	90%	Pathway-CL	$3,693	$7,975
Labor-nursing	89,359	95%	Pathway-NS	5,981	10,542
Labor-technician	15,944	100%	Pathway-TCH	665	1,927
Labor-admin/clerk	5,422	60%	Protocol-AD	237	454
Medical supplies	53,863	90%	DRG Weights	4,060	6,839
Subtotal	$211,342			$14,636	$27,737
Medical equipment	34,632		Depr Sch	259	453
Total	$245,974			$14,895	$28,190

STEP 5: ACCOUNTING FOR EXTERNAL COSTS Table 9-5 illustrates how the external costs are charged to the center. As previously explained, all these costs are external because they have been allocated to the production center from other cost centers. The staged implementation of ABC discussed in this chapter is particularly illustrated in this table. Activity based costing has been applied to the ED, while the external support costs are being charged using the traditional cost accounting system. As more and more centers are brought under ABC, the allocations would then be from two sources. The first source would be from the traditional accounting system, as shown here, for the nonintegrated centers (those that have not yet had ABC applied to them). The second source would be from those centers that have a newly implemented ABC system; in these cases, the centers will have already been integrated into the overall ABC system.

STEP 6: SORTING OF COSTS This is an incremental cost analysis, thus, inappropriate costs must be sorted out and disregarded before final steps are taken to assemble costs. This step involves a review of the information that has been assembled. Are all the line items appropriate for this center? Are the proper cost drivers used? Are the allocation proportions of the cost drivers to the cost objects (DRGs in this example) appropriate? Some facilities use a checklist for this step.

STEP 7: ESTIMATING THE COSTLINESS OF THE FACTORS This step is a spreadsheet calculation procedure. For example, if a factor increases by one unit, how much does the cost change? Spreadsheet formulas were used to arrive at the DRG cost columns in Tables 9-3, 9-4, and 9-5.

Table 9-5 External Costs Charged to ED by the Traditional Cost-Accounting System

Center Line Item	External Cost	% Variable	Cost Driver	DRG 236	DRG 486
Nursing	$7,316	70%	Nacuity	$954	$1,160
Operating room	9,665	45%	ORmins	1,012	1,805
Recovery room	4,149	55%	ORmins	531	947
Anesthesiology	5,342	70%	ORmins	870	1,553
Diagnostic radiology	5,672	30%	Radfilms	184	369
Electrocardiography	714	80%	EKGs	109	109
Pharmaceuticals	3,816	70%	Wtd procs	468	801
Central supplies	3,537	90%	DRG-wts	502	846
Clinical pathology	2,472	60%	RVUs	407	622
Anatomical pathology	650	10%	DRG-wts	11	18
Blood bank	981	90%	Bus	199	349
Pulmonary	805	40%	RTs	108	0
Immunizations	11,175	80%	Shots	0	0
Depreciation	65,366		Depr sch	5,100	7,450
Subtotal	$121,660			$10,455	$16,029
Corporate office	18,650		Pro-rata	815	1,330
Total	$140,310			$11,270	$17,359

STEP 8. AGGREGATING THE FUNCTIONAL COSTLINESS OF A UNIT OF SERVICE This final step collects all costs for a particular service. The report shown in Table 9-6 first presents the aggregate costs for each of the two DRGs, in total and broken into the three types of cost (direct, indirect, and external). The report then presents the incremental cost units for each of the two DRGs, again in total and broken into the three types of cost (direct, indirect, and external). Incremental unit costs represent the total aggregated costs for a service divided by the number of units or "quantity provided during period." This final report is the product of all previous steps.

Example Summary

This example provides the potential for an ABC system to be developed beyond the estimation stage as illustrated. Ongoing sequential upgrades would then allow even more accurate unit costs to be found through the same method. The ABC upgrade implementation method puts a cost-accounting system in place without disturbing the existing system, while creating and implementing an ABC-oriented system that can meet the cost-benefit test. The system can initially be put into place in a reasonable time frame, and its ABC capability can be sequentially upgraded in a rolling implementation subsequent to initial installation.

Table 9-6   **ED Departmental Aggregated and Incremental Unit Costs**

Service (by DRG)	DRG 236 Fractures Hip & Pelvis	DRG 486 Other OR Procedures for Multiple Significant Trauma
Quantity provided during period	10	18
Aggregated Costs by Service:		
Direct Departmental Costs	$14,913	$31,078
Indirect Departmental Costs	14,895	28,190
External Nondepartmental Costs	11,270	17,359
Total Aggregated Costs	$41,078	$76,627
Incremental Unit Costs by Service:		
Direct Departmental Costs	$1,491	$1,727
Indirect Departmental Costs	1,490	1,566
External Nondepartmental Costs	1,127	964
Total Unit Costs	$4,108	$4,257

CONCLUSION

Health care integration has a long way to go to achieve the fundamental changes necessary to demonstrate better care at lower costs. Activity based costing can support a delivery system's operations strategy by taking the guesswork out of service line costs throughout a continuum of care. This makes it an attractive initiative to support management goals.

KEY POINTS

- An ABC project requires managerial support.
- Managers are more likely to support an ABC project if they have had input into the project planning process.
- Management criteria must be taken into account when planning an ABC system design.
- Cost components will vary in different vendors' system proposals.

- Decision making in choosing a system is a series of trade-offs.
- Stages of implementation affect both capital expenditure and internal staffing hours.
- It is important to formally document both internal and external responsibilities for the system.
- To determine system detail, the actual method by which resources will be traced

and allocation in the new system must be perfectly clear.

- Actual implementation of an ABC system can be segmented into stages.
- Multiple-cost systems can be maintained, with one of the systems being ABC.

- An ABC system can be initially implemented and then upgraded in a sequential series of steps.

REFERENCES

[1] Kaplan, Robert S. "One Cost System Isn't Enough," *Harvard Business Review* (January–February 1988): 61–66.

[2] —. "The Four-Stage Model of Cost Systems Design," *Management Accounting* (February 1990): 22–26.

[3] Holmes, R. and R. Schroeder. "ABC Estimation of Unit Costs for Emergency Department Services," *Journal of Ambulatory Care Management* 19, no. 2 (1996): 22–31.

[4] *See* Finkler, S. A. and D. M. Ward. *Essentials of Cost Accounting for Health Care Organizations* (Gaithersburg, MD: Aspen Publishers, 1999); and Holmes and Schroeder, "ABC Estimation," p. 22.

[5] Holmes and Schroeder, "ABC Estimation," p. 23.

[6] Christensen, L. F. and D. Sharp. "How ABC Can Add Value to Decision Making," *Cost Management* (May 1993): 39.

Management Accounting Applications

Over the past half century, managers have evolved general decision models, cost-based management concepts, and application tools that have gained wide acceptance. Chapter 10 discusses the traditional method of measuring production costs for inventory valuations used in financial reporting while Chapter 11 discusses procedures for forecasting future values of variable of interest in analyses. Chapter 12 explains different types of budgets and the use of cost information in their preparation. Chapter 13 explains the use of cost-variance analysis in the control function; the appendix to the chapter discusses revenue variances. Chapter 14 discusses the use of cost-volume-profit analysis and an array of problems utilizing the concept of marginal cost. These chapters provide the reader the ability to use cost measures to support many decisions that are common to management problems in health care organizations.

CHAPTER 10

TRADITIONAL COSTING TO SUPPORT FINANCIAL ACCOUNTING

LEARNING OBJECTIVES

After studying this chapter, students should be able to:

1. Explain the uses of cost information in financial accounting and the differences from its use in management accounting.

2. Explain the procedures traditionally used to find the cost of health care organizations' outputs to include:

   a. Performing step-down service department cost allocations

   b. Using cost-to-charge ratio and RVU procedures to assign production department costs to individual products

3. Explain the relationship of the analysis of the cost of a patient's care to traditional "job-shop" costing in manufacturing organizations.

4. Explain the deficiencies in using traditional financial accounting costing procedures to support internal management decisions.

INTRODUCTION

Generally accepted accounting principles (GAAP) used to support preparation of financial statements demand that the full cost of manufacturing a product be attached to the product when its manufacturing is completed. This cost serves as its accounting value while it is inventoried prior to sale. When the product is sold, this full manufacturing cost is considered the cost of the good sold—an expense of the period in which the item is sold. Finding the cost of the item sold is, therefore, necessary in order to get an inventory value for the balance sheet prior to its sale. It is also needed to get the income statement expense associated with losing the item in the period of its sale. Basic accounting procedures for manufacturing organizations are also applied to service organization. A significant difference is that completed services are rarely inventoried; they are sold as they are performed.

The external users of financial accounting statements are primarily interested in the current financial position and the overall financial performance of organizations. One of the most used measures of future performance is the level of past performance. External information users are not in a position to choose the markets the firm will enter, the products it will produce, the technology it will use, the resources it will purchase, or the vendors it will use. They simply want to measure the aggregate benefit these decisions have produced as measured by the profitability and financial position of the firm. In the case of not-for-profit organizations, rather than profit, outsiders may look at services provided to its intended beneficiaries as well surpluses available to sustain the organization. The limited purposes of financial statements mean that cost information for financial reporting purposes can be less detailed than that used to support management decisions. Cost data used in financial accounting can be adequately served by simpler, less expensive cost analyses than those covered in the previous chapters. Analysis for financial accounting can be satisfied by highly averaged cost information.

Costing procedures for financial accounting became the traditional method of doing cost accounting. In the mid-1980s, many corporate executives became convinced that standard, traditional cost accounting did not give them product costs that were accurate enough to support pricing decisions and choices among alternative operating approaches. Investigating this problem led to the conclusion that the traditional methodology used for financial accounting was indeed inadequate for the support of many internal decisions.[1] The greatest fault lay in its failure to realize that many overhead costs should not be lumped together and allocated among products using a single basis for allocation. Revised costing methodologies to support internal management were devised; they focused on the cost of accomplishing activities needed to produce intermediate and externally sold services and products. The result was the development of activity-based cost accounting, as described in the preceding chapters. However, the traditional approach is still heavily used in health care organizations. Though it is adequate for measuring cost data for use in financial accounting, it is inadequate for management support. Unfortunately, it remains the approach specified by the Centers for Medicare and Medicaid Services (CMS) for Medicare reporting. This chapter will explain the traditional approach and some of the reasons why it is considered inadequate for management accounting.

Measures of Financial Performance

At the most general level, it is important to know the total cost of operating the organization. We have already examined this from two perspectives. First, we applied the concept of an expense to measure the value of resources consumed in order to gain the revenues of a period. The resources are valued at what was paid for them—their historical cost. Current financial accounting uses the amounts paid for the resources as its value for accounting purposes because they are objectively determined through transactions, verifiable, and free from bias. Evaluating the cost of the resources used to gain the revenues of a period is thought to give a more rational long-term measure of performance than simply using the amount of cash spent during the period. This is because, year in and year out, performance is held to be the difference between the value of resources consumed by the organization and the value of the products it provides.

Cash spent in a period may not represent the consumption of a resource in that period. Some of this cash may measure the acquisition of resources that will be used in a later period. Conversely, during a period, management might use a resource for which the company will pay during a later period, even though revenue from the sale of the product is received in the current period. These ideas are the foundation of the measurement of profit in an *accrual* financial accounting system. (The accrual basis of financial accounting is described in Appendix A at the back of this book.)

Financial accounting also considers the importance of understanding the actual *costs* of a period; that is, the amounts of cash exchanged for resources during the period. If these cash outflows are not matched by cash inflows, the organization may be threatened by bankruptcy. This is why *cash flow statements* are now a required part of periodic financial statements, in addition to the balance sheet and income statement. (Required financial statements are further discussed in Appendix A at the back of this book.)

DISCUSSION QUESTIONS

1. What are the primary purposes of cost accounting in support of financial statements?
2. How do these make the requirements of cost accounting different from those of management accounting?

TRADITIONAL DEPARTMENT-FOCUSED OVERHEAD COSTING

The health care industry has traditionally focused cost analysis on departments, rather than activities, when computing the cost of items it sells. These items were the products and services that are listed on the claim form, or bill, for a patient's episode of care and have been referred to as *billable line items*. Standard accounting procedure records the cost of each resource purchased by the organization in general ledger accounts that are specific to the departments that consume the resource. The total output of those departments is then valued at the sum of the cost of all resources they use. If a department's output is used by another department, the cost of that output is considered a cost of the receiving department. If the output is sold to an outside customer, its cost is an organization expense associated with the sales transaction. Tracing cost flows through the organization in this way creates two different categories of organization components: service departments and profit centers. This has prompted a two-step process for costing items that the organization sells. Figure 10-1 is a flow chart of this process.

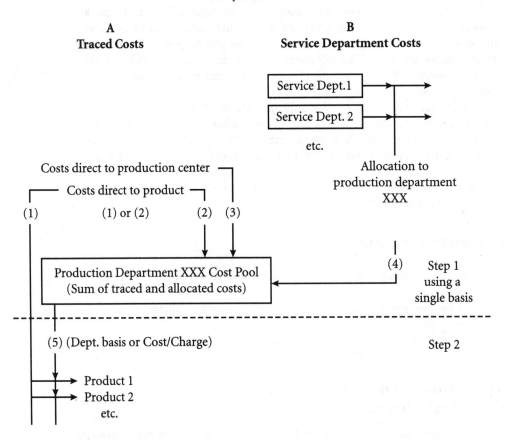

Traditional Production Center Cost Flows
The Department Focus

1. Traces direct product costs to the products.

   or

2. Puts direct product costs into the production center's cost pool (this takes less measurement).

3. Traces costs that are direct to the production center (but not direct to specific products).

4. Allocates service center costs to the production center's cost pool. These actions are Step 1 of the two-step output costing process

5. Allocates total production department costs to its different products. This is Step #2 of the two-step output costing processs.

Figure 10-1 **Traditional Production Center Cost Flows**

Step 1: Service Department Cost Allocation

First, there are departments whose output is not sold but is used by other departments within the organization. For instance in hospitals, biomedical engineering work is not a line item on patients' bills. The output of the biomedical engineering department is used by the laboratory, radiology, and other users of high-tech equipment to create products that do appear on patients' bills. The departments that have no billable output are referred to as *service departments* or *overhead departments*. (For governmental cost-finding purposes, they are referred to as *general service departments*.) These departments perform what are called organization and production sustaining activities in ABC analysis.

For each such service department, a single *basis* is found for allocating its total cost among the departments that use its output. The idea is to charge departments that use a service department's outputs the portion of the service department's costs that goes into the user's production. Laundry services present a rather straightforward example. The cost of running the laundry is usually distributed to other centers in proportion to their percentage of total pounds of laundry processed. If the surgical center uses 8 percent of the pounds of laundry processed, 8 percent of the cost of the laundry department is put into the surgical center's overhead cost pool. In this case, a measure of the output (pounds of laundry) is used as the *basis* of cost allocation. For some service centers, the basis is less obvious. The output of the housekeeping department is clean facilities, but probably no direct measure of quantities of cleanliness exists. In this situation, a satisfactory level of cleanliness resulting from housekeeping work is assumed and the cost the housekeeping department incurs might be distributed to the departments it serves in proportion to their floor area. In this case, square footage of floor space is a surrogate for the housekeeping department's output and is used as the allocation basis. Note that the bases used in traditional costing serve the same function as drivers in ABC. The difference is that one basis is used for all of a service department costs as opposed to the ABC method isolating separable activities within service departments and finding the driver for each one.

In the case of the biomedical engineering department, engineering hours assigned to work for other departments is a common basis. Here, the surrogate for the output of the service center is actually an input (engineering hours) to the services produced. For each service department, a variable that correlates highly with the department's total cost from period to period is found. These bases are arrived at through a logical examination of the department's outputs, the processes it uses, and its resource utilization. If several bases seem to be intuitively valid, a regression of total cost on the basis can be run for each one. The R^2 statistic will imply which potential basis is best associated with the variable portion of the service department's costs. Note that the basis of allocation of a service department's cost is determined in the same way that resource drivers are found for separable overhead activities in the ABC approach.

Departments whose output is sold to buyers outside the organization have been referred to as revenue centers, because the prices paid for the outputs are revenue to the organization. Because all departments have costs and these departments have revenue as well, they have also been called *profit centers* or *product centers*. The total cost of each service department is allocated among the profit centers according to each profit center's use of each service department's basis for cost allocation. After this is done, the costs of operating all service departments have been buried in the overhead pools of the profit centers. Several methods for doing this allocation are explained here.

ANOTHER INFLUENCE ON SERVICE DEPARTMENT GROUPINGS Financial accounting's generally accepted accounting principles have been discussed as a prevailing influence on the use of traditional departmental design in health care. However, another primary influence on traditional costing in health care must also be recognized: regulatory cost-finding and allocation principles. A contractual agreement (the participation agreement) is required when a hospital wishes to become a provider (and thus participate) in the Medicare program. One of the provisions in the participation agreement is that the provider agrees to file a cost report annually at the year's end. The Medicare cost report notes the annual costs of the hospital. It also allocates overhead to revenue-producing departments through an elementary allocation process. The cost-finding line items are generally departments and labeled as cost centers. These cost centers are grouped into five categories. The categories are illustrated in Exhibit 10-1. The general services cost centers are overhead only and do not produce revenue. The other four categories all produce revenue. Inpatient routine services cost centers include, among others, general routine care and intensive care units. Ancillary service cost centers include, among others, the operating room, recovery room, radiology, and laboratory. Outpatient service cost centers include clinics and the emergency department. There is also an other reimbursable service cost centers that includes such items as research, but is not involved in our present discussion.

Because Medicare cost finding has existed since 1966, the groupings and terminology have become embedded in health care traditional financial accounting. One must remember, however, when working with management accounting and segmentation by activities, that an activity-based "cost center" is not the same as a Medicare cost-finding "cost center." The step-down method of overhead allocation described in the following section uses the Medicare cost-finding technique.

Exhibit 10-1 **Cost Center Groupings for Medicare Cost Finding**

---

1. General service cost centers

2. Inpatient routine service cost centers

3. Ancillary service cost centers

4. Outpatient service cost centers

5. Other reimbursable service cost centers

STEP-DOWN ALLOCATION   The most simple method used in the traditional approach is called the *step-down method* of cost allocation. It is the method established by CMS, (formerly the Health Care Finance Administration or HCFA), for determining the cost of care for Medicare patients. It is probably best explained through a grossly oversimplified example. Assume an organization has two service departments, housekeeping and administrative services. Further assume it has two profit centers, the clinic and the laboratory.

Housekeeping costs are allocated using floor area as the basis:

> Admin. Services has 1,500 sq ft.
> Clinic has 10,500 sq ft.
> Laboratory has 3,000 sq ft.

Administrative costs are allocated using full-time equivalent (FTE) personnel as the basis:

> Admin. Services has 15 FTEs.
> Clinic has 30 FTEs.
> Laboratory has 5 FTEs.

The cost of housekeeping during the period was $13,000.
The cost of administrative services was $10,000.

First establish the order in which to treat the service centers. The rule of thumb is to first allocate those service centers that serve the broadest array of other departments. Under this consideration, housekeeping costs would be allocated before those of biomedical engineering. In this example, allocate housekeeping costs and then administrative costs. To format the problem, show both the service centers and the profit centers across a line, along with the costs traced directly to the service centers:

Cost Center	Housekeeping	Administration	Clinic	Laboratory
Direct Costs	$13,000	$10,000	———	———

The basis for allocating housekeeping is the square footage of its *using* centers: administration, the clinic, and the laboratory. These total 15,000 square feet. Of this total, administration has 1,500, the clinic has 10,500, and the laboratory has 3,000 of the total. They will, therefore, be assigned these fractions of the $13,000 total housekeeping cost. Expand the matrix to show this allocation:

Center	Housekeeping	Administration	Clinic	Laboratory
Direct Costs	$13,000	$10,000	———	———
Housekeeping allocation	└————→	$ 1,300*	$ 9,100	$2,600

*Note that 1,500/15,000 of $13,000 is $1,300.

The housekeeping costs are allocated to the three departments to its right in the matrix and will not be reconsidered. Next allocate the administrative costs to the centers to its right. However, we have just increased administrative costs to the sum of its direct costs plus those allocated from housekeeping, $11,300. (Remember that FTE personnel is the basis for allocating administrative costs.) In those centers to the right, the total FTEs are 30 for the clinic plus 5 for the laboratory or 35FTEs. Of the $11,300 amount, the clinic receives 30/35 (or $9,686) and the laboratory receives 5/35 (or $1,614). Expand the matrix again to show the new total cost of administration and its allocation to the clinic and laboratory according to the FTE fractions:

	Service Centers		Profit Centers		Total
Center	Housekeeping	Administration	Clinic	Laboratory	
Direct Costs	$13,000	$10,000	———————————————→		$23,000
Housekeeping allocation		$ 1,300	$ 9,100	$2,600	
Total administrative costs		$11,300			
Allocation of administrative costs			⌐———→ $ 9,686	$1,614	
Total costs allocated to profit centers			$18,786	$4,214 ——→	$23,000

If the allocation is done correctly, the total of costs allocated to production centers will equal the total costs of the service centers. Note that the allocation process stops when the costs of the last service center (the service center farthest to the right) has been allocated. It is meaningless to allocate any profit center's costs to other profit centers. To find the total cost for a profit center, add its costs allocated from service centers to the costs that were traced directly to it. This creates the profit center cost pool that must be further allocated to that center's outputs. Again, Figure 10-1 depicts this department costing flow.

RECIPROCAL ALLOCATION   An intuitively more accurate way of allocating service department costs to the profit centers is to recognize that each service department provides services to all other centers, not just those to its right in the flow matrix. The reciprocal approach allocates the first service department's costs to all other centers as is done in the step-down approach. However, in allocating the second service department's costs, allocations are again made to *all* other centers. In the example, this would mean that some administration costs would be allocated back to housekeeping as well as to the profit centers. After the first complete round of allocations from all of the service departments to other centers, some of each service department's costs will have been allocated to profit centers. That means that at the end of an iteration of allocations, the costs remaining in each service departments will be less than the beginning amounts. The allocation process can be taken through many iterations until the costs remaining in the service departments are so small as to make no material difference if they are simply distributed among the profit centers in arbitrary portions. For a large organization with many departments, this approach demands many calculations and lends itself best to computer software designed for the purpose.

Subjective View of Relative Cost Assignments

In this section, we look once again at the averaging problem and address proportional allocation.

THE AVERAGING PROBLEM REVISITED The costs of each service department are allocated using the relative amounts of a *single* basis appropriate for that service department. In doing this, financial accounting assigns overhead in a simpler, less expensive and more highly averaged way than does ABC. However, the costs involved in different subsets of services performed within a service department may not be the same. In addition, various production centers may not use these different activities in the same proportions; that is, in proportion to the single basis. Significant averaging of costs occurs in allocating service center costs to production centers by assuming there is only one activity using only one basis. This can create material misstatement of the relative amount of service department cost caused by different production centers. Biomedical engineering can furnish an example. Suppose the biomedical engineering department does equipment set-ups and maintenance of extremely sophisticated equipment and suppose its costs are allocated based on engineering hours used. One set of engineers, using rather inexpensive tools and equipment, does set-ups while higher salaried engineers using expensive test equipment handle maintenance. The allocation basis does not recognize these differences. The result would be that biomedical services to departments using larger-than-average amounts of sensitive, high-cost equipment that frequently needs maintenance would be undercosted. Departments whose primary use of biomedical engineering is for equipment setups would be overcosted. This is a weakness in traditional product costing that can be corrected by using ABC.

MANAGERIAL COST COMPONENT ALLOCATION PROPORTIONS To avoid using a single allocation basis for a service department, each department manager can estimate the proportion of each of a comprehensive set of general ledger account categories that are used by the department's internal customers. For instance, a manager may believe that by examining the general ledger, she can classify all costs charged to her department as either fixed salary, variable salary, fixed nonsalary, variable nonsalary, or capital costs (realize that capital costs are fixed costs). She also believes that she can estimate the percentage of each of these categories that is incurred to support each of the departments that use her department's services.

The service department costs can be allocated to profit centers by using these proportions in the general step-down or reciprocal approaches just described. Many analysts believe competent managers trained in subjective estimation techniques can establish more accurate allocation proportions than are derived by using a single basis. Increased accuracy is available because this approach recognizes that different categories of service departments' costs may be used in different amounts by various internal customers.

DISCUSSION QUESTIONS

1. Explain the basic steps in the traditional two-step approach to costing products. Why is it said to be department focused?
2. What is the difference between step-down overhead cost allocation and reciprocal allocation? Which is more accurate? Why?
3. Why do analysts contend that traditional service department cost allocation overaverages production center costs? Why is this undesirable?
4. What are the conditions under which subjective allocation scales can improve overhead allocation over the results of step-down or reciprocal techniques?

Step 2: Profit-Center Overhead Cost Allocation

The second step in costing specific products is to allocate each profit center's overhead costs pool to each of the outputs it produces. Hospitals have generally put product-direct costs in their profit centers' overhead pools rather than tracing them to specific products. This greatly simplifies the computation of product costs because it eliminates the need to trace any costs past the product center. When this is done, allocated service department overhead, direct-to-profit center, and direct-to-product costs are placed in a single profit-center cost pool. This pool is then allocated to specific products. As computer capabilities allow more detailed accounts, direct costs can be traced to more disaggregated sets of products. This allows Flow 2 in Figure 10-1 to replace Flow 1 and increases the accuracy of the product cost estimation. Whether the product-center cost pool contains all the costs flowing through the center or only the center's overhead costs, each center's pool must be allocated to its individual units of its products.

COST-TO-CHARGE RATIOS   The most common procedure for assigning profit-center costs to their outputs has been the use of each profit center's cost-to-charge ratio. At the end of a period, the total costs in the center's cost pool are divided by the total revenues received from the center's sales. This resulting figure is the *cost-to-charge ratio* (CCR, or sometimes as the ratio of cost to charges, RCC). To compute a cost allocation to any specific output from a profit center, the price charged for the output is multiplied by the CCR. A weakness of this approach to the second step of cost allocation is that the relative cost of different products is set by their relative prices, not the relative cost of the resources they use. It assumes that prices have been set by a consistent markup on the cost of producing each unit of output. This is not a valid assumption. In order to use a markup, one would have to already know the cost of the product. If this were the case, there would be no reason to use the CCR to compute the cost. The use of CCRs contributes to the overaveraging of costs and distorts the *relative* cost of outputs. Therefore, it cannot consistently tell decision makers which is the least expensive of alternative ways to reach the same objective. To make proper choices among alternative processes and protocols, understanding their relative costs is essential.

RELATIVE VALUE UNITS Profit-center costs can also be allocated among their products using relative value units (RVUs) as described in Chapter 5. However, the inaccuracies that evolve from using the relative amounts of direct costs to various products as the proportion of the profit center's fixed costs that the products consume may be significant. This is because fixed costs may be incurred in order to lower direct costs, if doing so will lower total costs at the expected quantities of output. For example, equipment may be used (resulting in a fixed lease cost) in order to reduce the material waste and technologist time used in a process. If this is the case, the process's output would have reduced direct costs while increasing its fixed costs compared to other products. An RVU allocation based on the proportion of direct costs used by different products would reduce the amount of fixed costs allocated to the product in question when it should be increased.

EXPERT JUDGMENT Subjective estimation techniques applied by experienced workers in a profit center can simplify estimating the amount of various overhead costs that should be allocated to specific products. For instance, a supervisor may be able to say with some accuracy what percentage of the use of various fixed-cost resources are used in the production of different outputs. A highly experienced manager may be confident in stating that one product needs twice the overhead support of another, a third product needs 80 percent of the support of the first, and so on. In so doing, the manager is subjectively establishing an RVU scale for allocating overhead costs to the center's products. Analysts can use this scale to allocate overhead costs among products or users. The dollar of cost per RVU is simply the total amount of a category cost divided by the total number of its related RVUs consumed in the period. The cost of a specific output is the number of RVUs assigned to it times the cost per RVU. This information, when combined with knowledge of the unit direct costs can produce fairly accurate unit cost for various outputs. These estimates, however, can be no more accurate than the accuracy of subjective RVUs on which they are based. The possibility of inaccuracies in these subjective judgments about relative usage of overhead resources is a weakness in the RVU approach.

DISCUSSION QUESTIONS

1. How are CCRs used to allocate profit-center costs among its products? What is the weakness in this procedure?
2. Why is it possible that allocations based on RVUs can reduce the problems caused by using RCCs? What are the weaknesses in using various RVU approaches to allocate overhead?
3. What are the advantages and disadvantages of using an ABC system rather than a two-step approach involving step-down allocations of overhead and RCCs?

A Summary of Traditional Costing Applied to Health Care

- The costs of each service department are measured by being traced through the general ledger to the department in question.
- Each service department's cost are allocated among the overhead pools of departments using its services by using a single, most appropriate allocation basis, or an RVU scale constructed by people experienced in the use of overhead resources within the center.
- Costs *traceable* to each profit center are also added to the individual profit center's cost pool. Costs direct to the department but indirect to its products are added to the profit center's cost pool. The sum of these costs and the service department allocations make up the profit center's overhead cost pool. In health care, costs traceable to a specific product are frequently added to the profit center's overhead cost pool and allocated to products as if they were part of the overhead pool. These direct cost could be charged directly to that center's products.
- Each profit center's cost pool is then allocated to its individual units of output using a single basis, a CCR, or an RVU system.

This two-step method, depicted in Figure 10-1, distributes all the production costs of an organization across its products. If the price charged for each product is greater than the cost assigned to it in this way, the organization will have a positive contribution from production. However, the usefulness of this truth is limited by the fact that, as competition increases among health care providers, prices are controlled largely by market competition, not the providers. Therefore, within a given organization, prices are rarely proportional to costs. This brings the commonly used RCC approach into serious question. The excessive averaging that results from both steps in this product-costing procedure has been found to cause serious misstatements of both the relative and absolute costs of products. This deficiency is extremely damaging when the delivery organization is attempting to select among equally effective intermediate products and protocols in order to maximize its efficiency. In today's highly competitive health care environment, efficiency is extremely important to the survival of the organization. The increased detail of applying RVUs subjectively estimated by experts in the overhead processes is believed to reduce these errors. There is a great deal of literature showing that ABC has the ability to greatly reduce the problem of inaccurate relative costs.[2] The disadvantage of ABC is that its data collection and processing require expenditures for software, hardware, and staffing. Because RVU scales based on subjective relative usage estimates are less expensive, the RVU approach is helpful when the additional accuracy of ABC may not be needed. This can be the case when the costs involved are low, good cost drivers cannot be found, or the level of usage of overhead among different products does not vary much.

EXAMPLE THE CLINICAL LABORATORY EXAMPLE

The example in Chapter 7 used ABC to compute the cost of four different laboratory tests. The traditional approach would have used less detailed data but the quantities for the data used would be the same. Service department overhead costs were:

Institutional overhead allocated to the laboratory

Maintenance	$ 46,284
Supply processing and distribution	8,510

Laboratory Direct Overhead Pool

Clerical services		147,000
Test set-up		
set-up labor	90,750	
set-up supplies	48,000	
set-up tools	16,000	
		154,750
Tools & equipment (for running tests)		30,856
Total laboratory overhead		$387,400

Other recorded information for the baseline period was:

Overhead allocation basis:	Direct labor hours (DLH)
Total DLH used in baseline period:	4,700 hours

The most commonly used traditional approach to costing the tests would use a single allocation basis to allocate the total laboratory overhead pool among its tests. A commonly used basis is direct labor hours (DLH). The cost of each type of test computed using the traditional approach is shown in Table 10-1. The allocations of service department costs (institutional overhead) are assumed to be the same as those in the ABC approach. This would indicate that no separable activities were found within the service departments. The direct costs per test were computed by dividing the amount of the cost traced to the type of test by the number of that type test produced as was done in the ABC approach. Then the allocation of laboratory overhead cost was added to the cost of each test by using the standard DLH for each test as a single allocation basis.

The differences between ABC and the traditional approach is in the categories of cost tracked to the various tests and the bases/drivers used to quantify their amounts. These are summarized in Exhibit 10-2. Note that the only differences between the traditional and ABC approaches have to do with overhead. The differences in the computed costs of the four tests when various costing approaches are used is summarized in Table 10-2. When using the traditional approach, test "Q" appeared to be overcosted by 17 percent and test "S" to be undercosted by over 7 percent. If patients in different categories use varying amounts of the tests, the cost per patient will be misstated. If these tests are sold competitively on the open market, test "Q" sales volume may well be suffering from price competition because its overcosting may well cause it to be overpriced. Test "S" is not as profitable as it appears, because its cost is about 7 percent greater than the traditional cost estimate.

Table 10-1 **Cost of Laboratory Test Using the Traditional Costing Approach**

Computed overhead allocation rate:			$387,400/14,700 DLH = $26.354 per DLH	
	Test specific direct cost*	+	overhead allocation	= total cost/test
Test	Materials & Supplies	+ Direct Labor	DLH (Overhead Rate)	
P	$ 5.00/test	$1.50/test	0.05 DLH($26.354/DLH)	$7.818
Q	3.20	3.00	0.10 DLH($26.354/DLH)	8.835
R	12.50	1.20	0.04 DLH($26.354/DLH)	14.754
S	2.00	3.00	0.10 DLH($26.354/DLH)	7.635

Exhibit 10-2 **Cost Assignment Driver/Basis for Each Line Item**

(A) Activity-Based Costing Method	Driver
Direct Costs	
Materials and supplies	
Labor	
Department Overhead	
Clerical support	Equally per test
Set-up	Test specific setups per test
Tools and equipment	Machine hours
Allocated Overhead	
Maintenance	Machine hours
Supply processing and distribution	Dollar amount
(B) Traditional Costing	Basis
Direct Costs	
Materials and supplies	
Labor	
Department Overhead	Direct labor hours

Table 10-2 **Comparative Results of Costing Approaches**

Test	Traditional Cost per Test	ABC Cost per Test	Difference	
P	$ 7.818	$ 7.550	− $0.268	− 3.43%
Q	8.835	7.330	− $1.505	− 17.03%
S	14.754	15.883	$1.129	7.65%
T	7.635	7.838	$0.203	2.66%

TYPES OF COSTING SYSTEMS

As mentioned earlier, the way management thinks about cost analysis in service-producing organizations has evolved from concepts of costing used in manufacturing industries. The traditional, department-focused approach has been applied to two different types of production: process costing and job costing. There is also a third type in health care called *operational costing*.

Process Costing

One type of production is the continuous production of one kind of product, such as the refining of petroleum, producing boxes of dish soap, or other products that lend themselves to assembly line manufacturing. This production uses what is known as *process costing*. In process costing, the costs of a steady flow of allocated and traced resources are measured for a production period. The quantity of the product output during the period is counted. The total resource cost is divided by the total quantities of output to arrive at a cost per unit of output.

Job Costing

The second common type of production is the "job shop." A *job shop* is a product center that responds to separate orders for quantities of a specific item. Items are not produced continuously, as on an assembly line but instead, batches of items are produced. The quantity could range from one to thousands. Each item produced in a job is identical. The cost of the job is the total of direct labor and direct materials that flow into the job plus the variable overhead assigned to the job and an allocated share of the producing organization's fixed overhead. The cost of a single unit of the item produced in a job is the cost of the job divided by the number of units the job produced.

Operational Costing

Health care organizations produce some services that resemble process costing (the assembly line) and other services that resemble job costing (by the batch). Therefore, a hybrid form of costing has arisen that is often termed *operational costing*. Operational costing contains elements of both process costing and job costing. The interaction is illustrated in Exhibit 10-3. The operational costing came about because of the large variety of health care services and products that are created and sold; this variety naturally involves multiple methods of production. This said, however, in the next segment we are going to take a closer look at job costing and the job shop.

Exhibit 10-3   **Three Types of Health Care Costing Systems**

Process Costing
$\updownarrow$
Operational Costing
$\updownarrow$
Job Costing

Job Shops and the Patient

This discussion continues the view of production as job costing.

JOB SHOPS   Job shops can produce intermediate products or products for sale. For instance, a clinical laboratory produces tests on order. At a particular time, a need for 50 of a particular type of blood test might exist. This would constitute a job with 50 units of production. The direct materials and labor involved in this job can be counted and the costs tallied. Determining the amount of sustaining overhead that should be allocated to each production center can be done in the traditional way. The center's overhead pool can then be allocated to its different jobs using the traditional processes. Hospitals have used single, rational, yet arbitrary bases for allocating the cost of service departments to production departments. Many hospital and clinic production department operate as job shops.

THE PATIENT AS A JOB   Thus far, we have discussed the job-shop approach to finding the cost of jobs such as a laboratory batch of identical tests. A "job," however, could consist of only one unit of production. In this sense, each patient cared for could be considered a job and the care delivery organization a job shop. Each patient's list of services shows the inputs to the job. Summing the cost of these services would give the cost of the job; that is, the cost of the patient's care. Care deliverers are increasingly paid under some sort of prospective payment system. These systems often pay a set fee for the discharge or other measure of categorized episodes of care. For instance, Medicare pays a set fee for the discharge of a patient based on the diagnosis-related group in which the patient is classified. In order to negotiate appropriate fee schedules, managers must understand how much delivering care to patients in each of these categories will cost. A corollary is that measures of these costs used by managers must avoid the errors in costing specific outputs that occur in traditional cost accounting to support the preparation of financial statements.

DISCUSSION QUESTIONS

1. How does process costing differ from job-shop costing? What are the factors that make one or the other appropriate?
2. What might cause some health care cost analysts to contend that health care deliverers manage job shops?
3. Why is it important for health care managers to know the relative cost of different jobs?
4. What differences in approach make ABC superior to traditional costing when attempting to cost a health care job?

Differences Between Financial and ABC Cost Accounting

Three differences exist between the traditional approach and the ABC approach. First, traditionally, the total cost consumed by a service department is allocated to departments that use its services; no attempt is made to look for separable activities within the service departments. Second, traditionally, a single basis is used to make each service department's allocation; no attempt is made to find specific drivers for different separable activities within the service departments. Third, traditionally, the allocations are made to the overhead pools of other departments; no effort is made to allocate overhead to the activities needed to create specific outputs of product centers. For instance, in the Chapter 6 example of costing diagnostic radiology tests, personnel service overhead was allocated according to the amount of its allocation basis to each of the activities needed to complete a test no matter in what department or production center the activity occurred. It was not simply allocated to the imaging center's overhead pool, which as we saw in Table 10-1 can lead to significant costing errors. These additions to the detail with which causal relationships between costs and the activities that demand costs are considered allow more accurate estimates of the differences in costs among different outputs.

DISCUSSION QUESTIONS

What are the differences between traditional costing and ABC with reference to:
1. The allocation of service department costs to profit centers of production centers?
2. The identification and use of allocation bases and cost drivers?
3. The handling of allocations of profit or product-center overhead cost to the center's products?

Key Points

- Financial accounting is concerned with the total expenses of an accounting period and the total portion of these expenses remaining in inventory.
- Health care organizations do not generally have significant inventories of products.
- Traditional cost accounting was designed primarily to support financial accounting, but it has greatly influenced management accounting practice.

- Traditional cost accounting focuses on tracing costs to departments, allocating service department costs to profit centers, and allocating profit-center cost to their products by using a single allocation basis in each case.
- The traditional approach uses a two-step process that collects profit-center costs in the first step and allocates them to the center's products in the second step.

- The first step is usually done using step-down or reciprocal allocations for organization overhead. Manager-estimated relative usage scales are now sometimes used.
- Costing can be done using process or job-shop based analysis. In health care, there is also a hybrid type called operational costing.
- Because revenue is earned largely through prospective payment systems that pay flat amounts for treating specific categories of cases, understanding the costs of caring for these different categories is critical to negotiating prices.
- Eliminating the overaveraging of costs among outputs is, therefore, critical to health organizations' financial performance and viability.

Exercises

PROBLEM 1

Step-down Cost Allocation

Service Centers:

Plant Maintenance and Engineering (PME). Allocation basis in square feet.
Administration (A). Allocation basis/full-time equivalent employees (FTEs).
Production Centers: Radiology (R), Laboratory (L), and Clinic (CL)

Assumptions Center	A	PME	R	L	CL
Direct cost	$600,000	$900,000	$800,000	$300,000	$2,500,000
FTEs	12	20	25	35	70
Square footage	3,500	6,000	3,000	2,000	15,000

Required: Perform a step-down allocation of service-center costs to the production centers.

PROBLEM 2

Step-down Cost Allocation

Service Centers:

Administration (A). Allocation basis/full-time equivalent employees (FTEs).
Plant Maintenance and Engineering (PME). Allocation basis in square feet.
Laundry (L). Allocation basis in pounds of laundry.
Production Centers: Diagnostic Radiology (DR), Physical Therapy (PT).

Assumptions

Center	A	PME	L	DR	PT
Direct cost	$400,000	$900,000	$200,000	$2,000,000	$1,700,000
FTEs	20	15	10	30	55
Square footage	2,500	3,000	1,000	3,000	6,000
Pounds of laundry	50	200	100	800	1,200

Required: Perform a step-down allocation of service-center costs to the production centers.

REFERENCES

[1] Cooper, Robin and R. S. Kaplan. "How Cost Accounting Systematically Distorts Product Costs" in *Accounting & Management: Field Study Perspectives*, W. J. Bruns and R. S. Kaplan, eds. (Cambridge, MA: Harvard Business School Press, 1987), p. 142.

[2] Kaplan, R. S. and R. Cooper. *Cost & Effect; Using Integrated Cost Systems to Drive Profitability and Performance.* (Boston, MA: Harvard Business School Press, 1998). *Note*: Extensive additional background is contained in the works referenced within the chapter notes of this book.

CHAPTER 11

COST PREDICTION

After studying this chapter, students should be able to:

1. Explain how ABC modeling is used in predicting costs.

2. Explain how trend analyses are used to improve cost prediction.

3. Explain the three basic requirements necessary in identifying causal variables.

4. Explain time-series regression analysis and seasonal correction.

5. Explain the use of exponential smoothing and moving average prediction models.

6. Explain the dangers in using trend analyses.

7. Explain the concept and use of learning curves.

8. Explain the general problems confronted in attempting to predict costs.

9. Explain how to evaluate the power of various prediction models.

INTRODUCTION

The fact that managers analyze the past in order to make decisions about the future was mentioned earlier. Data are historical as soon as they are measured. To make decisions about future activities, managers need information about future conditions. To forecast future financial viability, managers need to be able to predict future sales and their resultant revenue. Techniques to do this fall in the realm of marketing. In health care, demographic and epidemiological data are used to forecast potential demand. Then, estimates are made of the share of the demand that the organization can command. Revenue predictions are based on these sales forecasts and the expected prices for the services sold. Predicting revenue, therefore, requires understanding demand, market prices, price elasticities, and regulatory constraints on pricing freedom.

Financial viability also depends on costs being less than revenues. Therefore, forecasting the financial health of the organization requires forecasting the cost of providing the services the organization intends to bring to the market. Zero-based budgeting starts with the sales projections for the budgeted period and estimates all resource needs and their cost without using past cost experience. Experimentation with zero-based budgeting has shown that managers tend not to consider all the resources needed when they estimate future utilization without using recent experience as a starting point. They also tend to underestimate the prices that must be paid for the needed resources.

Budgeting experience indicates that starting with recent costs and projecting changes in the future is, in most cases, the most efficient way to estimate adequately accurate future costs. However, there are two dangers in taking this approach. First, inefficiencies occurring in the baseline analysis periods tend to be built into forecasts. Second, if the production technology or markets change significantly, old trends will cease and both costs and revenue will undergo sudden shifts. This is why periodic review of markets and technology is necessary. As markets and technology change more rapidly, this review must be done more frequently. In taking a change-analysis approach to forecasting costs, one assumes that adequately accurate cost measurements have been made recently. However, regardless of how accurately this has been done, decisions about continuing operations require that these costs be projected to the amounts they will be in the technological and market environment of the future.

FORECASTING COST

Two basic approaches to forecasting costs exist. The first involves finding the drivers of costs and the relationship between the amount of the driver and the cost in question. When this relationship is understood, the cost of a target can be computed if the amount of the driver that will occur in a future period can be known. This is essentially how ABC analysis is used in forecasting. The driver of a targeted activity is found and the cost of the activity per unit of the driver is determined. To do this, a combination of qualitative activity analyses and cost-behavior analysis is used, as explained in Chapter 4. The chart in Figure 7-2 gives an example. In that example, the clerical activity in the laboratory was found to be driven by the number of tests performed. Using past data, the clerical cost of a baseline period was divided by the number of tests performed. The cost per test was $0.60. If the number of tests is forecast for a future period, the cost of clerical activities can be forecast by multiplying the clerical cost per test by the volume of tests forecast. The second approach is to simply project historic trends in the lists of resources that will be used in the future.

Selecting Drivers

Finding the driver of a specific separable activity has been discussed in previous chapters. It requires understanding the processes within the activity and the causes of demand for the activity. This usually requires working with those who designed the production and those who perform the production activities. Appropriate questions are:

- What activity of users makes the company engage in the activity performed?
- What services demanded by the user makes the activity necessary?

The first question results in identifying the *activity driver*, such as requests for personnel actions driving a set of personnel department activities. The second identifies *resource drivers*, such as square footage of working space driving housekeeping costs. The cost relationship between possible resource drivers and the cost object is provided through cost-behavior analysis, as discussed in Appendix 3.

Because activity drivers are directly related to the activity being costed, the fit or accuracy of activity drivers is usually quite good. An exception will occur if the driver is used to allocate an activity's cost among users who demand different intensities of the activity. This would be the case if personnel actions requested by different activity centers within the organization demanded different amounts of inputs. As an example, if some personnel actions demand more data collection, interviews, approval authorizations, and documentation than others, the total cost of administering these actions will depend on the mix of the different types of actions as well as the their total volume. As discussed in Chapter 8, when this is the case, more accuracy can be gained by measuring the resources used for each type of action and developing an RVU system for the activity.

EXAMPLE

If management believes that overhead costs of personnel actions activities are proportional to their direct costs, direct cost RVUs can be used to allocate the total cost of personnel activities. Suppose direct resources used for a promotion action cost $300, for a hiring cost $2,000, for a firing cost $5,000 and for a voluntary separation cost $200. Assume that these were all the types of actions taken. The average direct cost of these actions would be ($300 + $2,000 + $5,000 + $200)/4 = $1,875. Administering a promotion would have a weight of 0.160 RVUs (300/1875). Similarly, a hiring would have a weight of 0.160 RVUs, a firing of 2.667 RVUs, and a voluntary separation of 0.107 RVUs. Assume also that, for a baseline period, the total cost of all activities related to personnel actions was $2,300,000, and the total number of RVUs for the actions taken was 1,060. The total personnel action cost per RVU would be $2,195 ($2,300,000 / 1,060). The personnel action cost allocation to a department having 4 promotions, 2 hirings, 1 firing, and 3 voluntary separations would be computed as:

Action	Quantity	RVU	Total
Promotion	4	0.160	0.640
Hiring	2	1.067	5.691
Firing	1	2.667	2.667
Voluntary Separation	3	0.107	0.320
Total department RVUs			9.318

Total personnel action allocation to the department:

$$(9.318 \text{ RVUs}) \times (\$2{,}195 \text{ per RVU}) = \$20{,}121.$$

A cost-behavior analysis of personnel action costs using these RVUs as the independent variable should have a much better fit (higher R^2) than one simply using the quantity of actions.

Whether the extra effort and cost of constructing an RVU system is warranted depends on:

- How much the costs of different actions vary
- The degree to which different users demand different amounts of the various actions
- The amount of cost created by the specific allocation in question relative to the total cost of the users

Using activity drivers to forecast the cost of a category of activity takes advantage of the increased understanding of resource usage gained by activity analysis. This understanding must include three relationships:

1. First, any changes expected from the current resources used by the activity in question.
2. Second, the future price of the each resource flowing into the activity being costed.
3. Third, the quantity of the driver that will occur in the forecast period.

DISCUSSION QUESTIONS

1. What are the factors on which revenue prediction is based?
2. Who is responsible for projections concerning these factors?
3. How are RVUs related to selecting a cost driver for a specific category of activity? Create an example.

Example | **229**

The Starting Points

Knowing the current prices of direct resources is not a large problem, because they are available in the records of recent purchase transaction or from vendors and trade associations. Knowing the cost of intermediate activities involves understanding the amounts and prices of resources used and the overhead needed. The overhead allocations are the result of top-down ABC analysis of sustaining, production center, and batch-level activities. The amount of activity-direct resources used requires analysis of flows into the activity. For instance, returning to the laboratory example in Chapter 7, understanding the cost of performing laboratory Test P (summarized in Table 7-2) requires measuring:

- the amount of supplies used, a direct resource cost
- the prices of supplies used
- the dollar amount of supplies used—as the driver of the cost of the supplying process
- the amount of technician labor used—as the driver of technician cost
- machine hours used—as the driver of both tool and equipment and maintenance costs
- the cost of the set-up
- average number of tests per set-up—to determine set-ups per test

The second and third requirements are highly variable. Prices change over time. Efficiency, even in stable technologies, also changes. The demand for activities will change as the quantity of their drivers varies. Therefore, the costs of input activities will probably change, and the changes, if significant, should be forecast. An advantage of activity analysis and ABC flow charting is that the relationships between the quantity and purchase prices of resources and the cost of specified cost objects are articulated. As price or efficiency changes occur, the changes can be made in the price and usage data input to the flow model, and the flow analysis will follow them through to the cost object of interest, as described in Appendix 5. The flow analysis will also work in reverse, because drivers are linkages between cost objects and their inputs. If the quantity of the cost object that must be produced is forecast, the quantity and total cost of any input can be projected. Forecasting the amount of clerical costs (as shown in Figure 7-2) is an example of the backward use of the charted flow relationships. If 1,000 Tests P are to be produced, this output will require $600 [(1,000 tests $\times$ $0.60/test)] of clerical support.

Therefore, activity analysis and ABC provide models for forecasting costs of products and hence total costs of operations. When cost flows are modeled as shown in Figure 7-3, forecasts for the total cost of producing Tests P can be made simply by forecasting the quantity to be produced. Total cost for any activity or set of activities can be computed by knowing the totals of the drivers of the activities. Using the information in Table 7-2, if the sales for a period are expected to be

180,000 Test Ps, 70,000 Test Qs, 100,000 Test Rs, and 5,500 Test Ss, the cost for the laboratory would be:

$$\$7.55(180,000) + \$7.33(70,000) + \$15.8825(100,000) + \$13.6880(5,500) = \$3,535,634$$

To repeat, the ease of forecast revision depends on accurate estimates of changes in the input variables. Changes in purchase prices and increases in efficiency in existing activities often follow trends, as do the volume of individual drivers. Techniques for forecasting trends are therefore useful supplements to ABC modeling. Similarly, cost drivers derived from ABC analyses give variables with which to project costs when technology and efficiency do not change but the level of activity does. However, in this case, future quantities of the drivers must be estimated. The example of personnel department costs caused by nursing services furnishes an illustration. If management understands that the cost of administering personnel actions is driven by the number of personnel actions requested, they must estimate how many of these actions nursing services will request in order to estimate the personnel administration component of the cost of nursing. The company must estimate the total number of personnel actions requested throughout the organization in order to forecast the resource use and cost of performing personnel actions in any future period. Trend analysis can be useful in making these quantity estimates.

Forecasting Trends

Some desirable trend information is available from trade associations and government agencies. For market analyses, demographic data can be had through the federal census bureau and state agencies. Epidemiological data is published by both state, federal, and in some cases, county agencies. Prices provided by trade associations and the federal Bureau of Labor Statistics are current sources. For productivity data, vendors are a ready, though biased, source. It is important that people within an organization's personnel and purchasing departments keep close contact with researchers in such organizations as the American Hospital Association, the Medical Group Management Association, and the Healthcare Information and Management Systems Society. Purchasers of supplies, equipment, and personnel should also take advantage of the information about potential change that is available at trade shows, through vendors, and by networking with colleagues. This is especially true in keeping abreast of important near-future changes in technology.

For information about trends in health care that is not available from public sources, several types of trend analysis can be useful.

DISCUSSION QUESTIONS

1. What are the starting points for ABC analysis of a specific activity?
2. What is the relationship of trend analysis to measurements that relate to these starting points?
3. What are sources of information on trends and related measurements?

TREND ANALYSIS

This section discusses regression, exponential smoothing, and moving averages.

Regression

The basic concepts of regression analysis and using statistical software are discussed in Appendix B. These concepts were applied in Appendix 3 when used in cost-behavior analysis. It was also used to verify the appropriateness of cost drivers assumed to be operating on activities.

REGRESSION SUPPORTING COST-DRIVER ANALYSIS   A brief review of how cost drivers are identified will help understand the difference between regression analysis done to help identify cost drivers and time-series regression done to describe trends. Finding the drivers of cost begins with analyzing an activity that incurs costs and asking what it is that necessitates the activity be done. Again, returning to the personnel department example, we asked why the department administered personnel actions. The answer was rather simple. It did so because there were administrative tasks associated with various personnel changes and the organization had the personnel department specialize in performing these tasks for all of its departments. The amount of resources used in the activity logically depends on the number of actions it is asked to administer. The cost of the activity, therefore, was driven by requests to administer personnel actions.

We repeat the logic behind proposing that the number of actions requested is the driver of the cost of *personnel actions*. First, a cause (the driver) must occur before the activity it is believed to cause. Second, there must be logic underlying the belief that a specific driver causes the specific activity to done. Management may notice that almost every time interest rates change, the number of personnel actions requested also changes. However, there is little logic in believing that personnel action requests are driven by interest rate changes. Third, if the driver causes the activity and the activity incurs costs, then the quantity of the driver and the amount of the cost must be positively correlated. This can be tested by regressing the cost of the activity on the potential driver. If this regression produces a high R^2 statistic, one can say that the regression model fits the data well.

The regression analysis quantifies the fixed cost of the activity and the amount at which the total costs increase each time the activity is performed. However, a good fit of the data to the regression line does not, by itself, establish that the driver chosen is the cause of the activity. In the example, the action request precedes the personnel action, it is logically related to the actions, and the fit of its relationship is good. These three facts constitute a strong argument that personnel actions are driven by requests for them. Finding the driver for many activities is not as straightforward as this example. For instance, the cost of maintenance in each of the various equipment-using activities is not as directly tied to the maintenance hours used in the activities.

TIME-SERIES REGRESSION   In time-series regression, rather than have a potential driver on the x-axis of the regression, the independent variable is time. Cost is plotted against time. The plot will show a trail of points reflecting the chronological variation of cost over time. The slope of this simple regression will indicate the periodic change of cost with time—or the trend. Time-series regression can be done on any price or usage to forecast its value at a future point in time.

Figure 11-1 shows a time-series regression plot that estimates a straight-line increase of cost over time. The y-intercept on a simple regression on this data will indicate the cost implied at the beginning of the period of analysis (as opposed to the fixed cost) and the slope will indicate the average change from one time period to the next (as opposed to the variable cost). The R^2 value will indicate how well the cost complies to a straight-line relationship. The methods of performing the regression analysis are the same as in cost-behavior analysis. The regression predicted number for a future quarter is computed in the same way cost was predicted given the amount of a driver when using cost behavior regression. From the situation in Figure 11-1, the cost forecast for the 15th quarter would be:

$$\$82,273 + \$13,881(15) = \$290,488$$

Studying a particular time-series plot may reveal a systematic variation around the straight-line solution. The variation may reflect seasonal changes. The regression will predict the value on the regression line. A seasonal correction can be added to that value. One way to do this is to average the past variations for a given month and apply it to the regression forecast for the month in question. Suppose that over the 3 years of data, the costs in December averaged 12 percent above the amount predicted by the regression line and the variation had the same general pattern each year. To forecast the cost for a given December, management would increase the regression forecast by 12 percent. If March costs average 9 percent below the regression line, the company would reduce the regression model's forecast for March by 9 percent.

It is important to remember that using regression analysis of historic data to predict quantities that will occur in future periods involves two important

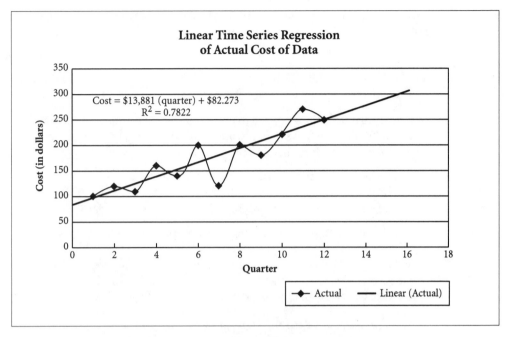

Figure 11-1 **Linear Time Series Regression of Actual Cost of Data**

assumptions. The first is that the future will change in much the same way changes have occurred in the past. The second is that the rate of change will approximate the average rate of change over the historic periods from which the data used in the regression analysis was collected. Many aspects of health care delivery are changing almost instantaneously, such as substituting lithotripsy for several surgical procedures. This makes the first assumption highly suspect in many situations. Relatedly, in many aspects of health care, recent rates of change may be more indicative of the future than are long-term trends. For these reasons, two other short-term prediction techniques are frequently used.

Exponential Smoothing

Exponential smoothing assumes that recent changes in the cost are more indicative of near-future forecasts than are long-term trends. However, it also assumes that there is some random variation in the amounts of short-term changes. It therefore assumes that the next period will be much like the past period; however, current trends and random phenomenon will change the cost. For instance, if the estimate for the last period was low, one could assume that the cost is rising above the last expectation but will probably not be as much higher than it was in the last period. Therefore, the prediction for the next period is set at the prediction for the last period plus a fraction of the last period's error.

EXAMPLE

Exponential smoothing applied to the data in Table 11-1 shows the forecasts for the fifth quarter based on the forecast for the fourth quarter and a proportion of the error in that forecast.

The forecast for the fourth quarter was $105,000.
The actual cost experienced in the fourth quarter was $160,000.
The error in that forecast was $160,000 − $105,000 = $55,000.

Exponential smoothing assumes that a portion of this error will exist in the next period. The size of the portion, "p," is determined from historic data and subjective beliefs about the near future. If past changes indicated that the successive errors average 20 percent of the prior error, the proportion could be set at 0.20. In this case, the forecast for the fifth quarter would be:

Forecast for Period "t−1" + [(Actual Cost for Period "t−1" − Forecast for Period "t−1") × Smoothing proportion] = Forecast for Period "t"
$105,000 + [($160,000 − $105,000) × (0.20)] = $116,000
Error in Period "t−1"

The exponential smoothing process can begin by setting the forecast cost for the first period at the cost experienced in the period immediately prior to it. Successive adjustments are made period by period from this starting point, as was done in Table 9-1. If there is believed to be an underlying trend in changes as well as imposed random variation, the smoothing proportion can be raised. Table 11-1 shows predictions based on p = 0.2 and p = 0.8. Realize that this prediction method makes forecasts only for the next period based on the forecast and the measured error of its immediate past period. It is not capable of projecting past the next period.

Managers may believe that there will be random phenomena that period by period create divergence from a generally accurate multiperiod predictions. If this is the case, the correction term, [(actual cost for Period t−1) − (predicted cost for Period t−1)](p), can be applied to the prediction made from the general forecasting model for Period$_{(t−1)}$ to predict the value for the next period. This approach includes trend information incorporated in the general long-term prediction model used, but also acknowledges short-term changes in the general trend. These changes would otherwise appear to be part of the random error. This is one of several variations from the standard exponential smoothing process that are available.

Example | **235**

Table 11-1 **Quarterly Time-Series Cost Data (without seasonality)**

Quarter	($) Cost	3-Quarter Moving Average Forecast	Squared Error	Exponential Smoothing p = 0.2 Forecast	Squared Error	Exponential Smoothing p = 0.8 Forecast	Squared Error
1	$100						
2	120			100	400	100	400
3	110			104	36	116	81
4	160	110	2,500	105	3,025	111	2,130
5	140	130	100	116	576	150	100
6	200	137	3,969	121	6,241	142	3,364
7	120	167	2,209	145	625	188	4,624
8	200	153	2,209	140	3,600	134	4,356
9	180	173	49	152	784	187	49
10	220	153	4,489	158	3,840	181	1,521
11	270	200	4,900	170	10,000	212	3,364
12	250	223	729	190	3,600	258	64
Sum of squared errors			21,130		32,757		20,053
Mean squared error			2,348		2,979		1,671

Moving Averages

The *simple moving average* uses the average cost over a set of recent periods as the forecast for the next period. The average can be taken over any number of contiguous, immediately past periods. This procedure makes a forecast of the next period at the beginning of the period. A set of moving average forecasts is also shown in Table 11-1. In this case a three-quarter moving average was used. For instance, to forecast the cost in the fifth quarter, an average of the costs in quarters 2, 3, and 4 was computed:

$$($120 + $110 + $160)/3 = $130$$

This is then the cost forecast for the fifth quarter. Similarly, the forecast for the sixth quarter was:

$$($110 + $160 + $140)/3 = $137$$

If analysts believe that recent trends are more indicative of the near future than those farther in the past, the more recent periods can be weighted more heavily. For instance, if analysts felt that each period had twice the forecasting power of the one before it, the three periods could be given weight of 1, 2, and 4. The total of these weights used in the denominator of the formula would be seven. This *weight moving average* computation for the fifth quarter would be:

$$[1(\$120) + 2(\$110) + 4(\$160)]/7 = \$140$$

Comparing this result with the simple moving average of $130 shows the effect of weighting the third month in the averaged set more heavily than the preceding two smaller values.

DISCUSSION QUESTIONS

1. Explain the differences between regression analysis done to understand cost behavior and regression analysis done to understand trends over time.
2. What are two assumptions made when using regression analysis to predict future conditions?
3. How can cyclical variations be handled when using a linear regression prediction model?
4. What are the differences in predictions using a regression model and those using exponential smoothing?
5. What is the purpose of the smoothing factor, "p," in the exponential smoothing process?
6. In what ways is the moving average prediction model similar to the exponential smoothing model? How is it different?
7. When should a moving average prediction model be replaced by a weighted moving average model?

Learning Curves

Costs of using newer technologies can be expected to decrease as the organization gains experience with their use. Similarly, costs can be expected to decrease as people gain experience in their work. A mathematical model of this decrease in cost with experience is called the *learning curve*. In analyzing cost improvements per unit of output during the rapidly expanded production of war material during World War II, industrial engineers discovered a surprisingly stable relationship. As production was doubled, the time to produce the last unit was a constant proportion of the time to produce the last unit prior to the doubling. The amount of the factor might be different for different outputs. However, for a specific output, it appeared constant over time.

Example 1

As an example, the cost of the 10,000th unit was $5,000; the cost of the 20,000th unit was found to be $4,000. This is 80 percent of the amount taken to produce the unit at half the volume. The discovery was that the time needed to produce the last unit at the next doubling of output (the 40,000th units) was $3,200, another 20 percent reduction. Because the unit produced at each successive doubling of output took 80 percent of the cost to produce the unit prior to the doubling, the production was said to be following an 80 percent learning curve.

Such relationships were found to exist generally across outputs, though the cost reduction factor might change from product to product. When man-machine processes are involved, the effect of production time on cost is limited by the maximum output rates of the machines. Learning curve analysis is, therefore, most helpful where machinery is not being used at capacity and forecasting cost changes in the early phases of output moving toward capacity is important.

Example 2a

As an example, suppose a company produced 10,000 diagnostic radiological tests. The costs are largely dependent on throughput time. The cost of the 10,000th unit was $20.00. If production follows an 85 percent learning curve, these costs for the 20,000th unit would be $17.00 (0.85 × $20.00). For the 40,000th unit, they would be $14.45 (0.85 × $17.00). For the 80,000th test, it would be $12.28 (0.85 × $14.45). The cost of products at various points in the total production volume is shown in Table 11-2 and plotted in Figure 11-2 for the 90 percent, 85 percent, and 80 percent curves.

Table 11-2 **Learning Curves When the 10,000th Unit Costs $20**

	Cost in dollars		
Unit Number	**90% Curve**	**85% Curve**	**80% Curve**
10,000	20.00	20.00	20.00
20,000	18.00	17.00	16.00
40,000	16.20	14.45	12.80
80,000	14.58	12.28	10.24
160,000	13.12	10.44	8.19
320,000	11.81	8.87	6.55

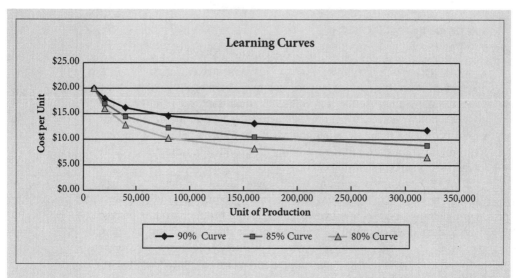

Figure 11-2 **Learning Curves**

Obviously, it will take longer and longer to achieve the doubled output, because it is reached over greater and greater amounts of additional production. However, in relatively early periods of the use of a technology, this learning can make significant differences in proper budgeting.

Example 2b

Using this example, assume that demand forecasts indicate that the output for the fifth quarter after reaching the total output of 10,000 tests will take the company from the 100,000 point up to the 135,000th test. Reading from the plot in Figure 11-2 and assuming an 85 percent learning curve, the cost per unit of the 100,000th unit would be about $11.95 and the 135,000th unit would be about $11.00. The average cost in this range would be about $11.475 per test ($11.95 + $11.00/2). Therefore, management would forecast this period's production to cost $401,625 (135,000 − 100,000 × $11.475). This is considerable less than the $700,000 (135,000 − 100,000 × $20.00) management would have forecast had they used the experience at 10,000 units of production and not considered the learning that would occur after that point. Looking at the leveling off of the curve, if output per quarter continues to increase, management would not expect much decrease in the cost per unit after about the eighth quarter, when total production will be near 300,000 units.

Learning curves do not include prediction factors other than learning. The example just discussed assumes that resource prices are stable and that no significant change in the technology being applied will occur. In doing more comprehensive cost prediction, it is common to use learning curves to predict the time needed for production and use other trend analyses to predict nonlabor-related resource costs.

DISCUSSION QUESTIONS

1. What is the theory underlying learning curves?
2. Why is the learning curve most useful in the early life of a production process?
3. What is the effect on costs of having a higher as opposed to a lower percentage learning curve operating in an activity?

EVALUATING FORECAST METHODS

In different situations, one approach to trend forecasting may give better results than others. Note that the exponential smoothing and moving average approaches only forecast the next period. Time-series regression can forecast farther into the future if there are no sudden changes in technology, purchase prices, or efficiency. The ABC model can be used for forecasting costs farther into the future if the costs of inputs to the activities that compose the model can be made for the future periods of interest, but these input cost forecasts are also dependent on understanding future technology and price structures. And, in our rapidly changing environment, the ability to foretell sudden changes in these things is limited. To the extent that trends are stable enough to allow analysis of recent trends to be projected into the future for a few accounting periods, the quality of different approaches can be compared by looking at how well they forecast in the past. A good measure of the relative quality of forecasts is to compare their mean square error. This statistic is simply the average of the squares of the errors in each forecast over a number of past periods. The squares of the errors are used so that large positive errors cannot cancel out large negative errors. Some other statistical advantages to dealing with squared errors exist, but are beyond the scope of this text. A comparison of the mean square errors for the moving average and exponential smoothing approaches is included in Figure 11-3. It indicates that in the example situation, exponential smoothing using a smoothing factor of 0.8 gives the best results. Readers may find it interesting to also compute the mean squared error of a time-series regression based on the same data. This data was used in the regression shown in Figure 11-1.

Examining Figure 11-3 gives some insight as to when one approach might be better that another. Notice that the moving average predictions were consistently

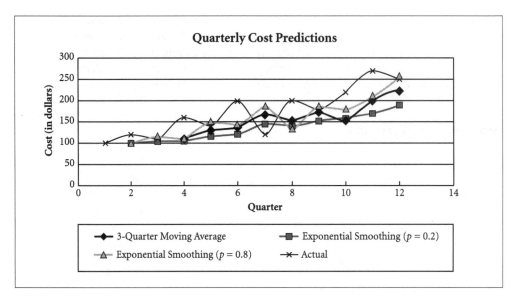

Figure 11-3 **Quarterly Cost Predictions**

low except in the two periods in which costs dropped radically. This is because there was a general increase in costs from period to period. Therefore, averaging past periods with the latest period tended to lower prediction for the next period. The moving average approach smoothes out random variation but does not adequately account for stable trends. Weighting the more recent data more heavily does partially resolve this problem. However, when trends are believed to be stable into the near future, regression analysis gives better projections, because it is not overly affected by recent, highly random events.

Exponential smoothing, as commonly described, puts heavy emphasis on the prediction for the first period of the chain of predictions made. To predict a value for the next period, it corrects the last forecast by a fraction of its error. If there is a stable trend in the quantity being predicted, this adjustment will incorporate that trend. However, the influence of the trend will be modified by random variations. If the trend is more significant over time than the amounts of the random variations, each prediction will be farther and farther off unless it is counterbalanced by a random change in the opposite direction of the trend. This tendency toward progressively increasing error is increased when the smoothing factor is small. In this case, only a small amount of the trend, which will cause a change from the last period, is incorporated into the prediction. Notice in Figure 11-2 that that predictions using the p = 0.2 curve is increasingly too low, though the curve is the smoothest. Also notice that the p = 0.8 curve better reflects the basic trend in what is actually happening. The problem with the large smoothing factor is that a large random change in the opposite direction of the trend (as in Quarter 7) causes a large error in the prediction for the following period.

GENERAL CONCLUSIONS

Several general conclusions about prediction tools can be made from this example. These conclusions vary as the forecasting situation varies. They are greatly dependent on rate of change in the working environment, the degree to which the nature of these changes is understood, and the accuracy of measurements used to analyze them.

Regression Analysis

When changes over time result from stable trends with some random variation superimposed, prediction based on regression analysis is helpful because it will recognize the trends. When the data used to do the regression analysis is plotted, the errors between the linear regression line and the data plots may seem to have a pattern. This phenomenon is discussed briefly in Appendix B. Methods of modifying the analysis to account for such patterns in errors are beyond the scope of this text, but managers should be aware that they exist. In predicting the amount of future quantities, it is important for managers to:

- Have the historic data plotted.
- Make judgment as to how stable the historic patterns of change will be in the future.
- Realize that statistical expertise can often be applied to nonlinear situations. It is frequently beneficial to request help from the information or industrial engineering group within the organization or from outside consultants.

Moving Averages

Moving averages put emphasis on relative recent past experience. Simultaneously, they prevent too much influence being placed on a large random error in the period immediately prior to the period being predicted, as happens when using exponential smoothing. They are also simple to compute. However, with the current ease of performing regression analysis, using a few recent periods as the data input (but one or two more than used in a moving average) in a regression will probably do a better job. Such a regression analysis focuses on recent events, picks up trends, and still avoids overemphasis on the immediate past period.

Exponential Smoothing

The effectiveness of exponential smoothing depends on both the nature of changes that are happening and the level of the smoothing factor "p" used. When there is a strong trend in the factor being predicted, exponential smoothing with a high smoothing factor picks up the trend over a series of predictions. Its weakness is that it is very sensitive to large random errors in the period prior to the one for which a prediction is being made. It is, therefore, best used in situations where trends are changing and random errors are not large. To prevent accumulated error in using the standard smoothing process, as done in the previous example, it is a good idea to periodically restart the prediction chain when successive errors in recent prediction have reversed their sign. When errors of the same sign increase from period to period, the smoothing factor is too low to detect the trend and should be increased.

DISCUSSION QUESTIONS

1. When is a regression, exponential smoothing, or moving average prediction model superior to the other two alternatives? Why?
2. Why should the data for a time-series regression analysis always be plotted?
3. What should managers do to assure that the benefits of regression analysis are available for decision support?
4. In situations where a moving average might appear to be preferable, what modifications can be made to regression analysis to give it competitive status?
5. In what situations is a high smoothing factor generally more predictive than a low one? What is the disadvantage of using a high smoothing factor?

FIXED-COST FORECASTING

Because drivers cause activities, the fixed costs necessary to perform an activity can be treated as if they are driven by the same things that cause variable costs. However, fixed costs are incurred in set amounts per period of time. As stressed earlier, an estimate of fixed cost per unit of driver is accurate only if the quantity of the driver does not change from period to period. Efficient use of fixed-cost resources depends on the degree to which they are used to their capacities. If more activity could be supported by the fixed-cost resources already available, the current fixed cost per unit of output could be reduced in the future.

Managing fixed costs, therefore, requires understanding:

- The volume of output demanded
- The kinds of fixed-cost resources necessary to produce the output
- The capacity of each type of fixed-cost resource
- The cost of each resource

The volume of future output is determined through the marketing function. Determining this volume sets the necessary level of capacity and is the beginning point of planning for fixed-cost resources. The specific fixed-cost resources necessary are identified by studying the production activities used. This involves analyzing the procedures used and identifying the resources that incur cost per period of time rather than per level of output. The cost of these resources can be determined from the documentation of purchase transactions. Their capacity, however, is not so easily understood.

Capacity can be defined as the number of units of output that a resource can produce at a sustainable rate during an accounting period. This assumes that analysts understand the normal work time of the organization, the rate of output of the resource when operated at acceptable levels of efficiency and wear and tear, and the normal downtime for maintenance when operated at those levels. Quantifying these factors involves some subjective judgments. Given these factors, estimating the capacity of a fixed-cost resource is done through theoretical analysis of how the resource is used and experience with its use under varying output demand. If the highest historical output is considered a resource's capacity, past inefficiency may be built into capacity estimates, or, at the other extreme, temporary unsustainable output may be considered normal. If an overly optimistic engineering analysis of potential output is used to set the capacity, output may fall short of expectations when demand increases. This could lead to efforts to find inefficiencies when none exist. The best estimates of capacity come from a combination of practical experience and engineering analysis. Analysts should keep in mind that normal capacity can be exceeded for short periods of time. Maintenance can be delayed and both people and equipment can be worked at higher than sustainable intensities. It may be appropriate to speak of 120 percent productivity for short periods of excessive demand. However, if that level of output can be sustained, output at 100 percent has been understated. In projecting the fixed cost per unit of output in future periods, it is helpful to assume that each resource will be operated at its capacity. Doing this defines the fixed cost per unit of output at maximum fixed-cost efficiency. A later chapter will discuss measuring the cost of underutilization should it occur.

To summarize fixed-cost forecasting, first the fixed-cost resources demanded for the type of output to be produced must be identified. The expected volume of output is divided by the capacity of a unit of each fixed-cost resource to determine how many units will be needed. For any future period, multiplying the quantity of each fixed-cost resource that will be needed by its cost and then summing these figures gives the total fixed cost for the period in question.

When resources are purchased, depreciation schedules convert the costs to a periodic expense. When purchasing, it is important to realize that estimates of fixed cost per unit are no more accurate than the estimates of the useful lives of the assets. Technological improvement can create great uncertainty about future cost when fixed-cost resources are bought or acquired through long-term leases.

EXAMPLE

Suppose a clinic bought a piece of equipment for $21,000 and expected to use it for 7 years. Using straight-line depreciation for the sake of simplicity, it would expense the asset at $3,000 dollars per year—a fixed expense. Let us also assume that, at the end of the second year of its life, new technology becomes available that makes the equipment obsolete. Though it can function as if it were new, clinicians have abandoned it for the improved equipment. This change causes an expense in the third year of the asset's life. Assuming that the equipment cannot be sold, throwing it away creates a $15,000 loss on the disposal of equipment, as opposed to a $3,000 expense in each of the 5 following years. Additionally, the new equipment must be acquired. Such a situation creates costs that were not forecast 2 years earlier.

This simple example demonstrates the risk in forecasting fixed costs too far into the future in organizations with rapidly changing technology. Similar forecasting problems exist when the market for services is changing. These problems can be reduced by having good information about technology and market changes before decisions about investment must be made. However, the ability to get such information is often limited, and this creates risk that financial outcomes may not be as planned. Because technology often changes in spurts, trend analysis does not help much when forecasting changes in fixed costs. Trend analysis may be helpful in forecasting market changes based on more gradual changes in demographics, prices, and tastes.

Forecasting fixed cost for the near future, for instance the budget for next year, is usually fairly easy, but forecasting for extended periods is extremely difficult. A factor that makes near-future fixed costs relatively easy to project is that they are usually fixed because of contractual arrangement or depreciation schedules. Next year's cost of a 3-year lease can be accurately forecast. However, if the lease expires during that year, forecasting the cost of the resource thereafter will demand estimates of the results of a renegotiation. The same is true of salaried labor. In industries such as health care, where technology and regulatory restrictions are changing rapidly, forecasting fixed-cost resource needed more than 4 or 5 years in the future becomes extremely difficult. The problem is that many of the technologies that will be used and the resources they require are themselves highly unpredictable.

When technology is stable, cost-behavior analysis can indicate the total fixed costs per period. To the extent that total costs of an activity have been isolated over a set of past periods, the fixed cost indicated by regressing total cost on the driver of the activity should predict the activity's fixed costs. If this figure agrees well with the fixed-cost amount determined by the analysis of the future just described, the separation of fixed from variable cost is confirmed. If this is the situation, forecasting fixed costs only requires adjusting the quantity of fixed resources needed to match changes in the quantity of sales. This can create one of two general situations. First, future sales quantities may be greater than the current capacity of fixed-cost resources. In this case, resources must be added. Second, resource capacity may be greater than demand; in which case fixed-cost resources should be reduced, if possible.

DISCUSSION QUESTIONS

1. Why is forecasting total fixed costs for the next budgeting period frequently easier than forecasting total variable costs for the same period?
2. Why is understanding capacity extremely important to forecasting cost per unit of output?
3. What is meant by 100 percent of capacity?

FURTHER OBSERVATIONS

The trend analysis techniques just described and commonly used to forecast future values of variables affecting cost and revenues are based on analysis and projection of historic data. Obviously, if the future is not going to be like the past, these tools are all of questionable value. Therefore, a primary role of managers is to envision the future and determine in what ways it will change and the speed of those changes. The general categories of potential change that must be continually examined are changes in the market, changes in technology, and changes in the culture and capabilities of the organization's workforce. Though it is helpful to divide change into these categories, they are not completely independent of each other. Changes in any of them will create changes in the products and services demanded and the resources used to meet those demands. Extremely rapid advancements in genetics, medical information technology, microbiology and biochemistry, and other aspects of clinical technology have the capability to radically change what constitutes health care within the practicing lifetime of today's young health care managers and practitioners.

This speed of change has several implications:

1. Major changes in technology, and hence resources demanded, can be expected in some aspect of care delivery almost annually.
2. Health care managers must keep themselves aware of the change environments in order to be prepared for the financial shocks some of these changes can create.
3. Trend analysis will not be of value in predicting these major changes. Other techniques must be used.

4. Trend analysis will be useful in predicting resource use and prices that are not affected by major changes. These could include such things as routine supplies, some labor rates, relatively low technology equipment, and relatively low technology contract services.

5. To the extent that the exact nature of major changes and their timing is unknown, the ability of managers to predict resource and cost structures past the near future is destroyed.

To stay as far ahead of major changes as possible, managers must assure that the organization is in close communication with the sources of these changes. This requires close contact and careful communication with vendors of equipment and their engineering staffs, providers of contract services, clinical scientists and their professional organizations, and any other sources of leading information. The necessity of this effort will be discussed further in the chapter on budgets.

KEY POINTS

- Future costs can be projected by estimating the amount of output to be produced, establishing drivers for the overhead activities, determining the quantity of each driver needed to produce the output, and establishing a cost of each input per unit of its driver.

- Whether RVU computation is worth its expense depends on the extent to which costs differ among different categories of the target, the degree of differences in demand among the users of the overhead activity, and the materiality of the costs involved.

- Using drivers to forecast costs demands understanding changes that will happen in the resources used to produce each overhead item, the future prices of those resources, and the quantity of the driver that will occur in the future period.

- Zero-based budgeting is excessively expensive and discards lessons learned from experience. However, periodically doing a zero-based analysis of a cost can prevent continuing waste of resources from unnecessary or inefficient activities.

- Estimating changes in input variables can be improved through awareness of trends.

- Trends of demands and prices of inputs are available from professional and trade organizations.

- Trends in organizations can be analyzed using exponential smoothing, moving averages, and regression analysis.

- Exponential smoothing and moving averages techniques are relatively quick and easy, but can only be used for only one period into the future.

- Exponential smoothing demands estimation of the fraction of the previous change that will carry into the future period. It is of limited value when a variable fluctuates significantly and frequently increases and frequently increases and decreases.

- Moving averages work best when there is a continuing increase or decrease in a quantity. However, in this situation, simple regression gives better results.

- Time-series regression on the relationship of a driver to the targeted cost enables prediction for several periods into the future.
- The quality of a regression forecast depends on the size of the R^2 statistic and the probability that the driver/targeted cost relationship will not change in the future.
- Systematic variation from linear regression models' forecasts can be identified by examining a plot of the data.
- Learning curves are helpful in predicting early changes in the resources use by new activities. Various types of activities have different learning curve percentage factors.

- Future unit costs will always be influenced by the degree to which the fixed costs of production are spread across units of production.
- The lower limit of unit cost is set by the capacity of fixed-cost resources, assuming that variable costs are minimized.
- Rapid technology changes make fixed-cost estimation farther than 4 to 5 years into the future very difficult.
- Trend analysis is useful when rapid changes (shocks) in resource use are not expected.

CHAPTER 12 — BUDGETS, BUDGETING, AND CONTROL

STRATEGY, PLANS, AND ACTIVITIES

In this book, understanding the market is considered the starting point for all management decisions. The purpose of an economic entity is to supply potential customers something they can use to their benefit—to meet their needs and desires. The general purpose of health care delivery organizations is to improve wellness in communities. They do this by performing morbidity-preventing and health-improving services or by producing intermediate products for use in those services. Statements of organization *vision*, organization *mission*, and *overall goals* define the market needs an organization intends to meet, the populations they

249

intend to serve, and their desired position within the competitive array of suppliers. *Strategies* are general approaches to realizing the vision or accomplishing the mission. It is important to realize that changes in strategy might be required because changes in market demand have made the current mission obsolete, a technology change has outdated the current production process, or specific products are now obsolete. Because these things can happen at any time and without much warning, strategic planning should not occur on a periodic schedule. Setting a strategy should be done when current or expected condition demand that the current one be abandoned.[1] Anthony (1988) combines these concepts in what he calls *strategic planning*. He states: "*Strategic planning* is deciding on the mission of the organization and the strategies for attaining it. Strategies are general approaches to accomplishing missions."[2]

For instance, an organization may establish its meeting the oncological needs of residents of an extended geographic area as its mission. Its vision may to become and sustain a reputation of being a world-leading oncology center. Its strategy may be to continuously maintain state-of-the-art facilities, do cutting-edge research, and attract the most expert clinicians. To do this, it must accomplish a hierarchical array of objectives. To measure whether it is fulfilling its mission, it could set a goal of establishing one of the three best records of patient outcomes in the nation. At a lower level, it could have a marketing strategy of promoting itself internationally with the intent of attracting well-insured and private-pay patients who believe that its services are worth their additional cost. If successful, this strategy would also enable subsidizing other patients. These mission and strategy decisions are made by executive management.

To implement a strategy, the executive management will have to focus management attention in specific areas. These could be research, oncological treatment concentrating on specific organs, promotion of its capabilities across potential payers and patients, and other areas for which technologies must be selected, processes determined, and resources marshaled. Within each of these focus areas, it is necessary to define objectives that must be reached, the activities that are needed to reach them, and goals to indicate that they have been reached. It is rare that executive management has the competence to do this alone. Activity analysis lies within the competence of operating (often clinical) managers. As discussed earlier, some of these areas conduct institutional-sustaining activities; others do production-sustaining activities and other produce intermediate or saleable products. Activities using related skills and resources are combined into organization units under managers with the appropriate knowledge and skills. These units may be service centers or production centers. Clusters of centers may be joined under a higher level coordinating unit. The example hospital might have a research department, a colon cancer center, a continuing clinical education program, and so forth. This breakout is done to gain the advantages of decentralization.

An important aspect of this view of strategies, activities, and organization units is that each unit is responsible for a set of activities. The cost of any output—whether a support service, an intermediate product, or a final sales product—

is the sum of the cost of the activities it requires. This is one reason that ABC is able to provide managers data that is better structured to help them manage. Because they must make decisions that are about activities, not departments as such, it presents costs of activities. By costing the activities that must flow to any output at any level of the organization, management can better understand the marginal costs of alternatives among which they can choose. By distinguishing between activities that are done in specific centers and those that flow to the centers, one can better evaluate the management of specific portions of the organization. Managers can be evaluated on the performance of activities they control and the efficient consumption of activities and resources they use.

A primary constraint on management is the costs of the activities they manage. Indeed, the general measurement of efficiency is relative cost. The efficient process or organization is the one that produces its outputs at the appropriate level of quality for the least cost. After the activities of an organization, its programs, and its centers have been specified, the organization needs to know what they will cost. Executive management must balance potential costs and potential revenue. Production managers need to know how much money they will have to produce the output expected from them. Establishing these cost figures for a period of time is known as *cost budgeting*, or simply *budgeting*. At levels of the organization to which revenue can be traced, revenue budgets can also be prepared. *Revenue budgets* are simply projections of sales revenues for specified periods of time. The length of the period over which a budget is constructed differentiates among *strategic, program*, and *operating* budgets. To some degree, defining strategic budgets by the length of the period they cover confuses the concept of strategy. Strategy concerns general approaches to missions. *Strategic budgeting* involves budgeting over the long periods for which management believes a given strategy will be used.

The standard duration of an operating budget is 1 year, which corresponds to the standard financial reporting cycle. A year also turns out to be an appropriate period to make detailed estimates of sales demand, and hence the demands for the operating activities. Program budgets usually cover the expected amounts and timing of costs over the life of project, such as a building construction program. An operating budget that is made for an accounting period, or periods, after the coming operating period can be called an *intermediate* or *extended* budget. Their format would be similar to that of any operating budget. Program budgeting may also refer to the costs and timing of a specific service. This is especially true when the activities needed to provide the service must be provided by separate parts of the organization. In this case, the revenues are traceable to the program but the costs are incurred in an array of centers whose activities must be coordinated. Program budgets are, therefore, often multiperiod budgets. Strategic budgets cover time periods in excess of a year. As one considers a hierarchy of budgets, strategic budgets would be defined as quantitative statement of strategic plans. The uncertainties surrounding the activities necessary to implement strategies a few years in the future make strategic budgeting rather hard to formalize.

To summarize, the planning function starts with estimates of market demands. An organization decides which demands it will try to satisfy and for which consumers. It then sets a strategy for doing this. To accomplish the market objectives using its selected strategy, the company must engage in a probably complex array of activities that demand an array of skills, facilities, equipment, and supplies. To maximize the efficient use of these assets in producing quality outputs, organizations decentralize management. The detailed planning of technologies and activities to implement strategies is delegated to managers who have the needed expertise in the activities concerned. At this point in planning, managers need to know what the probable cost of activities will be so that it can be compared to projected revenues. These estimates may induce several iterations of product specification, activity analysis, and cost/revenue estimations until a financially viable combination of product, revenue, and cost is reached. The cost segment of these estimates must, of course, be based on estimates of the total cost of the activities involved. When management is considering changes in operations, it must weigh the marginal costs against the marginal revenues.

DISCUSSION QUESTIONS

1. What are the differences in the meaning of the terms vision, mission, strategy, objective, and goal? How does one relate to the others?
2. What are the relationships among objectives, departments, activities, technologies, and goals?
3. What are the relationships of budgets to the factors in Question 2?
4. What is the relationship between activities and budgets?

OPERATING BUDGETS

Statements of the cost of implementing or operating a plan over a set period are called *cost budgets*. Budgets are not plans; they are the dollar-denominated restatement of plans. Budgets can be written for plans at any level. We will start by discussing operating budgets, because these are the building blocks for more aggregated budgets. *Operating budgets* are usually 1-year budgets. Their preparation should start with data from marketing managers about products and their levels of demand. Production management must furnish data on the activities needed to meet output demands and the resources needed to accomplish those activities. Operating budgets also use data from purchasing managers to estimate the prices that must be paid for material resources and data from personnel management on the costs of personnel. These are compiled to establish what the organization can expect a center's costs to be during the period of the budget. In building budgets for future periods, it is rational to assume efficient operation. This means that the cost data should reflect what the costs ought to be under expected conditions. The costs used in constructing budget are the organization's standards. Executive management must establish procedures for the coordinated collection, storage, and integration of this data.

Zero-Based Budgeting

As the name implies, zero-based budgets assume starting from zero; each activity and its resource demands are analyzed using new measurements on all of the variables involved. This approach guards against previous inefficiencies being perpetuated. When significant market and technology changes alter strategy, a thorough rethinking of activities may be in order. However, planning and budgeting in an organization with stable revenues and expenditures, assuming that very little will remain unchanged from previous periods, may be inefficient. Some activities are quite stable and the history of their costs is valuable costing data. Zero-based budgeting gained considerable attention in the 1980s as a mechanism to prompt abandonment of entrenched wasteful spending. However, it required detailed analysis, repeated effort, and time delays that sometimes appeared to be more expensive than the waste it was to correct. (Although to be fair, improper planning and control of the zero-based process by management often was the cause of the deficiencies just listed.) When completely new products or technology are introduced, zero-based emphasis is required by default, because there is no history. Zero-based budgets are also necessary in complete reorganizations or mergers of like entities, where labor forces and capital assets duplicate one another. For most situations, however, appropriate historical cost data is available and should be used as one of the inputs to the budget process.

Because zero-based budgeting may require too many resources for routine operating budget construction, its polar opposite is also of little value. Though using the last period's budget with adjustments for general monetary inflation and trends in dollar volume of output is fast and simple, it gives managers the information they need only in extremely stable marketing and production conditions. Because health care markets and technologies are extremely unstable, this approach should be considered inadequate.

Incremental Budgeting

In most situations, good budgets can be efficiently constructed by using historical data adjusted for expected changes. The future budget period should be analyzed for material changes in the products to be produced, the mix of products that will be demanded, changes in the technology and resources to be used, and the prices that will have to be paid for specific resources. After the output of an activity center is determined from market forecasts, activity analysis can be used to specify the types and quantities of resources that must be consumed. If the flow of activities and their resource needs is charted and programmed, the cost of any activity in a future period can be predicted. This ability is one of the great advantages of using ABC. However, ABC does not, by itself, create cost forecasts.

Information needed for an ABC cost-flow analysis for a future period must be appropriate to that period. There are two general types of cost information analysis that must be done to implement an ABC model for forecasting use. First, when analysis of the future indicates that technology will have changed, the effect of the change on activities, resources, and their costs must be quantified. If the technology is in use elsewhere, data on resource use may be available from those already using it. If not, management must implement a zero-based approach to projecting the effect of the new technology on costs.

Second, when the technology is stable, costs and usage rates of resources within the ABC flow model will still change because of trends in external variables and learning within the organization. Therefore, trend analysis is needed to forecast the values of independent variables in the model. Both of these forecasting actions are useful. Forecasting changes in the cost of operating stable technologies is assisted by trend and learning curve analysis. Forecasting technology changes and their effects on costs is much more difficult. It demands that the organization's clinical and other technical personnel maintain close contact with trade associations, vendors, research organizations, and their colleagues.

DISCUSSION QUESTIONS

1. What are the advantages and disadvantages of using zero-based budgets as opposed to inflation and volume-adjusted prior-period experience in constructing operating budgets?
2. What sorts of analyses are necessary when using an incremental approach to constructing an operations budget?

STEPS IN CREATING AN OPERATING BUDGET

Health care managers at all levels are involved in an annual budget preparation routine. An effective operating budgeting process should generally include the following steps:

1. The marketing staff makes estimates of expected demand in terms of categories of services. Services should be categorized in such a way that the demand for specific activities can be estimated from the service quantities forecast. Inpatient categorization could be by MDC or in more detail by DRG. The volume of outpatient visits could be categorized by APC, home visits by projected patients home health resource groups (HHRGs), and so forth. These estimates should be passed to both executive management and managers of the activities involved in the services demanded.

2. The initial reaction by the activity managers should be to determine if the quantities of outputs expected from them will demand more capital assets. If they will, this information should be passed to executive management so that capital spending can be reviewed to determine if funds will be available given the organization's overall capital structure plans. This requires working backward through the chain of activities leading to the product sold. As an example, nursing management may estimate that, given the caseload and mix predicted, a specific number of personnel actions will be required. This information must be passed to the personnel department so that it can determine its workload and the resources it will need.

3. Executive management should reconcile market estimates of demand to capital acquisition plans.

4. Activity managers should compute the kind and quantities of other resources they will need to meet the estimated demand and draft budgets for their activities.

Steps 2 through 4 generally involve a lot of crossdepartmental cooperation and coordination. Good management culture within the organization is extremely important to efficiently handle the levels of information sharing and coordination needed.

5. Outside the cost-budgeting function, marketing staff should estimate the revenue that expected sales in each service category would produce and pass this information to executive management.

6. When executive management has revenue estimates by services sold, cost estimated by activities and services sold, and capital demand estimates, it is ready for a first-pass review of the aggregated information. It must look for compatibility of the estimates made. This means making the following determinations:

- Does some of the input information need to be reanalyzed and revised? This especially applies to standards established for activity performance.
- Do the revenue projections cover the expenses and a profit/surplus that will enable survival?
- Do the capacities of some services need to be adjusted to bring capital expenditures into line with operations demands and longer term capital structure plans?
- Does the direction of services to be provided fit with the mission and short-term goals of the organization?

7. Executive management should then return budget information to the activity managers for appropriate revision based on executive perspectives and decisions.

It may be necessary to reiterate Steps 2 through 7 until executive management can approve a budget that appears workable to the activity managers. Budgets that are believed to be unattainable do not motivate people toward efficiency.

Uses of Operating Budgets

Operating budgets serve several purposes. First, as mentioned earlier, they restate short-term plans in terms of dollar values of resources needed. They, therefore, allow financial managers to know how much money must be available to purchase materials and pay personnel. When budgets are broken into monthly or quarterly cash flows, they facilitate the management of working capital by letting mangers know when operating shortfalls in cash are likely to occur and when surpluses for repaying short-term loans are likely to be available.

Second, they give managers of centers formal statements of the expectations of executive management. The budget process involves iterations of estimates of output demand, revenue, and production costs among managers affected by those variables. When this process is completed, senior management formalizes sales targets and acceptable levels of costs. Because these costs were developed activity by activity from the organization's operating plans, they can be assigned to the centers in which the activities are done. Operating budgets are statements of these costs for specific activities and centers. An operating budget can act as something of a contract between executive and subordinate managers. It informs subordinate managers of what is expected from their centers, but it also promises them that the budgeted resources will be made available.

Third, because operating budgets for all centers within the organization are available to all organization managers, they can also act as coordination documents. Managers are able to see the expectations and resource constraints placed on other managers with whom they interact. If budgeted amounts are built on realistic standards for efficient performance, they can also serve as quantitative targets of achievement and provide motivation. To have a motivating effect, personnel must believe that performing at budgeted costs indicates noteworthy performance for which they will be respected and rewarded. When budgets are set at virtually unachievable (as opposed to noteworthy) levels, they will probably be ignored. When this happens, the budget is interpreted as documentation of management insensitivity to workers and can become a source of internal conflict.

Fourth, budgets built on standards of appropriate levels of efficiency serve as benchmarks for the costs that should have occurred during an operating period. They can, therefore, serve as a basis of comparison for actual results. Differences between budgeted and actual costs indicated deviations from expected results. Analyzing and interpreting the differences is called *cost variance analysis* and is the subject of the next chapter.

CASH BUDGETS

After operating budgets are drafted, pro forma income statements can be written. These reflect expected revenues and expenses for a coming accounting period. However, revenue does not always produce cash inflow at the time it is recognized, and expenses do not always consume cash at the time they are recognized. The amount of cash flowing in and out of the organization during any time period and the amount on hand at any given time are affected by these timing phenomena. The timing of revenue receipt is dependent in credit policies and accounts receivable collection efficiency. Cash inflow associated with operations is also affected by short-term borrowing. The timing of cash outflows depends on the organization's payment agreements with suppliers and lending institutions.

A cash budget adjusts the figures in the pro forma income statement to reflect cash flows during shorter, embedded periods in order to indicate if the cash available will be adequate to meet short-term cash needs. When it is not, the cash budget allows creating a short-term borrowing schedule that assures adequate cash and minimizes the amount of interest that will be owed on the debt. Cash budgets are usually done for months of shorter time periods and show when short-term borrowing is needed, the amount, and when it can be repaid. Techniques for creating cash budgets are discussed in the appendix to this chapter.

DISCUSSION QUESTIONS

1. What are the implications of market demand estimates to long-term asset acquisition decisions made by executive and activity managers?
2. Why should operations budgeting be an iterative process?
3. What is the relationship between standard costs and budgeting?
4. Why are cash budgets necessary? What advantages do accurate cash budgets provide?

PROGRAMS AND STRATEGIC BUDGETS

Operating budgets state the expected costs for centers within an organization over an operating cycle, most frequently a year. They are written for both service and production centers. They contain considerably more detail than senior managers desire to know. However, the costs of any number of centers can be aggregated. Likewise, costs over a number of operating periods can also be aggregated. How aggregations are done depends on the information desired. For example, there may be several activity centers within the cardiovascular care product line. These budgets can be further broken out by categories such as labor, supplies, equipment rents, maintenance, and so forth if separate accounts for these cost categories are maintained in the ledgers. Summing these budgets over the component centers creates a product line budget. Such budgets can be consolidated to the level of detail desired by senior management.

When new programs are under consideration, the term *program budget* may be used to refer to the total cost of the program over a specified period of operation. This period can begin at program inception or the current time; it ends at the expected obsolescence of the long-term assets involved or demise of the market. These budgets often use cash outflows as opposed to expenses and include the cash flows necessary to obtain the long-term assets needed by the program. When these budgets are prepared using marginal cash flows, managers can evaluate the net benefits of the program by comparing the budgeted outflows with expected flows of revenue over time. The technique for doing this is called *capital budgeting;* it is covered more thoroughly in Chapter 14.

The term strategic budget is often used synonymously with long-term budget. In this context, it is the sum of operating budget numbers over the strategic time frame being considered. This implies that operating budgets can be constructed year by year to the strategic horizon. In a rapidly changing industry such as health care, this is extremely unlikely. The horizon to which existing operations will be stable is quite short. Markets and technology seem to change almost continuously. This means that the total set of organization activities will also change frequently. It is almost certain that in any budget period some of these changes will force changes in some services or programs. To the extent these changes can be foreseen, operating budgets for future periods can be adjusted. However, many cannot be predicted far in advance. The combination of the inability to forecast market and technology changes and the probability that each year some programs will be altered by such changes make organization-wide strategic budgeting extremely inaccurate. Because these changes are closely linked to changes in capital equipment needs, strategic budgeting places much emphasis on estimating the capital assets that will be needed. This is done because these assets represent future fixed cost with all the management problems associated with fixed costs.

Because change will force adjustments in some of a health care organization's activities, budgeting past the period of the operating budget may best be restricted to specific service lines or programs. Strategic budgeting is appropriate where reasonable estimates can be made of the duration of the demand for the product and the technology used to produce it. For these reasons, many large industrial organizations have virtually eliminated their central strategic planning units and delegated the initiative for long-term planning to decentralized management.[3] Managers near the resource markets clinical production technology appear to be better able to make these estimates. This long-term decentralized planning rests on the organization's mission and strategies established by executive management. It is done considering decentralized management estimates of the life of the products and technologies involved. Its primary quantitative analysis is based on projections of future demands for outputs and the capital assets that will be used to produce them.

This delegation does not mean that activity managers should avoid using the expertise of staff personnel. Demands for care beyond 3 to 5 years into the future depend on changes in demographics, technology, and epidemiology. Understanding demographic changes requires close analysis of population trends and coordination with civic planners. Projecting the technology that will be demanded by clinicians is helped by close communication with vendors, the health sciences community, and the organization's clinicians. Epidemiological changes within the population served will probably occur more slowly that the other two factors unless the socioeconomic mix of the served population changes greatly. Even so, planners should avoid being surprised by large changes in the composition of people within their drawing area.

Because the environment to be faced in the future is changing rapidly, the ability to budget accurately diminishes, as the budget period is farther into the future. One approach to being prepared for the future, but not deluded into overestimates of stability, is to prepare preliminary operating budgets for several additional periods at the time of preparing the operations budget for the next period. Each of these additional budgets attempts to reflect known or highly probable changes in the future. Because of uncertainties, each is also expressed in successively less detail. The later period budgets are revised in more detail in the following budgeting cycle. This process produces what is referred to as a *rolling budget* or an *operations* and *intermediate budget*. The term intermediate refers to budgets between the operations budget and the strategic budget.

DISCUSSION QUESTIONS

1. What are the differences between project and operations budgets?
2. What are the differences between operations and strategic budgets?
3. What are the primary problems in attempting to set strategic budgets?
4. What are rolling budgets and how are they related to strategic and operating budgets? What is the advantage of constructing them?

MARKETING, ABC, AND CONTROL

In order to assure an organization's movement toward its objectives, managers' awareness must extend well beyond the mechanics of control. For many, especially accountants, this control has meant budgetary control. *Budgetary control* involves determining what the revenues and costs should be if the organization is performing well, then measuring performance and comparing it to that which was planned. This concept assumes that the proper production processes are stable enough to allow input-output standards to be established. An example is knowing that a particular radiological diagnostic test should use a set number of machine hours, film frames, patient preparation minutes, and so forth. Budgetary control, therefore, requires countable output; for example, being able to know that 1,436 Procedures 501 were done during the budget period, knowing the standards for the amount of each resource used to produce one of these tests, and a standard price to be paid for each resource. These prerequisites exist at varying levels of precision for different outputs of various parts of the organization. They are most nearly satisfied when identical products are produced by a stable, continuing process or series of jobs orders.

If ABC analysis has been done for the activities necessary prior to production as well as the production activity for the product, it is relatively easy to update cost standards as inputs change at any point in the flow of resources to the product. When ABC software is applied to the flow analysis, a change to any input is automatically incorporated into a revision of the product cost. When inputs are set at their expected quantities and costs for a production period, a standard cost for that period can be computed.

A great advantage of budgetary control is that it is relatively simple. At intervals, measurements are made of outputs produced and compared to the planned production quantities. The cost of the production is measured and compared to what it should have cost according to the standards. Where discrepancies exist, management can attempt to isolate their causes. When the discrepancies are unfavorable, the causes should be removed. Conversely, managers can attempt to perpetuate favorable deviations from expectations.

It is often said that a completed operating budget results in a plan of operations for the coming year expressed in quantitative terms. It may be more accurate to say that the operating budget is the quantified documentation of the plan of operations for a coming period of time. This rewording attempts to clarify the scope and chronological order of budgeting activities. Budgeting begins with a marketing plan grown from the organization's basic mission and strategy. The marketing plan reveals the output demands that will be placed on the organization. From that, specific outputs are listed. Based on the types and quantities of output to be produced, the production processes (activities) to be used are specified and the resources to be consumed are estimated. Budgeted revenues and costs flow from this planning. We repeat this chronology at this point to emphasize that there must be considerable marketing effort involved in the early steps of the budget process.

ORGANIZATION STRUCTURE, PEOPLE, AND CONTROL

People control the activities of an organization. Specific people are held responsible for control of specific sets of activities or specific outcomes. *Responsibility accounting* is accounting to support and evaluate control by these designated people at selected locations in the organization. The locations are referred to as centers and are subunits of the organization. The people are the managers of the centers. A basic premise is that managers should only be held responsible for things they can control. Within an ABC management-accounting system, managers are held responsible for the efficiency of activities they manage and the quality of their outputs.

Determining if a manager within a health care delivery organization should be held responsible for profit or only for costs can be somewhat complicated. Assume a hospital laboratory responds to orders from the ward and outpatient clinic and the transfer prices are set by the hospital executive management—does its manager control its revenue? If the laboratory manager sets test prices, does the lab now control its revenue? If the lab not only meets the demands of the hospital but 25 percent of its business is from acting as a reference lab for independent clinics in its locale, can the manager manage the revenue? If the hospital is paid under a fee-for-discharge or capitated contract, does the lab manager have any control over revenues? In each situation, should the manager be held responsible for profit or simply for the cost of the lab meeting its demand? Questions such as these must be answered by senior management.

No matter how a given center is categorized, the total organization's budgets are broken into parts that cover the activities of each center. The center's performance is then compared against its budget figures. For profit centers, comparison is on profit; for cost centers, only costs are compared. To the extent that health care industry revenues come in the form of DRG-like prospective payments for discharge or capitated fees, the departments within a delivery organization do not have revenue traceable to them. For this reason, center managers are currently losing control of revenue and are being held accountable only for their costs. Only the total organization or large service lines with traceable revenue should be considered to be revenue or profit centers.

In summary, budgetary control rests on the broad philosophy that managers should be told what is expected of their units; they should be judged by aspects of the unit's performance that they can affect, and management of the center's activities should be largely left to its management. In each center, attention must be paid to the degree to which the manager can control costs and revenues.

DISCUSSION QUESTIONS

1. What is meant by responsibility accounting?
2. What must be considered in determining whether an activity center is a profit center or simply a cost center?
3. Why do management theorists often contend that departments cannot be controlled; that control refers to people?

CONTROL AND ACCOUNTING CAPABILITY

It may be meaningful to review a few ideas already mentioned and, for brevity, make a few bold assertions.

Different Perspectives for Different Decisions

We should reemphasize that financial accounting and management accounting are done for separate reasons. Simplistically, financial accounting is done because it is required for external parties; it is done the way GAAP requires that it be done. The process and reports are checked for compliance by AICPA-certified auditors. Tax accounting is similar except that the taxing authority sets the accounting rules and monitors compliance with them. Remember that income for tax purposes is not defined to reflect the financial performance of the entity but to determine its taxes. Management accounting is done to produce information managers want in order to manage, that is, to assure that the functions of management are performed using decisions based on sound information. For example, Tom, the management accountant for Giant Metro Hospital, needs to know the volume and productivity levels of Giant's emergency department. He is preparing a management report that will indicate the advantages and disadvantages of opening three off-site urgent care centers. The decision on this issue by the hospital's executive committee uses a marginal cost perspective. On the other hand, third party auditors see the emergency department as one part of the whole organization. They will examine its financial transactions to determine the full costs of its operations.

Computers and Databases

A common unpublicized fact is that with the support of computers, these three types of accounting can be done independently. There is no reason why the results of the financial, tax, or management-accounting systems should agree, even though they are generated from the same raw data. One usually has to think about this for a while before it becomes obvious. If the data needed for these activities is collected and stored in relational data bases, whatever is needed for a particular purpose can be called up and processed (computationally manipulated) in whatever way is appropriate to the purpose at hand. Some data elements may be used in all three activities. Some may be specific to only one. This ability to rather easily keep more than one set of books, or models for accounting information, is a marvelous gift of the computer age.

A similar truth exists for the two types of management-accounting models: those used for responsibility accounting and those used for making incremental decisions about the conduct of operations. For example, if management wants to evaluate how well a manager is controlling cost in a department, they compare the department's direct costs with the standard amount at its output. If they want to decide whether to add a service to the department's product line, they look at the total incremental cost that would result from the addition. These may be very different quantities. Hopefully, the data needed to compute each will be in the data base.

Profit Control Versus Cost Control

Now return to the idea of different types of responsibility centers. If profit (or surplus) is the best general measure of performance, why not consider all centers to be profit centers? However, to measure profit, one must measure both revenue and cost. As pointed out earlier, many centers simply do not have the revenue that results from the management or production performance of the center. If the revenue figures must be manufactured, the profit figures are automatically manufactured and have no real meaning. Also, much of the total cost of the center is allocated overhead.

Current changes in payment systems are compounding this problem for an increasing portion of total revenue. As more payers go to payment based on case category (as opposed to fees for specific line-item inputs), the concept of centers that produce intermediate products that can be profit centers within a care delivery organization loses its usefulness. All departments become cost centers. Payment is made for an aggregate of services used to furnish an episode of intervention. These services come from all over the organization. The laboratory, diagnostic clinics, and nursing services become cost centers. To attribute revenue to them, the payment must be arbitrarily divided among them. Therefore, if the financial performance of one of these centers looks bad, its management could legitimately place the blame on the way revenue and overhead costs are assigned to it, as opposed to the way it manages its activities. In this case, the value of responsibility reporting is lost.

Product Lines

Given this situation, what is the reason to have product lines? Decentralized management has advantages related to the proximity of the operating center to the processes, necessary expertise, and both the resource and product markets for the production. Additionally, there is evidence that significant motivation of managers and workers evolves from the feeling that they "own" their work and are rewarded for their performance. If ultimate performance is to be measured by financial performance, the most encompassing measure is profit (or surplus). Decentralization is, therefore, based on the belief that efficiency is maximized when general management by a single management group controls almost all aspects of a limited operation.

Product line management therefore attempts to place as much of the full array of marketing and production under one management unit as is feasible. If both the marketing (revenue) and the production (cost) aspects are in one center, that center can be treated as a profit center. Its general performance can be monitored through its profit. The array of products made by such a center is its product line. When the production and sale of some outputs produced by an organization are grouped under a single management unit, the organization is practicing product line management.

The primary reason for creating product lines is to improve operating management by focusing expertise, reducing response time, and facilitating coordination. Simplifying control by using profit to monitor their performance is an important, but secondary, consideration. Product line management does very little to improve the ability to determine or monitor the profitability of an individual product or patient unless revenue can be traced to the products or patients.

Cost Structure Implications

The cost structure (composition of fixed and variable costs) of the resources needed is important to the degree to which the benefits of decentralization can be gained. It is rational to want all the resources used to produce everything in the product line to be controlled by the product line management. This forces management to consider how those resources whose costs are fixed (regardless of the volume of production) should be managed. As an example, consider a cardiovascular care center. All the interventions and associated resources used in the care of cardiovascular cases are managed in this product line center by its product line manager. If the smallest number of beds that comprise an efficiently run ward is 20 and the center's caseload will fill that number of beds on most days, it is then reasonable for the center to have its own ward dedicated to nursing care of its patients. This ward could be under the complete management of the cardiovascular product line manager and staff. If, however, a fixed-cost resource cannot be completely utilized by patients from a single product line, that resource must either be utilized inefficiently or shared by other product line managers. In this case, at least one product line manager loses control of a needed resource and consequently should lose responsibility for the efficiency of its use. This problem in product line management demands attention to the capacity of fixed-cost resources. Where capacity of a fixed-cost resource cannot be fully used by a single product line, the issue of transfer prices (discussed in Chapter 5) must be faced.

DISCUSSION QUESTIONS

1. Why are relational data bases important to accounting's ability to support different demands for information?
2. What are the relationships among health care payment schemes, the designation of accounting centers, and control?
3. What are the criteria for establishing a product line? How does cost accounting relate to taking advantage of the benefits of product line management? How does the location of fixed-cost assets affect these benefits?

EXERCISE

Regarding the "different perspectives for various decisions" segment in the preceding section, what information necessary to next year's budget should be included in Tom's management report about the emergency department? What related information should he gather to create a projected budget for the proposed new off-site urgent care centers?

FLEXIBLE BUDGETS AND STANDARD COSTS

Flexible budgeting means that the budgeted amounts for an operating period are flexible with respect to the level of output of the period. Rather than saying that the ward's operating budget is $1,325,000 for the year (a static or deterministic budget), the company would say that it was $500,000 (for fixed costs) plus $128 for every patient bed-day provided. Realize that flexible budgets cannot be constructed unless cost-behavior analysis has been conducted to separate the variable and fixed components of the cost structure.

In the next chapter, we shall apply the information from cost-behavior analysis to flexible budgeting. Then we shall demonstrate how to quantify the amount of difference between planned and actual cost performance of a center in such a way that the probable location of problems, or superior performance, is indicated. The concept of standard costs is basic to these processes. This is true not simply because they are used in budgeting and cost centers' variance analyses, but because the concept of standards for the average resource use over large numbers of cases is becoming increasingly relevant to tactics for control of the cost of society's health care. As outcome measurement becomes more precise, researchers will be able to analyze which care protocols produce better outcomes. This effort is underway and the examination and use of benchmark protocols are gaining advocates. As protocols of care become standardized and the costs of the activities called for in the protocols are measured better, estimates of the average cost of caring for categories of patients will become more accurate. Because each patient's situation is different to some degree, a particular protocol may not be applicable to every patient in a given category. However, as patient categories become more refined, within category variations in protocols (and hence in cost) become smaller. For providers, the law of large numbers should cause prices negotiated on standard costs of caring for categories of patients to produce satisfactory total revenues.

Standard cost was defined in Chapter 3 as the amount a cost object ought to cost. The standard cost assumes specific levels of production efficiency, appropriate purchase prices for resources, and the use of fixed-cost resources at their operating capacity. Accounting for failure to use fixed-cost resources at their capacity is also discussed in the next chapter. Establishing standard costs is essentially forecasting the cost of items in the near future. Consider the near future as the period from the time of making the forecast to the end of the budget period of concern. The approaches to predicting costs discussed in Chapter 9 can be applied to establishing standard costs. Current costs analyzed using activity-based cost measurement can serve as the beginning point. These historic costs must be adjusted for changes in efficiency and resource prices expected in the period of the budget.

Adjustments must also be made for expected changes in technology. In producing standard costs for the next year, this may not be too difficult. The technology change has probably been planned already. The costs and changes in variable costs associated with it may be fairly easily found because the technology is already understood. Establishing standard cost for more distant periods demands forecasting and understanding the technology that will be used. This, as pointed out earlier, is much more difficult. The rate of change in technology used in interventions for specific health conditions is such that some planners contend that budgeting for health care interventions more than 5 years into the future is self-delusional. This is probable not true for some facets of the organization. Activities such as those used in preventive medicine, patient education, and administrative processes may change rapidly, but their capital cost probably will not. In such activities, the same people can be retrained and fixed-cost capital resources will probable remain nearly the same.

STATIC BUDGETS

A *static budget* is geared toward only one level of activity, and always compares actual results for the period against a budget of costs pegged at the original budget level of activity. For example, an annual static budget is not changed, or adjusted, over the course of the year. The budget figures remain the same—unchanged or static.

The static budget is easily compared with the flexible budget, because the differences are readily apparent. The flexible budget does not operate on a single level of activity; instead, it operates within a range of multiple activities. In addition, the flexible budget can (and should) be adjusted during the budget period. The flexible budget allows adjustment for a different activity level than the level originally planned and budgeted. This means management can first refer to actual activity levels achieved during a period and second can refer to the (adjusted) flexible budget to determine what costs should have been at that actual activity level. Thus, the flexible budget is *dynamic* rather than static.

DISCUSSION QUESTIONS

1. What are flexible budgets? What is the advantage in their use?
2. What are standard costs? Under what conditions can they be constructed?

3. How does ABC improve the ease and accuracy of construction of standard costs?
4. What is a static budget?
5. Can you give an example of a static budget and a flexible budget in your own experience?

KEY POINTS

- Mission statements define the products an organization intends to produce and the markets it intends to serve.
- Objectives are specific accomplishments that lead to performance of the mission.
- Strategy is the general approach to be used to reach objectives or, more broadly, to accomplish a mission.
- Goals are levels of measurable factors that indicate that the objectives have been met or the mission has been accomplished.
- Strategy should be changed when changes in the market or technology make the existing strategy obsolete.
- Budgets are plans expressed in monetary terms.
- Operating budgets state expected revenues and expenses for an operating period, usually a year.
- Zero-based budgets are operating budgets that are not based on adjustments to the budgets of previous periods. Although constructing them sometimes requires excess resources, they are useful for new projects and products and for complete reorganizations and mergers.
- Intermediate (or extended) budgets are operating budgets constructed for periods after the current operating budget. They are stated in successively less detail.
- Strategic budgets are statements of broad categories of revenues and expenses for

periods well in the future (in health care usually 3 to 8 years). They place strong emphasis on capital expenditures.
- Cash budgets convert revenues and expenses to cash inflows and outflows for short portions of the operating budget in order to isolate the timing of cash shortfalls that may require short-term borrowing.
- Creating operating budgets starts with analysis of the market. This is followed by analysis of resources needed to meet market demands. It requires iterative, closely coordinated efforts by executive and activity manager.
- Operating budgets communicate the distribution of funds within the organization to activity managers, promise resources to activity managers, inform all managers of expectations and resource constraints across the organization, and provide benchmarks for measuring financial performance.
- Program budgets are multiperiod, multiactivity budgets for specific projects of defined duration or separate segments of the mission.
- Budgetary control involves after-the-fact comparison of budgeted quantities to the quantities resulting from operations. The variances in these numbers are used to identify below standard performance for

correction and above expected performance that might be sustained.

- Budgetary control is dependent on constructing standard costs.
- ABC is a powerful tool in rapidly determining standard costs and keeping them accurate in a changing environment.
- Responsibility accounting involves holding activity managers responsible for quality and efficiency factors they can control. It is dependent on the ability to measure these factors at the level of the manager's activity.
- As health care payment systems tend to pay for episodes of care through prospective payment systems, health care organizations become profit centers and their component centers become cost centers. They lose the characteristics of profit centers.
- The ability of computers to store relational databases and manipulate specific data in them allows accounting to generate cost numbers appropriate to specific decision models used by specific decision makers.
- Flexible budgets take into consideration the fact that costs for future periods have both fixed and variable components.
- Static budgets remain unchanged when levels of activity change during the budget period.

References

[1] Mintzberg, H. *The Rise and Fall of Strategic Planning.* (New York: The Free Press, 1994), p. 240.

[2] Anthony, Robert. *The Management Control Foundations.* (Boston: Harvard Press, 1988), p. 10.

[3] Mintzberg, H. *The Rise and Fall of Strategic Planning.* (New York: The Free Press, 1994), pp. 79–101.

LEARNING OBJECTIVES

1. Explain the difference between costs and expenses and between revenues and cash inflows as well as why these differences are important to an organization's liquidity.

2. Explain the difference between cash and noncash expenses and how they are handled in a cash budget.

3. Be able to construct a cash budget, compute demands for short-term borrowing, and schedule short-term borrowing repayment.

In this book, we have not been careful to differentiate *costs* from *expenses* and *revenues* from *cash receipts*. These differences are important in financial accounting. By recognizing them, income can be attributed to specific periods of time. Revenue is considered to be earned when a sales contract is completed and delivery is made. This may not be the same time that payment is received. Consider the cost of the resources consumed in producing what was sold to be the expenses of the period of the sale. That is, attribute the expenses to the period of the sale, not to the period for which resources were paid. This allows financial statements to reflect income realized from the operations of specific periods. It does not reflect the net amount of cash gained or lost during the period. However, bankruptcy occurs when an organization cannot pay its bills, and this happens because of a shortfall in cash, not simply a lack of income.

Cash budgets recognize these facts, showing the timing of cash flows within operating budget periods and noting times at which cash shortfalls might occur. They, therefore, indicate times at which short-term borrowing might be necessary in order to remain liquid until adequate cash inflows occur. Analysis to produce cash budgets is done by adjusting the timing of expenses to the time at which the consumed resources are paid for, adjusting the timing of revenues to the time at which their cash collection occurs, and incorporating other inflows and payments of the period being analyzed. Doing this involves the following steps:

1. The amounts and prices of resources used to produce the sales forecast for the cash budget period must be estimated.
2. The time at which payment will be made for these resources must be estimated.

4. The timing of the receipt of cash for sales within the budgeted period must be estimated.
5. These cash flows along with nonsales-related cash flow must be aggregated for each cash budget interval to see what the net effect on cash will be.
6. When intervals of cash shortages occur, arrangement for short-term borrowing can be made.
7. When intervals will produce excess of cash inflows over outflows, existing short-term debt can be retired.

EXAMPLE

Constructing a cash budget for January through June of the coming year is described here. To recognize factors that affect a month's cash flows and yet keep the budgeting process reasonable, the following assumptions are made:

- Cash budgets are prepared for each month and all months are assumed to have 30 days.
- Materials are ordered so as to arrive 6 days before they are needed, and invoices accompany all materials. This means that invoices for 6/30th (or 20 percent) of a month's materials are received in the previous month. The remaining 80 percent are received in the month they are being paid.
- Fifty percent of invoices are paid in 10 days after receipt and the rest are paid 30 days after receipt. Therefore one third of the invoices received in a month are paid in that month; the remaining two thirds are paid the following month. (The reader may want to chart this flow to confirm these fractions.)
- Labor and related benefit plans are paid monthly, on the last business day of the month.
- Examination of patient billing and accounts receivable data indicates that 15 percent of patient net charges are paid at discharge, another 30 percent within 30 days of discharge, 40 percent more within 60 days, 10 percent more by 90 days, and the rest are never paid.
- A bond interest payment of $200,000 is due the end of each quarter: March 31, June 30, September 30, and December 31.
- Lease and contract services expenses are paid at the beginning of each month.
- Pledges from a recent charity drive total $100,000 to be paid by January 20, $40,000 by February 20, and $20,000 by March 20. Eighty percent of pledges are paid as promised.

- The organization has decided that it needs to maintain a minimum cash balance of $500,000.

Table 12A-1 shows the expected revenue along with labor, materials, and lease/contract expenses for the months in and around the budgeting period. Note that noncash expenses such as depreciation and amortization are not shown. This information is usually developed from monthly pro forma income statements.

Construction of the Cash Budget

CONVERTING REVENUE TO CASH INFLOWS The organization's credit and collection policies affect how long after billing that revenues are collected. Analysis of accounts receivable indicates that, for a given month, cash flows from revenues will be 15 percent of that month's net revenues, 30 percent of the previous month's net revenues, 40 percent of the revenues from 2 months previous, and 10 percent of those from the third month previous. The remaining 5 percent will never be collected and are written off as bad debt. Therefore, January's cash flow from revenue would be:

$$0.15(1,800,000) + 0.30(2,000,000) + 0.40(1,600,000) + 0.10(1,000,000) = \$1,610,000$$

February's cash flows from revenue would be:

$$0.15(2,500,000) + 0.30(1,800,000) + 0.40(2,000,000) + 0.10(1,600,000) = \$1,875,000$$

and so forth.

Table 12A-1 **Monthly Pro Forma Revenue and Expenses Figures (in $ thousands)**

	Oct.	Nov.	Dec.	Jan.	Feb.	Mar.	Apr.	May	Jun.	Jul.
Net patient revenue	1,000	1,600	2,000	1,800	2,500	2,700	2,100	2,000	2,000	1,600
Charity pledges				100	40	20				
Materials expenses	200	320	400	360	500	540	420	400	400	370
Labor expenses	300	480	600	630	875	945	735	700	700	520
Leases & contracts	640	640	680	680	720	720	680	680	680	640
Bond interest payments			200			200			200	

These computations show estimates of the cash receipts from patient revenues to be:

Jan.	Feb.	Mar.	Apr.	May	Jun.
$1,610,000	$ 1,875,000	$ 2,075,000	$ 2,305,000	$ 2,260,000	$ 2,010,000

CONVERTING MATERIAL EXPENSES TO CASH OUTFLOWS   We know the time lag between receiving invoices and making payment and we also know when invoices are expected relative to the time of using the material. Invoices are received for materials used in the first 6 days of a month in the prior month. If we also assume a steady flow of materials, this means that invoices are received for only 80 percent of the month's expenses, $(30 - 6)/30$. Invoices are also received for 20 percent of the next month's expenses. Therefore, January invoices received totaled:

$$0.80(360,000) + 0.20(500,000) = \$388,000$$

February's invoices for materials would be:

$$0.80(500,000) + 0.20(540,000) = \$508,000$$

and so forth.

These computations show the following amount of invoices estimated to be received in the budgeted months:

Dec.	Jan.	Feb.	Mar.	Apr.	May	Jun.
$392,000	$388,000	$508,000	$516,000	$416,000	$400,000	$384,000

Payment policy dictates that when trade discount of 2/10 net 30 are given, payment will be made on the 10th day. The rest will be paid 30 days after receipt. This common trade discount notation means that a 2 percent discount is given if payment is made within 10 days; payment is expected within 30 days. The organization has found that about a half of its material purchases have this discount. The dollar amount of the trade discount is not considered by the analyst as a matter of conservative accounting estimation.

Therefore, in any given month:

1. Half the invoices received in the first 20 days (two thirds of the month) will be paid that month (to take the 2/10 net 30 discount).
2. The other half of the first 20 day's invoices will be paid the next month (30 days after receipt).
3. All the invoices received in the last 10 days will be paid in the next month (either 10 or 30 days after receipt).

This means that:

1. $(1/2)(2/3) = 2/6$ of invoices received in a month will be paid in that month
2. $(1/2)(2/3) = 2/6$ of the invoice paid in a month will be from the previous month
3. $1/3$ (or $2/6$) of the invoices paid in a month will be those without the discount received the previous month

In a given month $2/6 + 2/6 = 2/3$ of the invoices from the previous month will be paid along with $2/6$ (or $1/3$) of the invoices from that month. Each month's payment for materials is computed as follows (the amount of the discount is not shown in these figures):

Payments made in January are:

$$0.333(388,000) + 0.667(392,000) = \$390,688$$

Payments in February would be:

$$0.333(508,000) + 0.667(388,000) = \$427,960$$

and so forth.

Cash payment estimates for materials in the months for which the cash budget is being built are, therefore:

Jan.	Feb.	Mar.	Apr.	May	Jun.
$390,688	$427,960	$510,644	$472,700	$410,672	$394,672

CONVERTING LABOR COSTS TO CASH OUTFLOWS We know that labor costs are paid at the end of the month in which they are incurred. Therefore, no conversion is necessary.

CONVERTING LEASE AND CONTRACT EXPENSES These are paid at the beginning of each month, so no conversion is necessary. Using the previous information, a monthly breakdown of cash flows can be made. This is shown in Table 12A-2.

COMPLETING THE CASH FLOW BUDGET To illustrate cash budgeting, assume that at the beginning of January the minimum cash balance, $500,000, was on hand. Assume also that revenues, material expenses, and labor expenses occur evenly throughout each month. We know that lease and contract expenses are paid at the beginning of the month. To be conservative, if a month is expected to have a cash shortfall, we will borrow the money at

Table 12A-2 Cash Flows by Month (in $)

	Jan.	Feb.	Mar.	Apr.	May	Jun.
Cash from sales	1,610,000	1,875,000	2,075,000	2,305,000	2,260,000	2,010,000
Cash from pledge	80,000	32,000	16,000			
Total inflows	1,690,000	1,907,000	2,091,000	2,305,000	2,260,000	2,010,000
Cash for materials	390,688	427,960	510,644	472,700	410,672	394,672
Cash for labor	630,000	835,000	945,000	735,000	700,000	700,000
Cash for contracts & leases	680,000	720,000	720,000	680,000	680,000	680,000
Cash for bond interest			200,000			200,000
Total outflows	1,700,688	1,982,960	2,375,644	1,887,700	1,790,672	1,974,672
Net cash flows	− 10,688	− 75,690	− 284,644	417,300	469,328	35,328

the beginning of the month. If a positive net cash flow allows loan repayment, it will be paid at the end of the month. Given the cash flows estimated, the timing of borrowing and paybacks can be charted as shown in Table 12A-3.

The table shows that after April operations, $417,300 is available after allowing for the minimum cash on hand. This can be used to reduce the accumulated borrowing. The $417,300 appears to be more than enough to pay back the accumulated principal and the interest due on it. Short-term borrowing contracts can be written many ways. A common approach is to pay the interest on the principal when the principal is repaid. Remember that we borrow at the beginning of the

Table 12A-3 Cash Budget (in $)

	Jan.	Feb.	Mar.	Apr.	May	Jun.
a. Beginning balance	500,000	500,000	500,000	500,000	541,80	1,010,908
b. Net cash flows	− 10,688	− 75,690	− 284,644	417,300	469,328	35,328
c. Cash at end of month (a + b)	489,312	424,310	215,356	917,300	1,010,908	1,146,236
d. Minimum balance	500,000	500,000	500,000	500,000	500,000	
e. Amount to be borrowed (c − d, where d > c)	−10,688	−75,690	−284,644	none	none	
f. Amount available for payback (c − d, where d < c)				417,300[*]		
g. Accumulated principal	10,688	86,780	371,424			
h. Amount of payback				375,720[*]		
i. Remainder				41,580[*]		
j. Ending balance (d + i)	500,000	500,000	500,000	541,580	1,010.908	1,146,236

[*] From computation on page A12-10

month in which additional cash would be needed and pay it back at the end of the month in which cash becomes available. Therefore, 4 months of interest is due on the January borrowing, 3 on the February amount borrowed, and 2 on the March amount. The $417,300 should be divided into the amounts to pay back principal, interest due, and the remainder (R) that will stay in the cash account. Assume that the money was borrowed at 6 percent per year (0.5 percent per month).

The computation is:

$$Amount\ available = [\ Interest + principal] + R$$
$$\$417,300 = [\$10,688(0.005)4 + \$75,690(0.005)3 + \$284,644(0.005)2] +$$
$$\$371,424 + R$$
$$\$417,300 = [\$313.76 + \$1,135.35 + \$2,846.44] + \$371,424 + R$$
$$\$417,300 = \$4,296 + \$371,424 + R$$
$$R = \$417,300 - \$4,296 - \$371,424$$
$$Amount\ available \quad Interest \quad Principal\ repaid$$
$$R = \$41,580$$

In this situation, the entire accumulated principal plus the interest on that principal could be paid back and $41,580 would remain after allowing for the $500,000 minimum cash balance. The ending balance would, therefore, be $541,580 ($500,000 + $41,580). This would, of course, also be the beginning balance for May.

ANOTHER SITUATION Let us change the situation in order to look at a slightly different problem at the end of a month. At the end of April, the available cash may have enabled paying off part of the accumulated principal, but not all of it. Because we want to reduce our interest expense, we would probably want to pay back what we could. Assume that at the end of April the amount available for payback was $250,000, not $417,300. This would appear to be enough to cover January and February's borrowing, but not all of the money borrowed in March.

The interest on the January loan would be: 10,688(0.005)4 = $ 314
The interest on the February loan would be: 75,690(0.005)3 = $ 1,135
The accumulated principal through February is: $86,780
The total to be repaid for January and February loans is: $88,229

Remainder after paying off the debt from January and February would be:

$$\$250,000 - \$88,229 = \$161,771$$

This remainder would be available to pay back part of the March borrowing. The question is how much principal and interest can it cover. This remainder after paying off the previous month's borrowing must cover:

Some of the principal borrowed in March: P
The interest on that principal: (P)(interest rate per month)(number of months P was borrowed)

Therefore:

$$\$161,771.00 = P + P(0.005)(2)$$
$$\$161,771.00 = P + P(0.01)$$
$$\$161,771.00 = 1.01P$$
$$P = \$161,771.00/1.01$$
$$P = \$160,169.00$$

This means that the amount of principal remaining from the money borrowed in March would be reduced by $160,169 to $124,475 ($284,644 − $160,169). The ending balance for April would be the $500,000 held as the minimum balance before determining the amount available for pay back.

Summary

In summary, cash budgets furnish managers the information they need to plan for continuous liquidity within budget periods when there are nonmatching variations of cash inflows and obligations to make cash payments. Monthly cash budgeting generally meets this purpose. It enables management to inform short-term lenders the amount and timing of borrowing. This allows lenders to prepare for the support the organizations will need. Establishing a track record of accurate prediction of the organization's short-term needs and repayment dates also builds confidence in the organization's understanding of its business and environment. This confidence in the banking community can facilitate negotiating favorable short-term interest rates.

This example outlines the basic approach to preparing a cash budget. Realize that other cash flows an organization may experience can be built into the analysis. These could include such things as tax payments, dividend payments, stock sales, capital equipment purchases, and investment earnings. These flows can be fit into the monthly breakdown at the times they will occur. The object is to create a picture of the organization's liquidity over the operating budget period so that the organization is not surprised by a lack of needed cash. When economic shocks that affect the flow of cash occur, the cash budget can also indicate the extent of the shock's impact on liquidity and possibly indicate approaches to recovery.

CHAPTER 13   **COST-VARIANCE ANALYSIS**

LEARNING OBJECTIVES

After studying this chapter, students should be able to:

1. Explain the purpose for doing cost-variance analyses to include the concept of management by exception.

2. Explain the characteristics of cost targets that are appropriate for cost-variance analysis.

3. Compute direct and overhead cost variances.

4. Explain the management actions appropriate in response to each type of variance, favorable and unfavorable.

5. Explain how capacity variance is different from volume variance and why it is useful.

6. Explain the limitations in using cost-variance analysis in the control function.

INTRODUCTION

In the previous chapter, the general approach to budgetary control of operations was outlined:

- Plans are made for the next period's operations based on the organization's strategies.
- Standard costs are used to build operating budgets based on planned requirements for activities and the resources they demand.
- At the end of the period, actual costs are measured.
- The actual costs are compared to the budgeted expectation.
- Action is then taken to correct the budgets if they are too tight or too loose, to eliminate unfavorable performance, and to perpetuate favorable performance.

The concept of standard costs is very important. This is true, not simply because they are used in budgeting and cost center variance analyses, but because the concept of standards for the average resource use over large numbers of cases is becoming increasingly relevant to tactics for control of the cost of health care. As outcomes measurement becomes more precise, researchers will be able to analyze which care protocols produce better outcomes. This effort is underway and the examination and use of benchmark protocols are gaining advocates. As protocols of care become standardized and the costs of the activities called for in the protocols are measured, estimates of the cost of caring for categories of patients will become more accurate.

The differences between planned and actual results are called *variances*. Cost-variance analysis looks at the amounts spent in each of the four general categories of cost (direct materials, direct labor, variable overhead, and fixed overhead) and analyzes separate variances for each category according to potential causes of unexpected cost performance. Cost variances can be computed for any activity that produces countable units of like products. Variances are shorthand signals about the degree, in terms of dollars, that the period did not go as planned. They flag apparent problems (unfavorable variances) as well as points of good performance (favorable variances). Variances are information tools that support the concept of *management by exception*. This is the idea that, in repetitious functions that lend themselves to standard costing, managers need not continually intervene in the work of subordinates if they can receive signals as to when it is appropriate to look at some aspect of the work. That is, as a control tool, variance analysis allows managers to intervene only when there is an exception to expectations. Initially, intervention should be to see if the exception was indeed the result of performance. The next step is to diagnose what caused the variance. Finding the cause should then prompt action.

In summary, cost-variance analysis is a control tool to save time for managers at all levels by identifying unexpected results and instigating research into their cause. It does not, in itself, find these causes though it does narrow the search for them.

DISCUSSION QUESTIONS

1. How are standard costs of use to health care managers?
2. How are cost variances used by managers?
3. What is meant by management by exception? What is its relationship to variance analysis?

DIRECT COST VARIANCES

Intuitively, one understands that when the company produces more output than planned, costs will be higher than planned. Hence, volume variances would exist. This means one needs to consider that costs will vary with volume of output. One can formalize this reality by thinking in terms of flexible budgets, which recognize that there are fixed and variable components to total costs. Realize that flexible budgets cannot be constructed unless cost-behavior analysis has been done (as explained in the appendix to Chapter 3) to separate the variable and fixed components of the cost structure.

When considering direct costs, there are essentially three things that could have caused the actual costs to be different from those planned:

1. The organization could have produced more or less output than it had planned. Cost variances caused by this condition are called *volume variances*.
2. The organization could have used more of the variable cost resource than it should have for the output it produced. These conditions are called *efficiency variances*.
3. The organization could have paid prices for the variable resources that were different from the prices it planned to pay. These conditions are called *price variances*.

It is helpful to divide the total variance according to the three possibilities just described because they tend to be the responsibility of three different sets of managers. Volume variances come from mistakes in planning (forecasting) sales volume. This is primarily the responsibility of the marketing managers. Efficiency variances tend to be the responsibility of activity managers. Price variances tend to be the responsibility of the purchasing department for supplies and materials and the personnel department for labor, although they can also be caused by using inappropriate levels of personnel within production activities.

Direct Material Variances

Direct material variances can vary in volume, efficiency, and/or price. Each type of variance will be discussed in this section.

VOLUME VARIANCE   Variance analysis begins with analyzing budgeted amount for the specific cost category. If budgets are built using standard costs, the budgeted amount will be the cost that should be experienced at the volume of output that was planned. Suppose management plans to do 1,000 surgical procedures that should use one sterile instrument set per procedure, and the standard cost of a set is $80. If 1,050 procedures were done, an additional 50 sets would be needed and their standard cost would be $4,000 (50 × $80), more than the budget allowed. This logic can be expressed in the formula:

(Budgeted volume − actual volume) × standard price = Material volume variance

$$(1,000 - 1,050) \times \$80 = \$4,000)U$$

If the actual volume is greater than the planned volume, the variance will be negative. In the vocabulary of variance analysis, negative variances are called *unfavor-*

able variances because the cost is higher than expected. Unfavorable variance amounts are indicated by a 'U' suffix, favorable by an 'F.' However, volume variances are caused by producing more than was expected. If this additional volume is sold, this is not an unfavorable situation.

EFFICIENCY VARIANCE From the set standards, management knows how much of each material should be used for a unit of output. Multiplying the volume of output by the standard amount of input per unit tells them how much material should have been used for the volume that was produced. If more was used, inefficiency would appear to have existed. In the example, the 1,050 procedures actually done should have used 1,050 sterile instrument sets. If 1,210 sets were used, the usage would be 160 sets (1,050 − 1,210) more than it should have been. At standard prices, this would have caused a $12,800 unfavorable *efficiency* variance ([1,050 − 1,210] × $80/set). Efficiency variances are also called *usage* or *quantity variances*, for obvious reasons. This logic can be expressed in the formula:

(Standard usage for actual volume − actual usage) × Standard price = Material efficiency variance
(1,050 − 1,210) × $80 = 12,800U

Again, if the actual usage is more than the standard usage, the variance isunfavorable.

Note that in computing both the volume and efficiency variances, the differences in the amounts of material involved are transformed to dollar amount by multiplying them by the standard price for the material. These cost variances are caused by differences in amounts, not deviations from standard prices.

PRICE VARIANCE The material price variance considers cost variance caused by not purchasing at expected prices; it is simply the difference between the budgeted cost for materials actually used and the cost actually incurred. The computation is done similarly to the preceding variances. If the hospital actually paid an average price of $78 per set, the price was $2 dollars below the budgeted price. The price variance was, therefore, $2,420 = ([$80 − $78/set] × 1210 sets used) favorable. It is favorable because the actual cost was less than the budgeted cost. This logic can be expressed in the formula:

(Standard price − actual price) × units used = Material price variance
($80 − $78) × 1,210 = $2,420F

Price variance can also be computed based on the quantities of resources purchased. When this is done, the variance is the difference between the standard price for the quantity purchased (as opposed to the quantity used) and what was paid for the purchases. This is a reasonable approach because if exceptional performance occurs in purchasing resources during a period, it affects the quantity purchased not just the quantity used. However, because the price variance is based on a different quantity than the other two variances, the sum of the three variances will not equal the total difference between the budgeted variable costs and the cost paid for the variable resources used in the period of analysis.

In summary, note that the budgeted amount was

$$1,000 \text{ sets budgeted} \times \$80/\text{set standard} = \$80,000$$

The amount actually spent was

$$1,210 \text{ sets used} \times \$78/\text{set paid} = \$94,380U$$

Therefore, the total material variance was $14,380, unfavorable.

This total variance is the algebraic sum of the three component variances:

Volume variance $	4,000U	
Efficiency variance	12,800U	
Price variance	<u>4,240</u>	<u>$14,380U</u>

This variance analysis divides the total difference between the amount of cost budgeted and the amount experienced into three components. The volume variance is the difference between the cost of materials that should have been used for the planned volume of output and the cost that should have incurred, given the actual volume. These costs assume standard usage and standard price. The efficiency variance looks at the effect of not consuming material at the standard rate. It computes the difference between the amount of material that should have been used given the actual volume of output and the amount that was used. Both amounts are valued at the standard price. The price variance simply measures the difference between the amount that should have been spent of the material used and the amount that was spent.

Consider these variances the differences between the following sequence of costs:

Cost of planned volume of output at standard usage and standard prices
↑
Volume variance
↓
Cost of actual volume of output at standard usage and standard prices
↑
Efficiency variance
↓

Cost of actual usage at standard prices
↑
Price variance
↓
Cost of actual usage at prices paid
_____

Again, note that the only time the prices actually paid enter into the computation is in finding the price variance.

Direct Labor Variances

Direct labor variances are computed in the same way as direct material variance except the units of labor (labor hours) are used instead of units of materials. The volume, quantity, and price variance mean the same thing with reference to labor as they did for materials. In the case of direct labor, the price variance is often called the *wage rate variance*. This parallel is illustrated in the example shown here.

EXAMPLE
Direct Cost Variances Example

Changeover Dialysis Clinic produces a single product, a dialysis treatment. The following standards have been established for that treatment:

Disposable supplies:	1 set per treatment
	standard set price = $19.50
Technician time:	1.5 hrs
	standard wage rate = $15.00 per hr
Variable overhead rate:	$2.00 per technician hr
Fixed overhead rate:	$25.00 per technician hr

Note that technician hours are used as the driver of overhead cost.

The clinic planned to do 6,000 treatments during the year.

At the end of the year, records indicated that the clinic had done 7,100 treatments. It had used 7,650 supply sets and paid $153,000 for them. It had used 11,950 technician hours for which it paid $242,000. For the period, what were the:

  a. Direct material volume, quantity (efficiency), and price variances?
  b. Direct labor volume, quantity (efficiency), and price variances?

Direct Material

Volume variance:

$$6,000 \text{ treatments budgeted} \times 1 \text{ set/treatment} \times \$19.50/\text{set} = \$117,000$$
$$7,100 \text{ treatments performed} \times 1 \text{ set/treatment} \times \$19.50/\text{set} = \underline{\$138,450}$$
$$\text{Volume variance} = \$\ 21,450U$$

Quantity variance:

$$7,100 \text{ treatments performed} \times 1 \text{ set/treatment} \times \$19.50/\text{set} = \$138,450$$
$$7,650 \text{ sets used} \times \$19.50/\text{set} = \underline{\$149,175}$$
$$\text{Quantity variance} = \$\ 10,725U$$

Price variance:

$$7,650 \text{ sets used} \times \$19.50/\text{set} = \$149,175$$
$$\$153,000 \text{ spent} \quad \underline{\$153,000}$$
$$\text{Price variance} = \$\ 3,825U$$

Direct Labor

Volume variance:

$$6,000 \text{ treatments budgeted} \times 1.5 \text{ hrs/treatment } \$15/\text{hr} = \$135,000$$
$$7,100 \text{ treatments performed} \times 1.5 \text{ hrs/treatment} \times \$15/\text{hr} = \underline{\$159,750}$$
$$\text{Volume variance} = \$\ 24,750U$$

Quantity variance:

$$7,100 \text{ treatments performed} \times 1.5 \text{ hrs/treatment} \times \$15/\text{hr} = \$159,750$$
$$11,950 \text{ hrs used} \times \$15/\text{hr} = \underline{\$179,250}$$
$$\text{Quantity variance} = \$\ 19,500U$$

Price variance:

$$11,950 \text{ hrs used} \times \$15/\text{hr} = \$179,250$$
$$\$242,000 \text{ spent} = \underline{\$242,000}$$
$$\text{Price variance} = \$\ 62,750U$$

DISCUSSION QUESTIONS

1. What basic circumstances can cause direct cost variances?
2. Why are separate variances computed for materials and labor and overhead?
3. Why are volume, efficiency, and price variances computed for direct costs?
4. Why are price variances sometimes computed on the quantities purchased rather than quantities used?

OVERHEAD VARIANCES

We continue the analysis of cost by examining indirect, or overhead, costs. Again, these are costs that cannot be physically traced to the cost target but must be incurred in order for the targeted activity to take place. The somewhat subtle difference between direct and variable costs is very important. Realize that a direct cost to one target (the lab chief's salary as direct to the lab) may be an indirect cost to a more disaggregated target (the lab chief's salary as an indirect cost of a specific lab test).

At this point, a few additional perspective setting remarks may help. First, assume that management has established the amount of overhead cost that is incurred by a production department and is dividing that cost (allocating it) among the units of output of the department. They then add the allocated overhead to the direct costs of the output to arrive at its full cost. We discussed earlier how traditional accounting allocates the costs incurred by departments that do not produce billable line item to departments that do (step-down allocations), in order for all the costs of the organization to be incorporated into the full cost of the total array of billed products.

Second, management would like to know the "full cost" of each service, or output. If the total amount of overhead is known, products can be priced so that it is covered without creating the myth that there is a knowable "true cost" to the organization for producing any one product. Traditional cost finding is simply cost spreading. Costs are spread over the outputs so that if all prices are set at or above each full cost, all costs will be covered. However, in the short run, prices are determined in the marketplace. All that traditional full cost does is to establish a set of baselines. If the company drops one price below its full cost, it must raise another above it.

Third, realize that determining variable overhead rates demands cost-behavior analysis; fixed overhead rates reflect an arbitrary chopping of the total amount of fixed cost for the period into the number of output units over which it must be spread.

In considering overhead variances, first aggregate all the overhead costs that are estimated to be used by a center into that center's overhead pool. One then does a cost-behavior analysis of overhead costs to differentiate the fixed overhead of a period from the variable overhead per unit of an appropriate driver. The driver one would like is units of production. Remember that management wants to estimate future costs (budget), so the variable overhead rate should tell them how much more or less overhead will occur if the company has more or less production activity. Suppose the hospital does both appendectomies and open heart surgeries. It would be hard to believe that each of these services creates the same amount of overhead costs. If the company had different mixes of these surgeries from period to period, the variable cost per unit (VCU) result of regression analysis would be quite unstable. They would have a poor fit with a low R^2 statistic.

Management, therefore, tries to find another driver that correlates well with total overhead cost. This measure frequently turns out to be an input such as machine hours, direct labor hours, total labor hours, wages paid, and so forth. They find such a measure by considering what aspects of the service cause overhead in its production activity. The company treats these as potential drivers. Management then regresses total overhead cost on each of these potential drivers until finding one whose measure of fit (R^2) is high. They use this statistical result and acknowledge that, as the driver increases, the overhead cost will increase at a rate equal to the slope of the regression line. Also, the constant, "a," of the analysis is used as an estimate of average historical fixed overhead cost. This must be adjusted for changes known to affect the budget period. This produces a standard for variable overhead per unit of driver and future fixed overhead future per period. Management then acts as if the driver causes overhead expenses.

Variable Overhead Variances

As with direct costs, one could incur more variable overhead by producing a greater volume of output than planned; hence, one could have a variable overhead volume variance. The company could also suffer too much overhead cost because it used too much of the driver. This creates demand for overhead that should not have existed. This difference is called the *variable overhead (VOH) efficiency variance*. Realize that the efficiency reflected is not the efficiency of managing variable overhead costs but rather is the efficiency of managing the utilization of the driver. The company experienced more overhead because they used more of the driver of variable overhead than the standard amount for the output volume produced.

For each category of overhead and in any period, the company could also incur more variable overhead cost by buying (using) too many overhead resources (as opposed to units of the driver) in providing overhead services and or by paying too much for them. This difference is called a *spending variance*. The spending variance represents the efficiency of overhead managers in managing overhead costs, given the amount of the driver that production activities used. Realize that the volume and usage variances cannot be affected by the managers of overhead activities, but the spending variance, to a large degree, can. These variances may be more easily understood by the following example.

VOH EXAMPLE

Standards related to overhead:[*]

Standard units of driver per surgery	5 hrs
Standard rate VOH	$2.81/hr of suite use (from an overhead cost-behavior analysis)

Planned output	1,000 surgeries
Fixed overhead budgeted	$34,250/period
Output capacity of fixed costs resources	1,280 surgeries/period

Actual results were:

Output	1,012 surgeries
Hours actually used	5,473
VOH costs	$18,696.95
Fixed overhead costs	$32,000

*The overhead driver is surgical-suite usage in hours.

VOH VOLUME VARIANCE As with the other variable costs (direct labor and direct materials), one should expect variable overhead will be more than budgeted if the output is greater than budgeted. A difference in the overhead analysis is that the change in output volume must be converted to the change in the standard amount of the driver that it should induce.

In this example:

■ The 12 additional units of output should have caused 60 additional units of the driver (12 units $\times$ 5 hrs/unit).
■ These additional hours should have caused $168.60 of additional variable overhead (60 hrs $\times$ $2.81/hr).

This would be an unfavorable volume variance. Additional volume caused more to be spent than was budgeted.

The formula is:

$$\text{(Standard units of driver budgeted} - \text{standard driver units at actual output)}$$
$$\times \text{\$VOH/driver unit}$$
$$[(1{,}000 \text{ surgeries})(5 \text{ hrs/surgery}) - (1{,}012 \text{ surgeries})(5 \text{ hrs/surgery})] \times$$
$$\$2.81 \text{ VOH/hr} = \$168.60U$$

The volume variance is unfavorable because more units of the VOH driver were needed to support the actual volume than the planned volume.

VOH EFFICIENCY VARIANCE Creating too much demand (or less than expected) for overhead services causes a *VOH efficiency variance*. It is computed by multiplying the standard variable overhead rate by the difference between the amount of driver that should have been used to produce the actual output and the amount of the driver that was used. This amount is compared to the rate times the amount of basis that actually was used.

The formula is:

(Driver units that should have been used given the output −
driver units used) × $VOH/driver unit
[(1,012 units × 5 hrs per unit at standard) − 5,473 hrs used] ×
$2.81/hr = $1,160.5U

The efficiency variance is unfavorable because more overhead-causing suite time was used than the standard for the surgeries done.

VOH SPENDING VARIANCE Spending too much on VOH to provide overhead services induced by the quantity of the overhead driver that actually occurs causes a *VOH spending variance*. This is the difference between the amount spent on VOH items and the amount that should have been spent given the quantity of the overhead-causing driver faced by overhead managers. The latter is the standard VOH rate times the amount driver that occurred. This variance can be caused by paying too much for overhead resources or using an excessive amount of resources. Unlike the volume or efficiency variance, this variance is the responsibility of the managers of overhead activities.

The formula is:

(Amount of driver used × $VOH/driver) − amount spent on VOH =
VOH spending variance
(5,473 hrs × $2.81/hr) − $18,696.95 = $3,317.82U

This spending variance is unfavorable because the VOH cost was more than the amount that should have resulted from the amount of the driver used.

Fixed Overhead Cost Variances

FIXED OVERHEAD VOLUME VARIANCE Fixed overhead (FOH) is unrelated to the volume of output in the budgeted period and will not change as output volume changes. Hence, there is no additional overhead cost or savings by producing more or less than budgeted. An exception is when output is raised to the point that fixed cost resources must be added. This rarely is done within an accounting period without having been planned beforehand. Therefore, FOH volume variances do not occur in management accounting.

When standard cost systems are used in financial accounting, FOH is added to inventory cost throughout the period as the inventory is produced. The FOH portion is added at a rate equal to the budgeted FOH amount divided by the planned output (or planned amount of the driver). If there is more or less output produced than was planned, too much or too little FOH will have been added to inventory. These errors must be corrected by subtracting or adding them to the inventory balance as an adjustment when closing the books for the period. These adjustments are also called *FOH volume variances*. They are irrelevant to management accounting.

FOH SPENDING VARIANCE For FOH, the spending variance is an extremely simple concept. It is the difference between what was budgeted for fixed costs and what was spent. It is unrelated to the activity measurement because fixed costs are unrelated to activity levels. Because overhead is a mixture of various expenses under various managers, the spending variance is, in effect, a combination of an efficiency and a price variance. It is generally caused by contracts that incur fixed costs being renewed within the period at amounts that were not expected. Consider, for instance, a contract for salaried labor at wages higher than were planned.

Assume the FOH was budgeted at $3,425 and 1,280 units could be produced with the fixed resources available. Assume $2,191 was actually spent for these resources.

The fixed overhead spending variance would be:

$$\$3,525 \text{ budgeted} - \$2,191 \text{ spent} = \$1,234F.$$

FOH CAPACITY VARIANCE The FOH capacity variance is more abstract than the others because it deals with the fact that if fixed-cost resources are not used at their capacity, more production could have been done without an increase in fixed costs. One can say that the cost of the portion of these resources' potential output that was not used was wasted. This is called the *capacity variance*.

Using the fixed-cost data just established:

- Capacity is 1,280 units at a standard cost of $3,425 or $3,425/1,280 = $2.676/unit.
- Underutilization was 1,280 units at capacity − 1,012 units made = 268 units.
- The capacity variance was, therefore, 268 units × $2.676/unit = $717.11.

The variance is unfavorable, because any time the full capacity is not used, money is wasted.

A Complete Overhead Variance Analysis Example

The PT Clinic provides the following information on its overhead costs for 2002:

Direct therapist hours (DTH) planned	100,000 hrs
Standard DTH rate	2hrs/session
Standard VOH rate	$3 per DTH
Total planned overhead cost	$500,000
Clinic capacity	62,500 sessions
Therapy sessions provided	48,000
DTH used	97,000
Actual FOH cost	$202,000
Actual VOH cost	$297,000

Required: Compute the VOH volume, efficiency, and spending variances and the FOH spending and capacity variances.

VOH Variances

Volume variance:

$$100,000 \ DTH \ budgeted \times \$3/DTH = \$300,000$$
$$48,000 \ sessions \ provided \times 2 \ DTH/session \times \$3/DTH = \underline{\$288,000}$$
$$Volume \ variance = \$ \ 12,000F$$

Efficiency variance:

$$48,000 \ sessions \ provided \times 2 \ DTH/session \times \$3/DTH = \$288,000$$
$$97,000 \ DTH \ used \times \$3/DTH = \underline{\$291,000}$$
$$Efficiency \ variance = \$ \ 3,000U$$

Spending variance:

$$97,000 \ DTH \ used \times \$3/DTH = \$291,000$$
$$(\ Spent \ ) \ \underline{\$297,000}$$
$$Spending \ variance = \$ \ 6,000U$$

FOH Variances

Capacity Variance:

FOH Rate at capacity = $200,000 / 62,500 sessions = $3.20/session
Capacity used = $3.20/session (48,000 sessions provided) = $153,600
Therefore, FOH Capacity Variance was $200,000 − $153,600 = $46,400.

This indicates that $47,000 of fixed-cost assets were available for production but were not used.

Spending Variance:[*]

If 100,000 DTH were planned, and the standard VOH rate is $3/DTH
Total budgeted VOH was $300,000
If total budgeted overhead was $500,000
Therefore, budgeted FOH must have been $200,000
Therefore, FOH spending variance was:
$200,000 budgeted − $202,000 spent = $2,000.

LIMITATIONS

Budget variance analysis has been criticized for being inflexible and overly negative in its approach; inflexible because it does not recognize changes in the operating environment during the budgeted period and negative because it is used to locate inefficiencies, so that managers can correct (reprimand) guilty workers. Both these complaint can be warranted if cost-variance information is not used properly.

Cost-variance reports allow managers to practice *management by exception* for routine activities with countable, standardize outputs. It is these types of activities for which standard costs can be established for periods in which technology is not expected to change. It is important to remember that cost variances do *not* identify the part of the organization in which a problem (or unusually good performance) exists. They save management time by identifying the centers that are the most probable source of a problem, and therefore, the first place to look when trying to correct them. A brief example should illustrate this point. A diagnostic radiology laboratory might have extremely large unfavorable material and labor usage variances. At the same time, the purchasing center could have a highly favorable price variance. If management assumes that errors have been made in the laboratory and demands an explanation of the inefficiency from the laboratory director, great harm could be done to morale in the lab and future working relationships. This would be the case if it were later found that inferior materials had been purchased to save purchase costs and that this material caused many test to be repeated. Management would, at best, be embarrassed if it complimented the purchasing center on its favorable price variances before inquiring into the unfavorable material usage variance. A rule of thumb in using cost-variance reports is to always allow the management of a center with a significant unfavorable variance to explain them before criticizing the center's performance.

A related issue is determining how large a variance must be before management intervenes to investigate its cause. Because so many things affecting costs vary randomly, one cannot expect to hit the budget exactly. There will always be some variance from expectations. If it is uncontrollable, over time it should vary between favorable and unfavorable in reasonable amounts. What amount is reasonable is a management judgment. However, a steady trend of increasing size in a variance almost always warrants investigation.

DISCUSSION QUESTIONS

1. Why should VOH and FOH cost variances be analyzed separately?
2. Why is a fixed cost volume variance meaningless in management accounting?
3. What information is conveyed in the capacity variance?
4. Whose performance is reflected in the VOH spending variance?
5. What efficiency does the VOH efficiency variance measure? Who is responsible for this variance?

Key Points

- Cost-variance analysis requires standard costs for inputs to countable outputs.
- Cost variances assist managers in locating activities whose financial results are not as planned. They identify the possible existence of a problem and suggest the first place to look for it. They thereby support management by exception.

- Cost variances do not identify the location of operational problems with certainty.
- Direct cost variances from budgets can be caused by the volume of output, the efficiency of the resource used, or the prices paid for resources not being as planned.
- Volume variance is caused by errors in

sales forecasts.
- Efficiency variances generally are the responsibility of activity managers.
- Material price variances are generally the responsibility of the purchasing activity and labor price variances are generally the responsibility of the personnel department or scheduling activity.
- Standard VOH rates are generally determined by regressing overhead costs on the appropriate driver, as done in cost-behavior analysis. The results of the regression analysis on historic data should be adjusted for changes in overhead resource costs foreseen for the period of the budgeting.
- Resource drivers can be used for overhead costs when VOH analysis done by regressing costs on units of output gives poor R^2 results.
- VOH volume variance measures errors in

sales forecast, as do direct cost volume variances.
- VOH efficiency variances measure the efficiency of the use of the driver/basis, not the efficiency of managing overhead activities.■
- VOH spending variances reflect on the efficiency of providing overhead activities.
- The FOH spending variance indicates the degree to which FOH was not as planned.
- The FOH capacity variance indicates the amount of fixed resource expenses that were wasted by not using the resources to capacity. It measures the cost of overcapacity.
- How large a variance must be before it triggers management intervention is a matter of management judgment.

EXERCISES

PROBLEM 1

DIRECT COST VARIANCES

Hill Diagnostics prepares its budgets on the basis of standard costs. A responsibility report is prepared monthly showing the differences between the master budget and actual costs. In addition to reporting material price variances on the material used, material price variances are also computed on the amounts purchased.

The following information relates to the current month:

Standard cost per diagnosis:

Direct material:	1 film at $10/film
Direct labor:	2 hrs at $14/hr

Planned number of diagnoses per month: 2,000
Actual data for the month:

Material purchased:	3,000 films at $9.45/film
Material used:	2,100 films at $9.45/film
Labor used:	3,200 hours at $15/hour
Diagnoses done:	1,900

Required: Compute the volume, quantity, and price variances for the direct materials and labor.

Answers:

DM volume	$1,000F	DL volume	2,800F
DM quantity	2,000U	DL quantity	8,400F

DM price   used   DL price   3,200U
            1,155F
            Purchased $1,650F

PROBLEM 2

OVERHEAD COST VARIANCES

Klean Company produces prosthetic devices and applies manufacturing overhead using standard direct labor hours. The company estimated that it would take 36,000 standard direct labor hours to produce 7,200 devices during 2004. At the 7,200 unit level, which is its capacity, the budgeted manufacturing overhead is:

Variable portion	$ 50,400
Fixed portion	$162,000
Total	$212,400

Actual production during 2004 was 7,000 devices and 36,000 direct labor hours with the following actual costs:

Variable manufacturing overhead	$ 52,300
Fixed manufacturing overhead	163,000
Total	$215,300

Required: Compute the standard overhead cost variances.

FOH Variances:

FOH spending variance: $ 1,000 U
FOH capacity variance $ 4,500 U
Hint: Capacity rate computes to $22.50/device

VOH Variances:

VOH volume variance	$1,400 F
VOH efficiency variance	400 U
VOH spending variance	$1,900 U

PROBLEM 3

GENERAL COST-VARIANCE ANALYSIS

Med-Sup, Inc., makes one product, IV supply sets. The following events took place last month.

Produced and sold	50,000 sets
Direct materials purchased	110,000 lbs at $1.20/lb
Direct materials used	110,000 lbs
Direct labor	6,000 hrs at $14/hr
VOH	$28,000
FOH	$83,000

Standard variable costs per set were:

Direct materials	2 lbs at $1/lb
Direct labor	0.1 hrs at $15/hr
VOH	0.1 DLH/set at $5/DLH
Planned fixed overhead	$80,000
Planned production	42,000 sets
Capacity	55,000 sets

Required: Compute volume, quantity, and price variances for the direct costs; efficiency and spending variances for VOH; and the spending variance for FOH.

Answers:

DM volume $16,000U	DL volume 12,000U
DM quantity 10,000U	DL quantity15,000U
DM price 22,000U	DL Price 6,000F
VOH volume 4,000U	FOH spending 3,000U
VOH efficiency 5,000U	FOH capacity 7,273U
VOH spending 2,000F	

LEARNING OBJECTIVES

1. Explain the concepts of unit, product, and total contributions.

2. Explain why revenue variances can be analyzed by analyzing contributions rather than profits.

3. Explain the information contained in market size, market share, product mix, and sales price variances.

REVENUE AND CONTRIBUTION

One assumes the deviations from planned profit that are caused by variations from planned costs are captured in cost variances. This leaves the revenue component of profit as the second potential cause of unexpected profit variation. Because cost variances are analyzed separately, when computing revenue variances resource use and costs are assumed to be at standard amounts for the output produced. The significance of this assumption is more clear when one looks at the relationship among cost, volume of output, and profit:

$$Profit = \sum_{i=1}^{n} (P_i - VC_i)Q_i - FC$$

Where: P = price

VC = variable cost

FC = fixed cost

i = subscript for specific saleable outputs

One assumes that the variable costs for each product are at their standard amounts because cost variances are analyzed separately, as discussed in Chapter 11. Therefore, the only thing that can affect the $(P_i - VC_i)$ quantity is changes in output prices. The quantity $(P_i - VC_i)Q_i$ is called the *contribution* of the product. Because the costs are assumed to be the standard amounts, the contribution will change only if the price or sales quantity changes—and profit will change only with changes in contribution. Fixed cost can, therefore, be dropped from the equation when examining *changes* in profit. These facts allow revenue variances to be analyzed by examining changes in the sum of the contributions across products sold. The underlying formula reduces to:

$$Total\ contribution = \sum_{i=1}^{n} (P_i - VC_i)Q_i$$

Where: P = price
VC = variable cost
Q = Quantity sold
i = subscript for specific product

If only one type of product was made and sold, the variable cost amount would not be needed, and revenue effects on profit could be measured by considering only prices and the volumes of products sold. However, if many different products are sold, profit for a period can vary because of the relative volume of different products and the fact that each has a different contribution.

CAUSES OF PROFIT VARIANCES

There are four revenue (or sales-related factors) that could make the profit diverge from the budgeted amount. The first two factors can create a difference between the budgeted and actual volume of sales.

1. The market demand could have been different from that estimated for the period.
2. The organization's share of the market could have differed from expectations.
3. Assuming that different products have different contributions, the mix of products could have been different from that expected.
4. Sales prices could have been different from those expected.

If market analyses are made primarily by projecting changes in the organization's historic volume of output, the first two conditions are analyzed together. Management simply says that the organization's market demand was different from expected.

REVENUE VARIANCES

To separate revenue variances caused by from these different factors, the following computations are made:

Market Size Variance

Step 1. Total contribution is computed using the expected market demand, expected share of the market, standard contributions ($P_i - VC_i$), and the expected product quantities Q_i. This is the *budgeted contribution*. The expected relative quantities of different products constitute the expected product mix. One first assumes the expected mix. This means that the budgeted contribution of each output must be multiplied by that output's expected quantity, and these product contributions summed.

Step 2. Next, the contribution is computed as in Step 1 except that the *actual* markets demand it used instead of the expected one. The expected share of the market and product mix is still used. The difference between Steps 1 and 2 is the *market size variance*.

Market Share Variance

Step 3. Total contribution is then computed using the actual market size and the organization's actual *share* of the market. The expected product mix is still used. The difference between Steps 2 and 3 is caused by the organization's share of the market not being as expected. This is called the *market share variance.*

If total demand and share of the market are not known, expected demand is compared to the actual demand in one step. Market size and market share variances are merged into an *organization demand* (or *output volume*) *variance,* as in the example that follows. The contribution from the *expected* demand, prices, and mix is compared with the contribution from the *actual* demand at expected prices and mix.

Product Mix Variance

Step 4. To compute the product (or service) mix variance, total contribution is computed using the actual quantities of each product. This reflects the actual mix. Product contributions are still computed using standard sales prices. The *product mix variance* is the difference between the contributions computed in Steps 3 and 4.

Sales Price Variance

Step 5. Finally, the computation made in Step 4 is repeated except actual sales prices are used rather than the expected prices. The difference between the amount computed in Steps 4 and 5 is the *sales price variance.* It is, of course, important to distinguish between sales price variance and cost variances due to prices paid *for* resources.

EXAMPLE

The situation:

1. Don't know the market demand.
2. Don't know the organization's share of the market.
3. Do know the planned output by product.
4. Do know the actual output by product.
5. Do know the planned and actual sales prices. Therefore, one knows the contributions, given the standard variable costs for each product.
6. The products are discharges categorized by DRG. The total output was in three DRGs.
7. The planned volume of cases was 500.
8. Contributions were DRG1: $500/case; DRG2: $200/case; and DRG3: $400/case.
9. Planned mix was DRG1: 50 percent; DGR2: 30 percent; and DRG3: 20 percent.
10. Actual volume was 450 cases.

Contributions were DRG1: $475/case; DRG2: $250/case; and DRG3: $470/case.

The mix was DRG1: 65 percent; DRG2: 20 percent; and DRG3: 15 percent.

Solution:

1. Budgeted contribution: Budgeted sales volume at budgeted mix × budgeted contribution

$$DRG\ 1: 500p \times .50 \times \$500/p = \$125,000$$
$$DRG\ 2: 500p \times .30 \times \$200/p = \$30,000$$
$$DRG\ 3: 500p \times .20 \times \$400/p = \underline{\$40,000}$$
$$\$195,000$$

2. Budgeted contribution at actual volume: Actual volume at budgeted mix × budgeted contribution

$$DRG\ 1: 450p \times .50 \times \$500/p = \$112,500$$
$$DRG\ 2: 450p \times .30 \times \$200/p = \$27,000$$
$$DRG\ 3: 450p \times .20 \times \$400/p = \underline{\$36,000}$$
$$\$175,500$$

Answer for Market demand (or volume) variance:

$$\$195,000 - \$175,500 = \$19,500 \ U$$

Actual demand was less than budgeted demand.

3. Budgeted contribution at actual volume and actual mix: Actual volume at actual mix $\times$ budgeted contribution

$$DRG \ 1: 450p \times .65 \times \$500/p = \$146,250$$
$$DRG \ 2: 450p \times .20 \times \$200/p = \$ \ 18,000$$
$$DRG \ 3: 450p \times .15 \times \$400/p = \underline{\$ \ 27,000}$$
$$\$191,250$$

Answer for Sales mix variance:
$$\$175,500 - \$191,250 = \$15,750 \ F$$

4. Actual contribution: Actual volume at actual mix $\times$ actual contribution

$$DRG \ 1: 450p \times .65 \times \$475/p = \$138,938$$
$$DRG \ 2: 450p \times .20 \times \$250/p = \$ \ 22,500$$
$$DRG \ 3: 450p \times .15 \times \$470/p = \underline{\$ \ 31,725}$$
$$\$193,163$$

Sales price variance:

$$\$191,250 - \$193,163 = \$1,913 \ F$$

Note that this difference in contributions must be due to differences in sales prices because the standard variable cost per DRG was used in all of the computations.

In this example, the overall revenue variance was $1,837 U ($195,000 − $193,163). The most significant cause was the fact that the volume of cases was 10 percent lower than expected. With everything else as expected, this would have caused a $19,500 revenue shortfall. However, this demand shortfall was partially compensated by the facts that the actual mix contained a greater proportion of high contribution DRGs and the prices received on two of the products were higher than expected. This should lead management to investigate whether more emphasis should be put into general promotion and advertising and the degree of sensitivity of specific categories of admissions to pricing.

CHAPTER 14

CLASSICAL COST-BASED DECISION MODELS

LEARNING OBJECTIVES

After studying this chapter, students should be able to:

1. Explain the use of contributions in analyzing changes to profits when operations are changed.

2. Explain the use of cost-volume-profit models to solve short-run operating choice problems.

3. Explain the relationships among marginal, relevant, and sunk costs.

4. Explain why money has a time value and how that makes decisions to buy expensive long-term assets different from other expansion decisions.

5. Solve short-term choice problems using cost-volume-profit and contribution analysis.

INTRODUCTION

Cost factors relevant to a specific decision must be interpreted according to the specific operating situation at hand. Collecting and using measurements appropriate to making specific decisions demands an incremental perspective. A decision should be analyzed at the *margin* of current activity. Measurements should answer the question: What will be the additional revenue and additional cost if a specific decision is made? If, when considering both short-run and long-run effects, the additional revenues are greater than the additional costs, the decision is most likely a sound one. The challenge is to make accurate estimates of the future marginal revenues and costs resulting from a decision. When choosing among alternative actions, decisions rest on the marginal profitability of the alternatives available.

Analysis of revenue is more closely related to marketing than to accounting. *Revenue* is the sum of the price charged for each product times the quantity sold. Variation among these factors is the content of economics analysis of decision situations. This book focuses on measuring and understanding the behavior of costs. It will assume that market analysts have produced appropriate sales information.

MARGINAL, RELEVANT, AND SUNK COSTS

Many short-term marginal analyses hinge on whether particular cost is or is not marginal. The emphasis on marginal costs focuses on decisions that have to do with choices among alternatives. Choosing any of an array of alternatives will most likely change the income from its current level. From a financial perspective, this change is the issue with which the organization is primarily concerned. This difference can be called the *alternative's marginal profit*. Because it is dependent only on marginal costs and marginal revenue, only the marginal costs are *relevant costs* in the decision process.

If an alternative involves producing a good or service, all the variable costs of the output are marginal costs. By definition, if the organization can make one more unit of the product, its variable cost is added to the total cost. (Problems come in being sure that specific costs are or are not marginal.) We have already mentioned the importance of determining whether labor is a fixed or a variable cost. We must also determine whether specific fixed costs are marginal to the alternatives under consideration. If a fixed-cost resource will no longer be needed as the organization changes products or procedures, it is marginal to the alternative and therefore relevant to the decision. Taking the alternative will eliminate that cost. Conversely, if a previously unneeded fixed-cost resource must be acquired, its cost is marginal to the alternative. It must be added.

There is a special type of fixed cost that is not relevant to decisions but is especially troublesome to managers. It is not troublesome because it is hard to classify as irrelevant to a choice, but, rather, because it is sometimes hard to admit that it is irrelevant. These are *sunk costs*. Suppose a hospital has just paid cash for an expensive piece of equipment. One month after its installation, a new type of equipment comes on the market that will produce much better outcomes at a lower cost. Physicians are so impressed by this new piece of equipment that they will not admit some types of patients to a hospital that does not have it. Therefore, the choice is to keep the old equipment and radically lower revenue from the procedures that use it or buy the new equipment, thereby increasing cost but maintaining (or perhaps increasing) the current number of cases served. Whether or not the newer equipment is purchased, the cost of the older equipment will not change. It has already been experienced, though it has not been expensed (depreciated). It cannot be recovered; it is sunk. The issue with reference to replacing the older equipment is simply a comparison of future revenue and future cost if new equipment is purchased as opposed to if it is not. Note that the sunk cost of an asset is the cost that cannot be recovered. If the asset has some salvage value, only the amount not salvageable is sunk.

CATEGORIES OF MARGINAL COST PROBLEMS

There are five common categories of problems for which marginal cost analysis is helpful. These are operations changes, price discounting, outsourcing, dropping products, and adding products. The specific costs that are relevant to these problems depend on the specific situation at hand.

DISCUSSION QUESTIONS

1. What makes a cost marginal? In what circumstances are the differences between marginal costs and cost figures for financial accounting purposes important?
2. What makes a cost relevant to a decision?
3. Why are sunk costs not relevant to decisions?

THE COST-VOLUME-PROFIT MODEL

Cost-volume-profit (C-V-P) problems involve short-term changes in operations. To determine whether a suggested new approach to operating is an improvement, the marginal changes in profit under the revised situation are computed. If the profit from the revised situation is higher than the current profit, the change is probably desirable.

We have explored the concept of cost behavior and realized that, for an accounting period, some costs will vary as output varies and some will not. The former are called variable costs; the latter fixed costs. One should note that most fixed costs are the result of past purchases of long-term assets and contractual arrangements such as rental agreements and labor contracts. The important implication is that, in order to produces anything, a certain level of fixed cost must be incurred.

In addition to fixed costs, variable costs must also be incurred. The total of these variable costs will increase as the volume of output increases. Such things as supplies, labor that is paid only when it is producing, and the cost of VOH activities are variable costs. The natural measure of variable costs is dollars per unit of output. Obviously, if every item that is produced causes a specific amount of cost, total production cost will vary from period to period as the output varies among periods. If one assumes that the variable cost per unit is the same at any level of production, the total cost for a period can be expressed as it is in Figure 14-1.

Referring to Figure 14-1, revenue in a one-product business would be the product's price times the quantity of the product sold during the period. Where price is P, and Q is the quantity sold, revenue can be expressed as:

$$Revenue = P(Q)$$

Revenue for any output volume, Q, is represented by the heavy line. Because profit is the revenue minus cost, algebraically profit can be expressed as:

$$\begin{aligned} Profit &= Revenue - total\ cost \\ &= P(Q) - [VC_u(Q) + FC] \\ &= (P - VC_u)Q - FC \end{aligned}$$

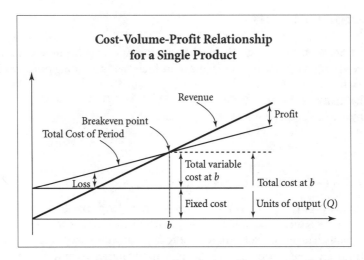

Figure 14-1 **Cost-Volume-Profit Relationship for a Single Product**

Where:

VC_u = Variable cost per unit of output

FC = Fixed cost per period

This form of the profit equation highlights some interesting relationships among profit, price, and the two components of total cost, variable costs and fixed costs. The difference between the price and the variable cost per unit of output is called the *unit contribution*. If one multiplies the unit contribution by the quantity of units produced and sold, $(P - VC_u)Q$, we get what can be called the *product's contribution*. The question is: Contribution to what? If one manipulates the equation slightly, the answer is obvious.

$$(P - VC_u)Q = Profit + FC$$

The product contribution goes to covering the fixed cost and profit. Obviously, the fixed cost must be covered before profit exists. However, after achieving a volume of sales whose contribution is great enough to cover the fixed cost, the contribution from all the following sales is profit. If one knows any four of the variables in this last equation, one can compute the fifth. Management can use the equation to solve several types of short-term problems.

Breakeven Analysis

Breaking even means that the organization neither makes a profit nor loses money. In other words, the profit is zero. If management knows their price, variable cost, and fixed cost, they can compute the level of sales necessary to break even. This is the volume of sales that must be reached before beginning to be profitable. To do this, enter the known variables in the equation, substituting zero for profit and solve for Q. Similarly, if management knows the costs and the quantity the organization can produce and sell, they can solve for the breakeven price. This is the minimum price that must be received so as not to lose money. These breakeven amounts are useful in considering the feasibility of new products or production processes.

As previously discussed, breakeven analysis is a target analysis where the target profit is zero. Breakeven is thus a special case of target analysis.

Target Analysis

Given the amount of profit that is expected from a product, the equation on page 306 allows one to see what combinations of price, costs, and sales would achieve the profit target. Examples follow.

EXAMPLES

A fitness center has leased space on the ground floor of a medical arts building and is promoting wellness and prevention with its programs. The fitness center has measured the following costs from its most recent experience:

Membership price per month: $95   Variable cost per month: $18/member
Fixed cost per month: $120,000   Last month's client volume: 1,400
Capacity: 4,000 members
Last month's profit: − $12,200 (a loss)

Example 1: Breakeven Quantity

At this cost structure, how many clients must the center have in order to breakeven?

$$Zero = (P - VC_w)Q - FC$$
$$= (\$95 - \$18)Q - \$120,000$$
$$0 = \$77Q - \$120,000$$
$$Q = 120,000/77 = 1,559 \; members$$
$$(assume \; no \; fractions)$$

A rational question to ask the center's marketing staff is: Can they get a clientele materially larger than 1,559 members?

Example 2: Breakeven Price

If the marketing staff contends that the sales staff can reasonably expect to sell 1,500 memberships, what price must be charged in order to breakeven?

$$
\begin{aligned}
\text{To breakeven:} \\
Zero &= (P - VC_u)Q - FC \\
0 &= (\$P - \$18) \times (\$1{,}500 - \$120{,}000) \\
0 &= \$1{,}500P - \$27{,}000 - 120{,}000 \\
\$1{,}500P &= \$147{,}000 \\
P &= \$98 \text{ per member/month}
\end{aligned}
$$

Example 3: Target Profit

Let's assume the marketing staff wants to make a profit of $20,000 per month. To reach this target profit, set the profit variable at $20,000.

$$
\begin{aligned}
\$20{,}000 &= (P - VC_u)Q - FC \\
&= (\$P - \$18) \times (\$1{,}500 - \$120{,}000) \\
&= \$1{,}500P - \$27{,}000 - \$120{,}000 \\
\$1{,}500P &= \$147{,}000 \\
P &= \$147{,}000/1{,}500 \\
P &= \$98 \text{ per member/month}
\end{aligned}
$$

Example 4: Cost and Price Changes

A business relation's consultant tells you that if you spend an additional $10,000 per month to increase the luxury of the facility and lower the price to $70 per month, he can find employers who will guarantee an additional 800 members. Should this be done? If it is:

$$Profit = (P - VC_u)Q - FC$$
$$= (\$70 - \$18) \times \$2,200 - \$130,000$$
$$= \$52(\$2,300) - \$130,000$$
$$= \$114,400 - \$130,000$$
$$= -\$10,400$$

Compared to the last month's results, this is even worse. A follow-on question for the marketers would be: Can you reach a volume under this price/cost arrangement that would yield a $20,000 per month profit? To do that, the volume must be:

$$\$20,000 = (\$70 - \$18)Q - \$130,000$$
$$\$52Q = \$150,000$$
$$Q = 2,885 \ members$$

Can we expect a market of 2,885 members at a price of $70 per month? If we cannot, a $20,000 profit is impossible at that price.

C-V-P Exploration

This type of probing around the C-V-P relationship allows decision makers to analyze the results of various assumptions about the market and the product. It is dependent on managers understanding their cost structure (their variable versus fixed costs) and the demand for the product in question. The quality of the decisions to which these models lead is no better than the accuracy of the assumptions that are used.

C-V-P analysis is considered a short-term tool because it assumes that the variables will remain at the same values over an unspecified number of future periods. This is usually only the case for a short number of periods. It also assumes that there are no additional large investments necessary that would incur opportunity costs by tying up capital. This is often not the case for major changes in an organization's products or its production processes.

DISCUSSION QUESTIONS

1. Because we realize that any organization without readily available charity or grant support must make an accounting profit in order to survive, why are we interested in breakeven analysis?
2. What must be known about a product in order to find its breakeven point?
3. Why is C-V-P analysis considered a short-term tool?

Price Discounting

Price discounting is really a special case of the short-term operations C-V-P analysis. We have seen that for each product

$$Profit = (P - VC_u)Q - FC$$

However, analysis of the total fixed costs (FC) may indicate that some parcels of these costs can be eliminated if a specific product or product line is dropped. Figures associated with a specific product line are given a subscript; the general subscript indicator is "i." Across an organization's products, total profit would be the sum of the contributions from each product line less the remaining allocated fixed costs.

A product line contribution can be expressed as:

$$Contribution_i = [(price_i - variable\ cost\ per\ unit_i) \times sales\ quantity_i] - fixed\ cost_i$$
$$= (\ unit\ contribution_i \times sales\ quantity_i) - fixed\ cost_i$$
$$= Product\ contribution_i - fixed\ cost_i$$
$$Total\ contribution\ from\ product_i$$

$$Total\ profit = \sum_{i=1}^{n} (Product_i\ contribution) - (total\ allocated\ fixed\ costs)$$

Where $\sum_{i=1}^{n}$ means the sum of the product contributions over "n" different products, which can be named Product 1, 2, and so forth to Product n.

The issue is, if prices to specific purchasers are discounted, will total profits be increased? In this situation, one assumes that neither variable cost per unit of output nor fixed cost is changed by the discounted sale. This implies that, without these sales, the producer has excess capacity. Therefore, as long as the discounted price is higher than the variable cost per unit, profit is increased by the amount of that difference. As noted earlier, the difference is called the *unit contribution*. As shown in the equation, a product's unit contribution times the number of units of the product sold is called the *product contribution*. The sum of all the product contributions is the organization's *total contribution*. The mathematics of price discounting are rather simple, but the marketing and revenue aspects are not. Before an organization accepts a payer's offer to raise its total sales volume by selling at a discounted price, management should consider at least three factors:

1. Will the reduced price provide an adequate contribution from the additional sales?
2. If other customers hear of the discounted sales (and such things are extremely difficult to keep secret), will they also demand the same discount or buy elsewhere? If this is the case, profit might drop, perhaps even turn to a loss.

3. Will the increased sales volume cause an increased need for fixed-cost assets? If this is the case, profit will be lowered by the amount of fixed-cost increase necessary. This could perhaps wipe out the additional contribution.

Excess capacity and the purchasing power of third-party payers have made these factors important in the health care industry. HMOs, government payment programs, and casualty insurers have played providers against each other to gain significant discounts. This has happened to the extent that *list* (or *charge master*) *prices* are almost meaningless, because few pay them. The only prices that are meaningful to financial viability are the contracted sales prices. These negotiated prices in the case of managed care organizations (or "allowed charges" in the case of the Medicare and Medicaid programs), which are often expressed in terms of a discount from the list prices. These discounted prices are the amounts that are collectable by law or by regulatory authority. (In health care accounting, the discount is commonly called *contractual allowance*.) The gross charges, which are the sums of list prices, are not collectable and do not constitute revenue according to law or to GAAP. Although, mathematically, an organization is better off if it can get some contribution from an additional sale, it must carefully investigate the follow-on consequences of discounted prices. When the total capacity of health care resources within a region is well-matched to the demand, payers for care lose much of the bargaining power that now allows them to achieve purchase prices that produce low, or negative, contributions. When a community's health care resources are being used near their capacities, buyers can no longer successfully threaten to take their business elsewhere if the discount they demand is not met. There is no elsewhere.

At times, the use of *loss leaders* (the technique of selling a few products at a loss in order to access customers who will also buy other, more profitable, services) may be wise. However, outside this tactic, providers must be sure that discounts do not lower prices below the variable cost of production. Obviously, producers cannot protect against this unless they know the variable cost of the products. When a provider is under extreme price pressure and has excess capacity, any price that produces a contribution will, in the short run, improve profit. In the long run, of course, prices must be high enough on average to produce contributions that also cover fixed costs, or there will be no profit.

Example 5: Price Discounting

A company has installed an ABC system that provides cost data on their high-volume, high-cost DRGs. The company has developed a reputation for high quality care on a specific DRG and has significant excess capacity in resources used to care for patients in this DRG. A managed care organization (MCO) approaches the provider to negotiate a price per admission to care for all of its members who would be in this DRG. Cost measurements indicate that, at the current volume of 1,100 patients, fixed cost is $6,000 per patient with the variable cost at $2,000 per patient. This is a total cost per patient of $8,000. The current remuneration is $8,700 per patient, which provides a profit of $700 per patient.

The MCO believes it has estimated the provider's costs rather well and offers a price of $4,000 per discharge. It will make the provider the single source of care for its members categorized in this DRG. This should, on average, provide 400 more cases per year, which would provide an additional $800,000 contribution per year (400 [$4,000 − $2,000]). The fixed cost associated with this DRG is covered by the contribution ([$8,700 − $2,000] 1,100 = $7,370,000) from its current patients. Therefore, the additional contribution will all be additional profit. If you do not agree to this price, the MCO will find another hospital with which to contract. The question is should you agree to this arrangement?

Analysis of the Arrangement

- You first analyze the facility's capacity to see if it can increase utilization by 400 cases per year without increasing the fixed cost. You estimate that it cannot, you determine it would have to incur $150,000 more fixed costs to handle the increased caseload. This reduces the potential increase in contribution to $650,000.
- You then look at the nature of the savings from an agreement with this MCO compared to other payers who currently have similar contracts. This is considered because you want to have a reason for not giving the current payers this large price reduction when they learn the provider has given such a low price to a new customer.
- Of the total of 1,100 patients per year in this DRG, about 950 patients per year are from similar sole-source contracts. The contribution from these contracts is $6,365,000, (950 [$8,700 − $2,000]).
- You next try to determine what price the current payers will demand when they discover the lower price to this MCO. Your negotiating team believes that within a year the provider will have to lower the prices for these payers to about $5,500 per patient or lose them. This means agreeing to the $4,000 MCO price will reduce contributions from the current payers, after a year, by about $3,520,000, ([$8,700 − $5,500] 1100) in order to gain the short-run contribution increase of $650,000. This makes the agreement highly questionable.
- At this point, it would be interesting to see what price would give all payers the benefit of your increased utilization of capacity.
- You have determined that the fixed cost needed for the proposed total volume of 1,500 patients is $6,750,000.

- The current profit is $700 per patient. For 1,500 patients, this would be $1,050,000.
- The variable cost per patient is not expected to change; it will remain $2,000.
- Therefore, from the C-V-P model:

$$\$1,050,000 = (\$P - \$2,000) \, 1,500 - \$6,750,000$$
$$1,500P = \$1,050,000 + \$3,000,000 + \$6,750,000$$
$$1,500P = \$10,800,000$$
$$P = \$7,200$$

- This means that the price for all payers can be set at $7,200 and the hospital will make its current profit per patient. The patients added by the new MCO contract would increase profits by $280,000, ($400[$700]). The price to existing patients would be decreased by $1,500, ($8700 − $7,200), but this price is still $3,200, ($7,200 − $4,000) higher than the MCO's offer, and would be unacceptable to them.
- If you feel that a profit margin near that gotten from current business is justified and that charging old customers considerably more than a new customer is not, this analysis gives you a window in which to negotiate. This would be between the $4,000 offered to the $7,200, which provides the same margin across all buyers, given the increased utilization of fixed costs that the additional contract provides.
- If you settle on a price less than $7,200 per patient for the new business, you must determine how much higher than this the current payers can be charged and still keep their business.
- You should then redo the profit computation based on the prices probably acceptable and see if the provider is better off by contracting with the MCO.

Note from this example that, in the short run, any sale at a price greater than the variable cost of the product sold will increase profits by the amount of the unit contributions. This is true whether or not the price covers the full cost. However, that short-term additional profit may not be worth the longer term changes it may cause. These longer term implications should be examined thoroughly. C-V-P analysis helps in doing this examination.

One must realize that this analysis is impossible without fairly accurate measures of the fixed and the variable costs of the products involved. Equally important are estimates of the reactions of other buyers to accepting a greatly discounted price for one or more of them. Total profitability must be the prime consideration. Many of these estimates are subjective. They depend on the general level of understanding of health care markets and individual payers. This, in turn, depends on the degree to which the organization remains in close contact with its market participants.

DISCUSSION QUESTIONS

1. What is the difference between a unit contribution, a product contribution, and the total contribution?
2. What are the advantages and dangers in accepting a special contract that provides a contribution but does not cover full costs?
3. What are the components of a product line's contribution?

OUTSOURCING

In deciding to purchase an intermediate product rather than produce it within the organization, it is necessary to be sure that the cost of purchase is less than the marginal cost (as opposed to the current full cost) of producing it. The full cost probably contains shares of fixed costs that cannot be eliminated if the product is outsourced, because these resources are needed to produce other outputs as well. This joint use of fixed-cost assets influences the marginal cost relevant to a specific outsourcing decision. Therefore, each such decision demands its own analysis. Analyzing the possible outsourcing is done by determining what costs are marginal to its production within the organization. These are the costs that will be saved if it is purchased from an outside source. If it can be purchased for less than the marginal cost of producing it, the product is a strong candidate for outsourcing.

Example 6: Make or Buy

BASIC DATA   Get-Cheap Clinic makes admission kits for its patients. An outside company has offered to supply these kits for $6.00 each. In order to evaluate this offer, the clinic's accountants have gathered the following information relative to its cost of manufacturing the kit internally. This data came from the full-cost analysis used for financial statements. The clinic uses 15,000 kits per year.

Cost Analysis for Admission Kit Production	Per kit ($)	Per yr ($)
Direct materials	4.00	60,000
Direct labor	2.00	30,000

Variable production overhead	0.80	12,000
Admitting dept. supervisor's salary	1.00	15,000
Hospital-allocated fixed overhead	10.00	150,000
Total cost to make	$ 17.80	$267,000

SITUATION 6-1 Assume that the clinic has no alternative uses for the facilities now being used to produce the kits. The marginal cost of producing the kits is:

Direct materials	$4.00
Direct labor	2.00
Variable manufacturing overhead	0.80
Total	$6.80

The supervisor's salary and hospital is allocated fixed costs and will exist whether or not the kits are produced. Because the cost to purchase is only $6.00, savings from outsourcing would be:

$$[(Marginal\ cost\ to\ produce) - (cost\ to\ purchase)] \times (volume)$$
$$(\$6.80 - \$6.00) \times (15,000\ sets/yr) = \$12,000/yr$$

Outsourcing appears to be a good decision.

SITUATION 6-2 Now assume that the direct labor cost component comes from salaried employees who produce the kits at slack periods in their other work. In this situation, direct labor is no longer a marginal cost. Therefore, the marginal cost to produce a kit is reduced to $4.80 per set. If the clinic purchased the kits for $6.00 per set, it would raise their cost by $1.20 per set ($6.00 − $4.80). At a volume of 15,000 sets, this would increase the clinic's costs by $18,000 per year. Under these circumstances, outsourcing would be unwise.

This example highlights the importance of understanding the activities involved in producing internal products and the importance of the capacity utilization of the resources used. Full-cost data that may be readily available from the accounting system usually does not meet managers' needs when examining the advisability of outsourcing.

Example 7: Make or Buy

BASIC DATA In a hospital, a certain specialized laboratory test is done approximately 15 times per month. The full-cost analysis is as follows:

Direct labor (1.5 hr at $13/hr)	$19.500
Direct materials	8.500
Variable dept. ovrhd (by DLH)	0.750
Fixed dept. ovrhd (by test)	0.800
Variable svc. dept. ovrhd (by DLH)	1.200
Variable corporate ovrhd (by DLH)	0.015
Fixed corporate ovrhd (by test)	0.055
Full cost of test	$30.820

The test can now be purchased from a reference laboratory in the city for $25.50 per test.

SITUATION 7-1 Should the hospital continue to make the test or buy it?

- The fixed department and corporate overhead are not marginal costs; they will exist whether or not the test is outsourced. Therefore, the marginal cost of producing the test is $29.965.
- The outsource price is $25.50. Therefore, by outsourcing, cost would be lowered by $66.975/month, ([$29.965 − $25.50] 15 tests/month), or $863.70/year.

SITUATION 7-2 Management learns that the lab technicians are salaried employees who work 35 hours per week, regardless of work load. Does this change the analysis?

- If the technicians worked in a pool that could be managed so that they were paid only when there was work for them to do, the previous analysis would be correct. However, because they are salaried for a set number of hours per week, they will be paid whether or not this small number of tests are produced. The labor cost is, therefore, not marginal, and the marginal cost is reduced to $10.465 per test.
- Outsourcing would then cause an additional $225.525 cost per month, ([$25.500 − $10.465]15), or $2,706.30/yr.

SITUATION 7-3 If third-party payers want to use the hospital as a fee-for-service source for this test, given the laboratory test information, what is the lowest price for which the hospital can sell more tests and not lose money? Assume that the additional sales will not affect the prices of the existing business.

- The hospital must assure that it does not have a negative contribution from each sale.

- This means that management must price the test at or above the variable cost of production.
- If production uses a technician pool, that cost is $29.965 per test.
- If labor is from the excess time of salaried staff, the marginal cost is $10.465 per test.

SITUATION 7-4   If management believes that, instead of 15 tests per month, the laboratory will soon be called on to do 110 tests per month, does this change the analysis again? Technicians are salaried and, therefore, are a fixed cost.

- This significant increase in the quantity of tests could cause a change in the fixed costs that could be eliminated by outsourcing. Investigation shows that the FOH costs created by the department will not change. However labor costs might be affected. The labor time that could be eliminated by outsourcing would be 1,980 hrs/yr, (110 × 12 × 1.5). One technician works 1,750 hrs/yr (35 hrs/wk × 50 wks/yr) and is paid for 1,820 hours for year (35 hrs/wk × 52 wks/yr).
- Because more than this amount of technician time would be eliminated by outsourcing, the lab could eliminate one technician position and thereby save $23,660/yr (1,820 hrs × $13/hr).

The total annual savings from outsourcing would then be:

Marginal costs per test eliminated	12 × 110 × $10.46	$13,814
Technician salary saved		23,660
Less the cost to purchase	110 × $25.50 × 12	−33,660
Total savings		$ 3,814

In this higher volume situation, it would appear to be appropriate to buy the tests from the outside source.

SUBJECTIVE CONSIDERATIONS

As with any decision, quantitatively analyzable factors are not all that should be considered. Managers may tend to avoid an alternative whose expected marginal profit is determined to be better than others because of factors that are not or cannot be measured in monetary terms. It is fairly common for vendors to offer favorable prices when opening negotiations to sell a provider intermediate products. Providers should attempt to learn if the vendor has a pattern of raising its prices after its customers have shut down their ability to produce the item.

Because providers give up a great deal of their ability to control the quality and the detailed specifications of products after outsourcing, they should also check the vendor's quality history with other customers. For intermediate products such as diagnostics, providers should be sure that the vendor can and will respond with adequate speed to emergency orders. Making accurate judgments about these and similar factors related to the intermediate product in question is critical to good outsourcing decisions. The vendor's current customers and trade associations are good sources of this sort of information.

DISCUSSION QUESTION

What is the biggest analysis problem in determining the marginal cost of continuing to produce an intermediate product you are thinking of outsourcing?

Dropping Products

Determining whether to drop an apparently unprofitable product or product line also requires a marginal profit perspective. When deciding how much will be saved by no longer making a product, the cost portion of the analysis is much the same as the cost analysis in the outsourcing decision. The product's full cost extracted from financial accounts may contain allocations of fixed cost that will not be eliminated when the product is dropped. If these are included in the costs saved, savings are overstated and the decision to drop may be incorrect.

Examples

Example 8: Keep or Drop a Product

Discount Laboratory operates three product lines. The laboratory manager is considering the elimination of Product Line 2 because product line specific income statements consistently show a net operating loss for that center. The centers' operating performances during the past year were as follows (shown in dollars):

	Product Line		
	1	2	3
Sales revenue	345,600	230,400	576,000
Costs:			
Direct product costs	224,640	172,800	345,600

Direct product-line expenses	34,560	28,800	57,600
Variable overhead assigned	6,048	4,032	10,080
Product contribution	80,352	24,768	162,720
Fixed overhead allocated	60,480	40,320	100,800
Net income	19,872	(15,552)	61,920

Note: In analyzing these operating results, the laboratory accountant determines that a product line specific fixed marketing cost of $25,760 is the only fixed overhead that can be avoided if the Product Line 2 is terminated.

To decide if the product line should be dropped, its marginal profit (or its product line contribution) must be found. Of the itemized costs for Product Line 2, fixed sustaining overhead is one that might not be reduced when the product line is dropped. This depends on the extent that other product lines use the fixed service activity assets. The note indicates that $40,320 of such costs are fixed sustaining cost allocated to Product Line 2. Normally these costs cannot be eliminated when a product line is dropped because they are used to support remaining product lines. However, in this case, $25,760 can indeed be eliminated through advertising and promotion cost reductions in the marketing department. The remaining $14,560, ($40,320 − $25,760), of fixed costs would still have to be allocated to the remaining two products because they are not eliminated when Product Line 2 is no longer produced. If the product line were dropped under current conditions, the marginal changes would be a loss of $230,400 in revenue, which means a $24,768 loss of product contribution. Because $25,760 of fixed sustaining overhead can be eliminated, there would also be a cost reduction of that amount. These reductions would create a net gain of $992, ($25,760 − $24,768). This creates a close call. If management believes that this product line also creates business in other product lines, it would definitely not want to drop it, because it is doing a bit better than breaking even.

The amount of analysis justified to determine how much of the cost allocated to a product will actually be eliminated when the product is dropped depends of the volume of the sales involved. If this were a large-volume product, it would be appropriate to see if eliminating it would justify eliminating other service department resources, such as a payroll clerk or an equipment maintenance technician. These secondary results of abandoning a product create the need to analyze the overhead costs farther up the activity chain than the center that completes the product's production.

Example 9: Keep or Drop a Product Line

A rural health system operates a 95-bed hospital, an outpatient surgery center, two primary care clinics, a home health organization, and a hospice service. The long-term care and home health organizations are for-profit subsidiaries of the system, which is itself a not-for-profit county-owned institution. The last financial statements are reflected in the following information. The amounts are shown in thousands of dollars.

When the board reviewed these figures, it noticed that the system had a 1.85 percent overall profit margin but was carrying three components with financial loss. It also noticed that this pattern had been roughly the same over the past 4 years with the same three losers. It has asked you to investigate the viability of these three units and the effects of dropping them.

- Each of the three centers showing a loss has been charged with institutional fixed overhead that will exist even if the center ceases to operate. When these costs are not charged to these centers, only the centers' marginal costs are considered. Analysts then find that Clinic 1 provides a $1,000,000 contribution and the hospice provides a $1,500,000 contribution, but the home health center has a $4,000,000 negative contribution.
- If all three of these centers are dropped, the change in contribution will be $−1,000,000 − $1,500,000 + $4,000,000, which is an increase of $1,500,000.
- If only the home health center is dropped, contributions will increase by $4,000,000 because the centers with positive contributions have not been dropped.
- A more informative presentation of a summary of profit center results would be (in dollars):

	Hospital	Clinic 1	Clinic 2	OP Surgery	Home Health	Hospice
Net patient service revenues	220,000	18,000	14,000	52,000	11,000	8,000
less:						
Direct labor	130,000	11,000	7,000	20,000	6,000	4,000
Direct materials	20,000	1,000	3,000	8,000	3,000	1,000
Fixed overhead						
direct to center	40,000	3,000	1,000	10,000	2,000	500
system allocated	10,000	2,000	1,500	4,000	1,500	2,000
Variable overhead	15,000	2,000	1,000	3,000	4,000	1,000
Net income	5,000	− 1,000	500	7,000	− 5,500	− 500

	Hospital	Clinic 1	Clinic 2	OP Surgery	Home Health	Hospice	Total
Net patient service revenues less:	220,000	18,000	14,000	52,000	11,000	8,000	323,000
Center marginal costs	205,000	17,000	12,000	41,000	15,000	6,500	− 298,000
Center contribution less:	15,000	1,000	2,000	11,000	− 4,000	1,500	26,500
System fixed overhead							21,000
System Profit							5,500

This clearly shows that only the home health center is hurting the system's profit.

The critical part of the analysis of a decision to drop a product or product line involves finding the costs that will be eliminated if the product line is dropped, that is, the marginal costs of the product line. The revenues that will be lost from that product line are rather easily derived from sales data. Revenues that may be lost from business associated with the product line in question are much more difficult to estimate and usually rest on highly subjective judgments. When examining available cost data, the first move is to consider direct-to-product center costs as marginal. The next move is to assume that fixed overhead allocated to the product center is not marginal. This assumption may not be totally valid. There may be portions of fixed service center costs that can be reduced when a product line is dropped. It may be that demands on the personnel department may be reduced to the point that some of its salaried workers can be eliminated. Similarly, capacities in fixed-cost equipment and labor may be reduced in other service centers when products involving many activities and large quantities are dropped. In these cases, the assumption that all allocated fixed costs will remain in the system should be checked.

ADDING PRODUCTS

The general approach to analyzing these opportunities is to determine if the marginal revenue over the life of the product will exceed its marginal costs. This is more complicated because it is not rational to assume that the marginal revenues and costs will be the same in each year of its life. Adding a product line usually demands acquisition of long-term assets that will be expensed over a period of time.

It also usually creates additional sales volumes that vary over time. This causes a different mathematical problem than the one faced when dropping a product and losing the same contribution annually over what had been the planned life of that product. The difference is caused by a phenomenon called the *time value of money*. Money has a time value because the sooner it is in hand, the quicker it can be reinvested to earn more. If one can collect $100 now or 5 years from now, the money should be collected now and invested. This way, it can grow to a larger amount over the 5 years. The formula for computing the amount to which an amount of money now in hand can grow at a given interest rate over a given length of time is:

$$FV = PV(1+r)^n$$

Where: FV is the future value

PV is the present value (the amount invested)

n is the number of periods the PV will earn interest

r is the interest rate per period that will be earned

If the $100 were invested at 10 percent per year for 5 years, it would grow to $161.05 or $100(1+0.10)^5$. Receiving the money now as opposed to 5 years from now allows the recipient to have $61.05 more at the 5-year point.

By manipulating the formula, we see that $PV = FV/(1+r)^n$. Using this formula, the amount of money that would have to be invested now (time zero) to grow to a given future value in a given number of periods at a given interest rate can be computed. To reverse the situation, if 10 percent can be earned on an investment, how much would one be willing to invest in an arrangement that promised to pay $161.05 at the end of 5 years?

$$PV = \$161.05/(1 + 0.10)^5 = \$100$$

This formula can be use to solve for the present value of the net cash gains in each year of the investment. If the present value of the future years' gains is greater than the investment, the addition is profitable. Because solving the problem deals with a calculation that involves raising a quantity to a power, pencil solutions are somewhat complicated. Fortunately, there are quite inexpensive calculators available that can solve this formula by simply entering the three values that are known and requesting a solution for the unknown fourth amount. (These calculators are usually labeled as *business calculators*.)

Example 10: Capital Investment

Suppose it will take $100,000 of capital investment to start a new product. Analysis of expected sales and annual costs indicates that the product's life will be 7 years. At the end of the 7 years, the fixed assets involved can be sold for $8,000. The cost of the $100,000 needed will be an interest rate of 10 percent per year. Estimates of the excess of revenue over operating costs each year is shown in the "Money Flow" column in the following table. The "Present Value" of each flow is shown in the last column. Again, this is the amount of money that would have to be invested at time zero in order to have that year's return of cash if the present value earned the stated interest rate per year. The interest rate, "r," used in this present value computation is 10 percent, the amount the organization must pay for the invested capital. This is used as the discount rate because one assumes that, if it must be paid to get the money, the company could loan the amount of the investment to someone else and get that return. The 10 percent return is treated as an opportunity cost. If a company is to invest in a new product, they want it to return at least what they could earn by simply investing it with a borrower whose risk of losing the money is no greater than their risk of losing it in a failed new product.

Year	Money Flow	Present Value	Notes
0	− $100,000	− $100,000	(the needed investment in new assets)
1	5,000	4,545	(annual marginal net cash flows)
2	20,000	16,529	"
3	40,000	30,053	"
4	70,000	47,811	"
5	70,000	43,464	"
6	70,000	39,513	"
7	50,000	25,658	"
7	$8,000	4,105	(the salvage value)

Note: Total present value (PV) of future inflows at r = 10 percent is $211,678; net present value (PV of future inflows less the investment) = $111,678.

The present value of the future flows from the investment is $111,678 more than the present investment, so the investment is profitable. Another way to view this result is that, if a company knows it can earn 10 percent per year by investing money somewhere, the cash flows shown could be pro-duced by investing $211,678. However, with this investment, the company need only invest $100,000 to get the same future inflows. Therefore, this is better than opportunities that return only 10 percent. Business calculators can also compute the actual percentage return on the investment made. In this case, it is 35.71 percent, which is considerable better than the 10 percent interest that must be paid to acquire the money for the investment.

Adding products and product lines commonly demands making capital invest-ments. Analyzing these situations falls under the heading of *capital budgeting*. We discuss adding products at this point for two reasons. The first is to explain why this type of decision is more complex than short-run decisions. This is because it involves an initial investment that could be made in another venture, and there will be different amounts of inflows and outflows in different future periods over the life of the investment. The second reason is to introduce the concept of the time value of money. More detailed discussion of time-value analyses for long-term additions to business and other capital investments is contained in texts on financial management.

Management accounting is important to product-addition analysis because in order to do the analysis, estimates must be made of the marginal costs that will be incurred year by year by the expanded activities. This estimation demands analy-sis of historic costs and projection of costs into the future. The difference between good and bad capital budgeting rests on the accuracy of these estimates. This ac-curacy depends on how well the analysts understand the technology to be used, the markets to be served, and the markets for the resources needed. The quantita-tive analysis itself is quite straight forward. Making accurate estimates of the cash flows involved is not.

DISCUSSION QUESTIONS

1. What is the greatest analysis problem in determining the contribution of a product line?
2. What phenomenon gives money a time value?
3. Why do long-term product line decisions demand a different analysis ap-proach from short-term decisions?

KEY POINTS

- Because managers' work usually deals with changing an existing situation, decisions should be based on measures of change, referred to as marginal measures.
- Therefore, marginal costs are the relevant costs for most decisions.
- Sunk cost, because they cannot be changed in the future, are not relevant to decisions.
- The cost-volume-profit (C-V-P) model is useful for short-term decisions in which the time value of money is not important.
- Profit is increased by achieving contribution, which is the difference between revenue and variable costs that can be applied to fixed costs and profit.
- Think in terms of unit contributions, product contributions, product-line contribution, and total contribution. Each concerns a greater level of aggregation of products.
  1. Unit contribution is the contribution from making and selling one unit of a product.
  2. Product contribution is the contribution from making and selling a quantity of a product.
  3. Product line contribution is the total contribution from a set of products that make up a product line. It is the sum of this product set's product contributions less the fixed costs that are incurred solely to produce the product line.

4. Total contribution is the sum of product line contributions.
- Breakeven analysis can provide low-end thresholds for factors relevant to short-term decisions.
- When giving a price discount for special contracts or sales, managers must be certain there will be positive contribution and that other buyers are not offended by the discount given to a new customer.
- Some price discounts that eliminate the products contribution may be justified by the support the product gives to other sales, as in completing a product line.
- In outsource decisions managers must be sure that only the costs that will be eliminated by outsourcing are considered in the analysis.
- For a specific decision, different situations will cause different cost elements to be relevant.
- In decisions concerning adding or dropping products, the total contribution of the product or product line is the relevant cost to consider.
- Decisions about adding products that require acquisition of expensive long-term assets must consider the time value of money. These are referred to as capital-budgeting decisions.

Exercise

PROBLEM 1

C-V-P: A Single Product Problem

Assume FC = $10,000, VC_u = $2, P = $3.
In January, the production unit made
   13,000 units, which were sold.
Total Profit = ($3 − $2) 1,300 − $10,000
   = $3,000.

   a. Suppose an opportunity exists to
      rent better equipment that will re-
      duce wastage and save labor, but
      raises fixed costs by $1,500, such
      that:

   FC = $11,500
   VC_u = $1.80
   P = $3.00
Q is estimated to remain at 13,000 units per
   month.
Should the company rent the equipment?
   Check: Profit is raised to $4,100. Do it.

   b. What if the new equipment only re-
      duced VC_u to $1.90?
      Check: Profit drops to $2,800. Don't
      do it.

PROBLEM 2

C-V-P: Preventive Medicine

Your preventive medicine section has been
asked by the state to serve as a sole source for
giving flu shots to elderly citizens in response
to a spreading epidemic. The variable costs
(needles, vaccine, etc.) will be $13 per shot.
The fixed costs necessary to run the project
(added salaries, equipment rental, etc.) will

be $9,000. The state expects you to give
20,000 shots.

   a. The state offers to pay you $13.25
      per shot. From a purely financial
      standpoint, should you take the
      project? Why?
      Check figure: $4,000 loss
   b. The state says it wants to furnish the
      additional equipment needed, which
      is $4,000 of the $9,000 fixed cost.
      However if it does, it will only pay
      $13.20 per shot. Should you accept
      these terms? Why?
      Check figure: $1,000 loss
   c. You are afraid that the equipment
      the state would furnish would not be
      up-to-date and would lower your ef-
      ficiency, so you reject that proposal
      regardless of the profit computed.
      Using the original costs, what price
      would you have to charge in order to
      breakeven on the expected 20,000
      shots?
      Check figure: P = $13.45 per shot

PROBLEM 3

Outsourcing

Your supply section makes the tubing sets
used in your clinical lab. It is considering
purchasing them from a very reliable plastics
products firm. If it does, it can rent the space
used for this purpose for $14,000 per year.
The lab's capacity is 120,000 connectors per
year. The supply section's labor is salaried on
a weekly basis and works on an array of fabri-
cated products in addition to the tubing sets.
The following information on the connectors
is available from the standard cost sheet:

	cost/connector
Direct materials	$0.60
Direct labor	1.40
Variable overhead	0.30
Fixed overhead traceable to connector production at capacity	0.70
Fixed overhead allocated to connector production at capacity	0.40
Total	$3.40

The plastic products firm has offered to make the connectors for $1.70 cents per connector.

   a. What is your relevant cost of producing a connector when making a make-or-buy decision? Assume 120,000 produced per year. Check figure: $3 gain

   b. If you outsource the connectors, how much will you gain (or lose) per year in comparison to continuing to make them yourself if your actual production were 110,000 sets for a year? Be sure to state whether the change is a gain or a loss. Check figure: $150,000 gain

PROBLEM 4

DROP OR DISCOUNT A PRODUCT, DRG ANALYSIS

Cost analysis of a DRG indicates (in dollars):

Current payment: $4,500 per discharge

Variable cost: $3,500 per discharge
Allocated fixed costs: $5,800,000 per year
Fixed costs traceable to the DRG:
   $1,200,000 per year
Current discharge rate: 850 per year
Given current utilization, capacity for the
   DRG is 1,300 discharges per year.

   a. What is the current contribution from this DRG to the hospital allocated overhead and profit?
      Check: $350,000 loss

   b. What is the volume that will give a zero contribution?
      Check: 1,200 discharges

   c. Should the DRG be dropped? Why? Why not?
      Check: It depends

   d. An HMO offers to make your hospital a sole provider. They have averaged 400 patients in this DRG per year. However they want a 10 percent discount from your current $4,500 price charged other payers. Should you accept the contract? Why? Why not?
      Check: Contract will add $220,000 to the contribution

   e. Assuming that the contract is accepted, what price could be set for all payers so that the DRG would not have a negative contribution? Why is this price hard to compute given what we know?
      Check: $4,460 assuming no other changes

PART

4   Performance and Reporting

Measurements, no matter how accurate and relevant, are of little value to decision makers unless they lead to the performance desired. In order to support wise decisions, measurement and the information they create must be efficiently conveyed to the appropriate decision makers.

Chapter 15 discusses perspectives from which performance can be measures and basic performance measurements. It also discusses management insights available from these measurements. The appendix to Chapter 15 gives examples of common performance measurements.

Chapter 16 discusses the structure of reports for use by managers. It emphasizes the concept of *balanced score cards* and gives examples of graphic support for reported management reports.

Chapter 17 summarizes the ideas presented in this text and reviews aspects of the health care industry that will cause changes of both measurement and reporting of managerial information in the near future.

After studying this chapter, students should be able to:

1. Explain the perspectives from which managers should view the organization when measuring performance.

2. Explain the relationships among those perspectives; that is, how conditions discovered through analysis from one perspective affect another.

3. Explain the performance measures available from financial statement data and the limitations of these measures.

4. Explain the attributes patients, physicians, third-party payers, and suppliers want in health care organizations with which they do business.

5. Explain the nature of exchange between physicians and hospitals or clinics.

6. Explain why third-party payers are instrumental in setting prices in health care.

7. Explain situations in which health care providers may want to terminate relations with specific physicians and payers.

8. Explain why learning and growth are important to an organization and should be managed.

9. Explain why management of equipment and supply acquisition should go beyond finding low prices.

10. Explain the measures that can be used to evaluate performance from each of the nonfinancial analysis perspectives.

11. Explain the sources and uses of organization and industry standards.

INTRODUCTION

Managers' jobs involve assuring performance that sustains the viability of their organization. In this book, we use the following set of definitions. The *mission* of the organization articulates why the organization should exist; it states the societal needs the organization intends to satisfy. Its *strategy* describes the general approach it plans to take. Strategy lays out broad sets of activities the organization intends to accomplish in order to perform its mission. Its *vision* specifies the place it sees for itself at points in the future within the markets it plans to serve. *Objectives* are specific intermediate accomplishments that must happen if the mission is to be achieved. *Goals* are thresholds on measures that indicate whether objectives are being reached. If goals are met for the sequence of objectives established by the organization, the mission will be accomplished. This assumes that the planning of strategy, objectives, and goals is appropriate.[1] Among management accountants, one frequently hears the opinion, "If you can't measure it, you can't manage it." In this chapter, we will view the measurement of organization performance from a broad array of perspectives and varying degrees of measurability.

As we have stressed in prior chapters, an organization's performance is the aggregate result of all of its activities. Kaplan and Norton propose a set of four perspectives from which managers should view their organization's objectives and activities: *customer, internal, learning and growth*, and *financial*.[2] We would add the perspective of the *supplier*. To fully understand an organization's performance, its performance must be measured from each of these perspectives.

First, the perspective of customers must be understood. If not, there will be no definable mission, appropriate products, or sales. The organization must also take an internal perspective that leads to efficient production of quality products with which to serve its customers. Efficiency is linked to the costs at which it acquires its resources and the skill with which they are used. Quality demands skilled application of processes and keeping pace with the technology needed for state-of-the-art care. Optimal technology, in turn, demands continually enhanced knowledge and skills. This requires learning within the workforce, including management itself. The ability to use appropriate inputs acquired at appropriate costs requires attention to suppliers. The financial perspective summarizes success within the other four perspectives. It is critical to the external confidence that is required to sustain necessary flows of outside capital. The performance of the organization is, therefore, dependent on understanding the organization from all five of these perspectives. Understanding the levels of performance demands measurement.

FINANCIAL PERSPECTIVE

The measurement of financial performances is covered in financial accounting and financial management literature. The financial accounting perspective involves measures of performance revealed in the income and cash flow statements and measures of financial position revealed in the balance sheet. These statements are able to give a picture of the organization's history expressed in a common denominator, money.

Income Statements

From an operations standpoint, the income statement provides the primary measure of financial performance. Revenue, broadly defined, is the lifeblood of an organization. In a for-profit organization, revenue is dependent on sales. Profits from sales are the principal factor in assuring a continued flow of capital. Retained earnings are themselves a source of capital. Concurrently, if future earnings are not expected, the firm has little chance of raising either debt or equity capital. The amount of profit or surplus that can be raised from a given level of revenue is, of course, dependent on the level of expenses. Measures of performance relative to cost control are, therefore, also relevant to financial performance. Though not-for-profit organizations may raise a smaller portion of their capital by retaining surpluses, they should produce value for their communities in order to maintain a flow of grants and contributions. These flows are surrogates for equity capital raised by for-profit organizations through expectations of future earnings.

Frequently used income statement measures of financial performance start with profit and include other derived variables such as:

- Profit margin—profit divided by revenue as a measure of the ability to achieve profit from sales.
- Revenue variances—discussed in Appendix 13.
- Cost variances—discussed in Chapter 13.

Measures of revenue tend to focus on total market demand, share of market, prices, and product mix, as discussed in Appendix 13. These measures give some indication of where revenue problems exist and where management action, especially marketing action, may be productive. Performance measures related to cost focus on cost variances in repetitive production processes for which standards can be set. As discussed in Chapter 13, they are helpful in spotting the location within repeated activities of performance that is not producing planned results. This makes them valuable tools. They support a management by exception approach with reference to the use of resources.

Balance Sheet

The balance sheet is thought to provide measures of financial position at a point in time. Short-term financial health is indicated by the relative amounts of current assets and current liabilities. These are represented in measures such as the:

- Current ratio—the ratio of current assets to current liabilities. This indicates the ability to pay short-term liabilities as they come due.
- Quick ratio—current assets less inventories divided by current liabilities. This indicates the ability to pay short-term liabilities if inventories are not turned to cash.

Long-term indicators of financial position include balance sheet ratios that indicate the organization's ability to meet its future obligations and to raise additional capital. These include comparisons such as the:

- Debt-to-equity ratios—a comparison of long-term capital from creditors to that from providers of equity. This indicates the organization's ability to suffer losses without affecting creditors' returns.
- Debt-to-assets ratio—a comparison of debt to the book value of total assets. This gives an indication of the ability of the organization to sell off assets in order to pay debt.

Joint Measures

Relationships between income statement numbers and balance sheet numbers provide more powerful measures of financial performance and status.

Greater insight to performance is gained from measures such as:
- Return on assets (ROA)—profit as a percent of the assets used to produce it.
- Return on investment (ROI)—profit as a percentage of the equity furnished by investors.
- Market value added (MVA)—the market value of equity less its book value.
- Economic value added (EVA)—operating profit less the total cost of capital.

These numbers can point out strengths and weaknesses in financial performance period by period relative to the investment made, which is the perspective on performance of basic interest to investors. These measures focus on the history of short-term profitability. Multiperiod reports can show trends in financial performance. Trend measures in turn indicate whether or not progress is being made.

Short-term financial position is indicated by:
- Days cash on hand—the amount of cash and cash equivalents divided by average daily cash expenses. This indicates how long the organization could pay its expenses without acquiring additional cash inflows.
- Days inpatient accounts receivable—the amount in accounts receivable divided by the average daily patient revenue. This indicates the ability to turn accounts receivable into cash for paying short-term liabilities.

Long-term position measures using both income statement and balance sheet numbers include:
- Times interest earned—income plus interest expense divided by interest expense. This indicates how well earnings before paying interest were able to cover the interest expense.
- Debt service coverage—income plus depreciation and interest divided by principal payments plus interest. This indicates how well cash generated from operations was able to cover the total obligations from debt.

The financial perspective has probably been the one most analyzed. It is reflected in volumes of accounting and financial management literature, security, and exchange legislation and GAAP. An organization that produces inferior products and attempts to sell them at prices above those of its competitors can exist until it runs out of money. Organization viability is, therefore, financial viability. When an organization fails to pay its debts, it will die. Financial measures are valuable to those who furnish capital to the extent that it helps them to foretell future insolvency, given little expected change in operations. They are valuable to managers for the same reason. The value of these measures to managers would be greater if they could also show why the profits needed to maintain solvency are not flowing from operations. Unfortunately, financial measures do not provide much of this type of information.

One must also keep in mind that these financial statement measurements are historical. Basic problems exist in using historical information as the basis for decisions about the future. Actions to correct mistakes or inadequacies of the past might not be appropriate for a changed future. Because these issues are more the focus of financial accounting and financial management than of management accounting, we leave more comprehensive coverage to other texts. We know that the environment of health care delivery is changing rapidly; the ability to estimate what these changes will be is critical to management's decision making. Reacting to indications of financial weakness in a changing environment demands information from perspectives much broader than financial information provides. However, financial performance measures act as summaries of past performance. Because past performance, especially under the same management, is considered a strong indicator of future performance, these measures are valuable.

DISCUSSION QUESTIONS

1. Why is the relationship of the financial perspective to the other four perspectives suggested for use in analyzing the performance of an organization?
2. Why might one contend that revenue is the lifeblood of an organization? What other factors are required for financial viability? How do they relate to revenue?
3. What are some of the measures of financial performance and position that help analysts understand a health care organization? What specific information is contained in each one?
4. What are the limitations of financial measures as inputs to managers' decisions?
5. Why is it necessary to use both balance sheet and income statement figures to construct these measures?

CUSTOMER PERSPECTIVE

Revenue is dependent on customers. In a competitive environment, customers' perception of an organization's performance is critical to sales. Satisfying customers generally involves three somewhat different factors. The first is delivering services that are desired. Second, the customers must be convinced that services being provided are of acceptable quality. Finally, the prices of the services must be competitive. The combination of quality and price is often referred to as *value*, however, we will discuss these separately. In the case of many health care delivery organizations, examining customers' perceptions is complicated by the fact that there are at least three distinct sets of customers: the patients, the physicians who refer or admit them, and third-party payers.

Patients

From the perspective of patients, at least four attributes seem to be important in their decision to use a given care provider: (1) their specific needs for health care services; (2) access to the services needed; (3) the perceived quality of the services provided; and (4) to a lesser degree, price. To attract patients, providers should be able to evaluate these.

SERVICES For existing care deliverers, the health care services they have chosen to provide should be revealed in their mission statement. Epidemiological and current facility availability measurements are discussed in Appendix 13. These are needed to establishing total demand within the drawing area and the organization's expected caseloads. Organizations should periodically examine the total demand in their drawing area and the facilities currently available to meet that demand. If adequate capacity exists currently, patient perception of quality of care relative to the competition is of major importance. If there is not adequate capacity, creating that capacity is potentially profitable. In this case, measures of fixed costs involved and patient volumes to assure high quality care are important. Research indicates that high technology interventions produce higher quality outcomes when they are performed frequently by the provider.[3] In filling a need for expanded capacity for a high-tech intervention, a provider must match the number of interventions needed to produce competitive quality to the number of interventions that could potentially be requested. Measures of potential demands come from market analyses. Measures on the relationship of outcomes to frequency of use of an intervention are often available through specialty medical practice associations, hospital associations, and published research reports. Measures of the capacity of the fixed-cost assets involved are available through vendors, noncompeting providers, and trade associations. All three sets of measurements are necessary to determine if high performance levels can be sustained at competitive prices in high-technology services. This information can prevent situations in which low demand for a specific service causes low quality of care. Such situations increase costs and decrease reputation of the organization. The result can be a material reduction of profits.

ACCESS Access to services is an additional factor in patients' choice of care deliverer. The backlash of patients to the restrictions on the source of care required by HMOs would indicate that patients want to feel they have control of the source of their health care services. To the extent that they do, patient volume for a care deliverer is affected by patient perceptions of access-related factors other than the existence of the service they desire. Some such factors can be at least partially controlled by the care deliverer. These include the promptness with which admission can be scheduled, the ease of getting to the facility, and the time from entering the facility to the initiation of appropriate care.

Data on variables like these can be collected during the scheduling and admission procedures. Because many high-cost care interventions have relatively low demand, there is always a trade off between geographic access and cost per intervention. In order to reduce the number of installations to the point that they will be utilized near their capacity and thereby reduce cost per use, the installations must be placed farther apart. This forces providers to estimate the degree to which clients are willing to sacrifice geographic access for lower price.

The patient's ability to pay for care is, of course, an extremely important access problem. However, the ability to pay is largely a social policy problem outside the case-by-case control of the care deliverer. It is therefore outside the area of management accounting, except for the obvious relationship of greater efficiency leading to lower costs and the resultant potential for lower prices leading to greater financial access.

QUALITY Selecting specific aspects of performance that affect potential patients' perceptions of the quality of service can be determined from patient surveys. Patient satisfaction surveys have become common management tools. In constructing surveys, it is important that they produce actionable information. The information can be of two types. The first is responses to open-ended questions such as: "What could have made your experience here better?" An answer could be: "I had to wait too long to get a nurse to respond to my call for assistance." Questions of this type indicate variables that should be measured in order to help isolate causes of the failure to satisfy patient expectations, create standards, and track improvement. Some of these variables can be measures as part of clinical procedures. In this example, a timing mechanism can be constructed to measure the lapse between the call for assistance and the call indicator being turned off at the bedside. Information about this variable can become part of periodic management reporting in order to maintain attention to it. Some variables can be measured using the second type of survey question. One such question might be: "Did all staff members who assisted you introduce themselves, explain why they were with you, ask if you had any questions, and answer your questions satisfactorily?" Percentages of "yes" and "no" answers by patient type or ward can indicate where training is needed on this aspect of patient care. It is important to stress that patient satisfaction surveys should serve as sources of awareness of areas that need management attention as well as data on the level of performance on recognized aspects affecting patients' confidence in the organization.

Whatever the key factors affecting patients' opinions about the desirability of receiving health care services from the organization turn out to be, in order for managers to be able to use measurements related to them, the measurements must be actionable. This means that the measurement must indicate specific conditions that need management attention. In the previous example, if the survey had asked the patient to rate the nursing service on a 10-point scale, the responses would not lead management to any specific action. By first asking what could be done better and being told that response time was not adequate, managers have a specific performance factor to improve and a measurement to help them understand where improvement is needed. The second survey question is immediately actionable in that it indicates a specific area of patient interaction that may need attention and the personnel who need additional training.

PRICE The influence of price on patient volume is primarily indirect. Most care services are paid by third parties through contractual arrangements. The amounts on most patients' bills are set by these contracts in which potential patients have little direct influence. The charge master, or list, prices for line item services are only a reference point from which third-party payments are negotiated, often in the form of discounts from these prices. More realistically, the negotiated prices are set based on estimates of average costs for categories of patients or aggregates of care. DRGs, per diems, and APCs are examples of these pricing mechanisms. In today's health care market, providers of care are generally price takers due to private third-party payers' market power and the de facto monopsony of geriatric care held by the federal government. The pricing issue is essentially related to interaction with third-party payers, not patients.

DISCUSSION QUESTIONS

1. What are the sources of measurements to determine the demand for specific services that a care deliverer can expect?
2. What is the trade-off that affects potential patients' geographic access to care for a specific service?
3. What are the three measurements that are necessary prior to determining if high-technology services can be profitably sustained by a care deliverer? Why are they important to good acquisition decisions?
4. What measures would impress potential clients that a specific hospital is the one in which they want to receive care?

5. How can a care delivery organization discover what attributes of organizations like theirs impress potential payers?
6. Why does the price of services have limited effect on patients' choices of where they get health care?

Physicians

Physicians' perceptions as customers are important in hospitals. If one thinks of hospitals as the workplaces of physicians, a hospital's performance is judged by the physician according to the degree to which the hospital expedites the physician's work. As customers, physicians expect providers to supply the equipment and supplies they choose to use and skilled clinicians to provide ancillary services that support their medical and surgical interventions. They also expect high quality in hospital services supporting them and their patients.

SERVICES   One aspect of services to physicians is the availability of fixed-cost assets for physicians to use and for the hospital to fill physicians' orders. Quite rationally, physicians would like to have all of the best equipment and supporting assets they may want for the care of any patient they might admit. This creates two problems for hospitals. First, technology is changing so fast that to continuously maintain the latest technological applications necessitates frequent abandonment of equipment that is still functional. This can dramatically increase capital costs. For example, suppose a hospital has an $800,000 piece of equipment that it is depreciating over a 5-year period at $160,000 per year. At the end of the third year of use, a new, improved version of the equipment is available and the medical staff strongly desires that the hospital acquire it. If other hospitals are under the same pressure, the salvage value of the equipment may be only $20,000—or perhaps zero. This means that the hospital will have a $300,000 loss in the disposal of the old equipment. It is easy to see that, if this situation occurs very frequently, material losses can be incurred from equipment updates. These costs could be offset if the operating and depreciation cost of the new equipment is less per use than that of the equipment it replaces. This should be determined before any equipment replacement decision is made.

The replacement decision involves other consideration as well. These considerations center on why the physicians want the new equipment. It may reduce the time they must spend performing the interventions it supports and therefore increase their productivity and earning power. It may also significantly improve the quality of the intervention with reference to the wellness of the patient. This improves the physician's professional success, reputation, and probable patient volume as well as that of the hospital. Because physicians suffer no costs in replacements of equipment that they desire, there is no downside to replacements from their perspective. There is no reason they should not want the equipment replaced.

The financial effect of equipment replacement on the hospital is not always favorable. A reduction in the cost per usage would be beneficial to the hospital. The new equipment, if faster, may allow quicker throughput time for patients. This is an advantage if the hospital currently needs more capacity. If the hospital currently uses several of these pieces of equipment, the increased speed of the replacement could allow a reduction of the number of pieces of the equipment kept available. The hospital might also benefit if the new equipment increases quality of care from the standpoint of patients through shorter length of stay, less pain or embarrassment, and better outcomes. In these situations, there is no downside. The downside is in factors that would increase costs to the hospital without increasing profits in the short run through lowered costs or the long run through greater patient satisfaction.

The first potential downside from the hospital's perspective is if replacement causes a loss on disposal of the old equipment. The most obvious potential downside is if the new equipment costs more per usage than the old. There are two related operating phenomena that can also affect the hospital's cost of replacement. One is the fact that different physicians use different protocols for patients with the same condition. The other is that some physicians may want a transition period in which both the old and new equipment is kept operational. The first situation can mean that the operating costs of the old equipment will not disappear and salvage cash flows will not occur. The second means that realizing the disappearance of the old operating costs will be delayed.

These relationships mean that negotiation between physicians and the hospital administration will need measurements that indicate:

- The sunk cost of the replaced equipment—found from general ledger asset accounts. Though this amount is irrelevant to a specific replacement decision, its total over a period of time can indicate losses from a too rapid replacement of equipment. Large losses should prompt after-the-fact analysis of the advisability of past replacements and current replacement rates.
- The relative cost per usage of the old and new pieces of equipment—found from standard costs of procedures using the old equipment and estimates of these costs for the replacement equipment.
- The potential physician revenue increase from availability of the replacement equipment—found from estimates of physician revenue per hour of hospital work and additional work potentially billable.
- The change of outcome quality enabled by the replacement equipment, its affect on future physician and hospital patient volume, and related profits. Measures on the increase in quality are available from the equipment's vendor, but are highly biased. More accurate information about quality is often available from noncompeting users of the new equipment. Measures of the effect of the

improvement on future patient volumes are very subjective and may be limited to a simple "none," "good," or "very good" scale.

- The certainty that the new equipment, if beneficial to both the hospital and physicians, will indeed replace the old equipment. The risk of not disposing of the old equipment can be lowered by careful wording of the management's purchase-approval authorization.
- The cost to the hospital of losing patients the physicians will take elsewhere, if the new equipment is beneficial to the physicians (which it is or they would not request it) but not to the hospital.

Estimates on the last variable are subjective and complex. They deserve some discussion. If both the hospital and physicians believe that the replacement will significantly improve patient outcomes, both parties must evaluate its effect on their future. Physicians must estimate whether patients will notice the difference and become more loyal to them because of it. Hospitals must also estimate whether patients will notice the difference and become more supportive. They must also determine if payers will cover any additional cost of the improved outcomes. If the replacement will cause a reduction in hospital profits because of inadequate payment, hospitals must be able to support their estimate of lowered profit through acceptably accurate measures of the changes in costs and revenue. Current popular vernacular says that they must present *fact-based evidence*. If these cost estimates do not allow them to negotiate higher payments, they must attempt to gain physicians' agreements that the new equipment should not be acquired. Management's argument would be that such acquisitions will seriously damage the hospital's continued existence and the ability to agree to other requests for fixed-asset purchases.

The ability of the hospital to develop this argument depends on the accuracy of its cost estimates for specific protocols using specific resources. As explained in previous chapters, this accuracy depends greatly on the degree to which activity-based costing is applied. It also depends on the physicians' previous experiences and impressions of the degree to which the hospital administration conscientiously attempts to serve the best interest of its patients, physicians, and community, while maintaining its viability. It is not in the best interest of physicians and other clinicians to allow a good hospital to go into bankruptcy.

Another aspect of services provided to physicians is the level of skilled services to support them and fill their orders. Physicians as customers want highly competent people to perform the tasks associated with the array of services the hospital or clinic is equipped to provide. Furnishing these people in an efficient manner demands a trade-off between the cost of paying highly trained people and the need for high levels of competence across the labor force. The objective should be to have appropriately skilled people perform every task, but not pay for overskilled people to do any task. An example of this issue is the question of whether to have an all registered-nurse (RN) nursing staff or have a combination of RNs, practical nurses, and nurse's aids. Physicians may like the idea of an all RN staff because a highly skilled person would always be close at hand on the ward and the physicians do not have to bear the cost. However, the hospital would bear the costs of many nursing tasks being done by people who are overpaid for the specific work involved. The solution lies in intensity measures of workloads, matching labor classifications to the skills demanded, and an appropriate scheduling system.

QUALITY Specific measures that physician can use to evaluate their support from a provider are such things as wait time for admissions, the availability of medical records and ease of data entry, order response time, and the rate of unsatisfactory completion of orders. Maintaining data on such measures allows management to compare its performance to competitors in order to convince physicians to admit patients to their hospital.

PRICE When thinking of the prices paid by physicians as customers of a hospital or clinic, the exchange between the organization and the physicians is unlike most others. There is a mutual customer relationship. Physicians sell patients to care delivery organizations. Their price is the services the organizations perform for them. It is a barter arrangement. Physicians can withhold their product (patients) if the hospital does not pay a competitive price. As with any supplier, the hospital must hope that competition among physicians will prevent the price from becoming excessive. This happens when an organization's cost to supply a service is more than the organization is paid for performing the service. To manage profitability, hospitals should have measurements of the costs of services ordered by physicians and the total revenue from the patients they admit.

Care organizations can also affect some control of physician admission choice by competing for patients directly. Their recruiting efforts can be based on measures of service and outcomes communicated to potential patients through advertising and by their reputation built through patients' experiences. This can result in patients telling their physician which hospital or clinic they will use.

DISCUSSION QUESTIONS

1. What is the nature of the customer/client relationship between care delivery organizations and physicians?
2. How does that relationship create problems for hospitals in the efficient delivery of high-technology services? How does this relate to a physician's access to a workplace?
3. What are the variables a hospital must understand in order to address these problems? What are the sources of measures on these variables?
4. What are the differences in the quality of hospital or clinic services as seen by patient and as seen by physicians?
5. How is the price hospitals must pay to have physicians admit to their facilities patients set? How is it paid? How is the payment measured?

Third-Party Payers

Because most patients' charges are paid by third parties under some sort of insurance arrangement, these payers can also be considered customers of care providing organizations. The care provider furnishes services to the payer's clientele in return for payment. The care provider has a contract with the payer that specifies the payment structure. Over the past 20 years, the relationships among potential patients, providers, and third-party payers have gone through a series of changes.

Originally, the third-party payer was essentially a casualty insurer who paid for a client's health care according to an insurance contract. The payments were to cover fee-for-service care required under the contract. In the 1980s, HMOs became more popular in the private sector. The organizations served the casualty insurance functions but also took on care management roles. The intent was to reduce the cost of care by making payment only to providers who followed certain protocol restrictions and accepted the prices set by the payer. The objective was to control health care costs by eliminating unnecessary care interventions and putting competitive pricing pressure on providers. There has evolved an array of ways in which these organizations and contracts among the patient, payer, and provider are structured. The generic term managed care organization (MCO) is used to refer to these organizations that assume the casualty insurance function and attempt to influence some control over provider behavior and payments to providers. For the elderly and the medically indigent, federal and state governments have dominated arrangements for much of the care provided, using taxpayer funds.

SERVICES Third-party payers attempt to arrange for the services needed by their clientele. They compete for clients by offering a full range of services under an insurance contract priced competitively. The contracts generally cover both physician and other provider charges. The array of services covered, therefore, need to be those that are needed by both patients in the insured population and the physicians serving them. In the aggregate, these services must be profitable.

PRICES Current overcapacity among providers gives these payers strong bargaining power, because providers are competing among themselves to get the contributions that the payers can provide. Payers' negotiating strength comes from the ability to steer large numbers of patients to their selected providers and thereby reduce the fixed cost per patient episode for those providers. As discussed in Chapter 14, providers may be willing to accept prices that furnish a contribution but do not cover fixed costs. A provider might do this if it believes that capacity among its competitors will shrink. When capacity shrinks, payers will have limited alternate sources of care and the provider will have gained market power. The provider must, however, believe it can sustain the losses that will occur until that time. In this bargaining environment, it is imperative that providers understand the fixed and variable nature of the costs of providing various services and using various available protocols. To the extent that they do, they can underbid their competition without bidding themselves into receiving revenues too low to sustain their organization until better times. It is in support of this bargaining that the additional accuracy of activity-based information can justify its additional cost. A financial result for providers is that their prices can be established through data-driven negotiation with the third-party payers.

A provider may be able to negotiate price improvements if it can establish that being in the payer's provider system will increase the payer's client base simply by associating its reputation for quality care with that of the payer's. Measures that support such negotiation include high cure rates, high patient satisfaction, correct first-time billing, and expedited appropriate discharge planning.

PRICES CHARGED BY THE PAYER   The prices charged by third-party payers to those they insure depends on the risks born by the insured individuals and the cost of the mix of health care services they will demand. The implication for health care providers is that the payers are interested in maximizing their profits and, therefore, lowering their costs. This has been made more important because employers who pay a large part of the insurance premiums are putting increased pressure on third-party payers to lower premium costs. This pressure combined with the excess capacity just mentioned places extreme pressure on the ability of care deliverers to negotiate prices they desire. It adds to the requirement for them to build strong arguments to support their measures of operating cost and needs for capital.

DISCUSSION QUESTIONS

1. What is the difference between a health insurance company and an MCO?
2. In what sense are MCOs customers of other health care delivery organizations?
3. How do the services purchased from care deliverers by MCOs and government insurance programs differ from services desired by physicians? How is their form of payment different?
4. Why are MCOs and government insurance programs more instrumental in setting health care prices than patients?

DETECTING UNWANTED CUSTOMERS

The old saying that the customer is always right is not universally true. Some customers may not be right for some organizations.

Detecting

One of the weaknesses of accounting data is that grouping selling and administration costs as period costs provides no information about variation in profitability among customers. Indeed, there are some customers with whom dealing is more costly than others.

Doing business with any customer who requires nonstandard information, questions legitimate charges, and pays late is more costly than those who do not. If the contributions from such customers are less than the extra cost of doing business with them, providers are probably better off without their business. Third-party payers who demand prices with small unit contributions while providing few patients may be causing more transaction and other overhead costs than the total contributions from their business. In such cases, awareness of costs to sell and administer transactions with individual customers is needed if providers are to identify customers who are causing financial losses. Measures such as dollar-days of late payments and sales cost per dollar of revenue listed by payers can help identify individual third-party payers covering excessive costs. Measuring the ratio of the cost of selling and administrative activities to revenue by customer can provide evidence to justify renegotiating prices, changing services, or dropping the customer.

Physicians who consistently place more hospital orders than others for patients with the same diagnoses and severity may be causing total costs for caring for their patients that are higher than the payment received. Variable cost per dollar of net patient revenue helps identify admitting physicians causing unnecessarily high costs. Operating room minutes for standard surgical procedures benchmarked against other surgeons in the facility may identify physicians who tie up scarce operating rooms for excessive lengths of time. Percentage of dollar value of the unjustified prescription of high-cost drugs rather than generic equivalents may also identify high-cost physicians.

Terminating

Detecting the unwanted customer is often easier than terminating that customer. Terminating a physician is usually controlled by strict protocol. The chief of staff will make the final decision, and the arguments (and supporting data) have to be convincing enough to make the case for termination. Excessive mortality rates attributable to a single physician, for example, would make a strong case. If the physician is a specialist and the facility is closing down their service line for that specialty, then obviously termination can occur. Termination for excessive use of supplies, drugs, devices, or facility revenue-producing areas such as the operating room means the excessive use must be blatantly obvious, and the physician will probably be given one or more chances to reform before termination occurs. Meanwhile, the losses to the provider continue.

Terminating a payer is marginally easier. Each managed care or discounted fee-for-service payer generally has a contractual agreement with the provider, and these contractual agreements often have a renewal date or an expiration date. These anniversary dates are the point where termination can readily occur. Payers who contribute little allow an easy decision. The difficult decision for management occurs when the problem payer represents a large portion of the business of the provider. (It is virtually impossible to terminate either the Medicare or the Medicaid program, so greater efficiency is the only reasonable answer with these governmental payers.)

INTERNAL PERSPECTIVE

Activity-based approaches naturally support internal performance evaluation. Performance evaluation is concerned with performers, and activities are performed by people or people-machine groupings. Both control and improvement of performance involve decisions by people. Chapter 5 emphasizes that each activity occurs within an organization center with a responsible manager. ABC systems can allow the costs of an activity to be estimated by following the flow of resources and other activities to it. This essentially means treating necessary prior activities as resources. We have claimed that activities producing specific care interventions flow into the treatment and discharge of individual patients.

Using ABC to estimate the cost of caring for patient in specific categories, such as DRGs, allows providers to justify an appropriate payment for each such category. Similarly, patients in specific categories flow into the cost of capitated contracts. The cost of a future contract can be estimated if one knows the cost of each category of patient and if the patient mix from the population covered can be estimated. This, of course, demands actuarial analysis of demographic and epidemiological data. However, keep in mind that ABC analysis is expensive, and so the number of intermediate products that undergo ABC must usually be limited. The criterion is that the value of the increased accuracy in costing must be more than the cost of the analysis. It is also important to keep in mind that evaluation of *cost performance* demands measurements of activity costs for the period of evaluation and standards for those costs. Cost variances are measures of internal performance of production activities. Similarly, revenue variances are measures of marketing activities.

Organization Standards

Standards for cost performance evaluation can be established from two sources. First, the organization can establish quality, resource usage and acquisition costs for resources used in its activities and use these amounts to establish a standard cost for the activity. Using an ABC approach as described in Chapter 7, institution-sustaining overhead can be broken into activities that happen within service centers. The degree to which this should be done depends on the degree to which separate costs can be traced to different outputs of the center and the degree to which demands for these outputs differ among their users. Let us return to the example of the personnel department that realized it produced two different services, managing the payroll and processing personnel actions. If users of an intermediate output (such as payroll management) demand a measurable amount of the intermediate product's driver (such as people to be paid), the cost of the intermediate product can be traced to the user. If the user's outputs also require measurable amounts of the driver, intermediate product costs can be further traced to these outputs. The costs of these outputs, which now include parts of institutional- and production-sustaining overhead costs, then flow to discharges. To reemphasize, the increased accuracy of ABC comes from the finer grid of overhead cost allocations using more appropriate bases; that is, more accurate activity drivers combined with following the use of these bases by each activity needed to produce the cost object (as opposed to departments). Those overhead costs for which activity drivers cannot be identified are allocated using resource drivers. In the example, these could be personnel department costs that are not traceable to the payroll or personnel actions. They are therefore put in the personnel department's residual overhead pool and allocated using a basis such as *FTE* employees. In this example, FTEs are considered a resource driver because their variation correlates highly with changes in the remainder pool. This was discovered through a cost-behavior analysis regressing the remainder of the pool costs on the organization's FTE count.

Organization performance standards result when future activity costs are established using historical costs, experience, and production expertise to estimate what they *should* be in the future. Once standards are set, cost variances can be computed for any activities in the same way they were for department outputs in Chapter 13. These variances are performance measures.

Industry Standards

When evaluating the performance of an organization, benchmarks can be found in the results of other similar organizations. These are often made available by trade or professional organizations as well as commercial information-processing businesses. The American Hospital Association, American College of Pathologists, Medical Group Management Association, and the Healthcare Financial Management Association are just a few of these sources. Benchmark data range across measures such as the average length of stay for patients by DRG, the blind specimen test accuracy by test type, recruiting costs by clinical specialty, and the average time to collection for outpatient revenues. Note that this data include measures related to causes of costs, measures of the cost of activities, and measures of clinical quality variables. It is only through use of this type of comparison data that an organization can tell if it is keeping up with its competition in specific areas of its operations. Every organization should select a set of such variables that it believes are meaningful to its stakeholders. The set should provide a comprehensive look at its competitive position yet be small enough to be used by busy managers.

The fact that standards for periodic cost and revenue-variance reporting can only be established for stable processes has caused legitimate criticism of their use in rapidly changing processes. This criticism is related to recent criticism of strategic planning. The argument is that an organization cannot plan action over a long period of time if it does not know what its markets and technology will be. However, even with the rapid changes that health care is experiencing, change in a specific activity tends to be incremental and not occur in every accounting period. ABC is helpful because it examines the organization activity by activity. This analysis is done where the activity happens—in the center responsible for it and under the supervision of a technically competent manager. Standards based on projections of the cost of their component activities facilitate reacting to change. When change occurs that will affect costs, only the cost of the activities affected by the change need be analyzed. If the flow of activities leading to a specific cost target has been identified and charted, input data need only be changed where change occurs. When this is done, all the resultant changes in costs farther down the cost flow will be reflected. This makes ABC software extremely flexible and accurate when investigating the sensitivity of any cost target and its resource demands to any change in output.

We should note that when an organization meets standards established by benchmarks from current best practices, it is simply doing as well as its competition at the time. Our society expects progress, and the best performance will improve over time. Strategically successful organizations must make a conscious effort to continuously serve their markets better. The continuous quality improvement literature discusses this phenomenon at length.

Regulatory Standards

Governmental agencies also set standards for health care providers. These standards are often rigorous and national in scope. Thus, if the agency publicizes provider standings, a prime source of national benchmarks is available. (For example, in late 2002, the CMS began publicizing a rating list of skilled nursing facilities across the nation.) The disadvantage of regulatory standards is their rigidity. The advantage of regulatory standards is that they are uniform across many providers and thus provide a large sample for comparative purposes.

DISCUSSION QUESTIONS

1. How does ABC enable identification of physicians and payers who should be dropped?

2. What are some nonfinancial measures of health care organization performance needed for effective management? What are the sources of these measures?
3. What is the primary weakness in depending on industry standards to evaluate the performance of your organization?

LEARNING AND GROWTH PERSPECTIVE

Financial management literature emphasizes that the financial worth of anything is the present value of the future cash flows it can produce, as described in the discussion of capital budgeting. This applies to health care organizations as it does to any other entity. The ability of a health care entity to generate cash in the future is strongly tied to the knowledge and skills of its employees integrated with the capabilities of its facilities. To maintain competitive strength in an industry undergoing rapid technical change, health care organizations must assure that they are able to efficiently apply new learning and technology as it evolves. This means that the organization must be constantly learning and growing to be able to apply new capabilities as they come into existence.

Financial accounting procedures indicate whether capital assets have been increased. This gives some evidence of an organization's growing in order to utilize new technology. However, many organization attributes that contribute to its future competitive and financial position are not measured and reflected as assets on its balance sheet. In order for something to be called an asset, it must posses three characteristics: it must be the result of a transaction whose cost establishes its accounting value; it must be essentially owned or controlled by the organization; and it must have future value to the organization.[4] Training, advertising and public relations, and research and development costs can be shown as expenses when incurred. Unfortunately, their value toward future cash flows is not indicated at all on the balance sheet. This means that new measures need to be created if this important perspective on organization performance is to be managed.

To assure that the organization will perform optimally in the future, management should understand the future technological changes that will occur in heath care, understand the knowledge and skills that will be needed to apply that technology, and know the number of people who will need each skill. Full knowledge of these factors is impossible. However, the general direction of change in these factors can be estimated. Often the issue is not predicting the environment at the 10-year horizon but preparing for the application of technology that is close to becoming operational. In these cases, estimates of the equipment and personnel needs can be made fairly well and should be formally articulated. Once this is done, measures of progress toward possessing the new capabilities can be made and tracked. These measures can be such things as the percentage of needed personnel trained, the percentage of facility planning and installation completed, and the percentage of supplies and support activities located. Information of this sort is essential to managing toward efficient and competitive future operation.

DISCUSSION QUESTIONS

1. What measurements can assist managers in assuring that their health care organization will be ready for the demands placed on it in the future?
2. What analysis must be done prior to constructing these measures?
3. What factors can obstruct this readiness?

SUPPLIER PERSPECTIVE

The total cost of purchased and leased resources involves more than the purchase or lease prices. Costs can be reduced if an organization works with its vendors to:

- Establish resource specifications that can be met efficiently
- Set order quantities and delivery times that support logistical efficiency
- Limit the number of different item used for the same purpose

After working with vendors to optimize integration of the supply function with one's production activities, the following types of measurements can assist continuing management of supply efficiency:

- Percentage of on-time deliveries by vendor
- Percentage and dollar value of unaccepted items
- Lag time from change order to product change
- Percentage of price change per year

Tracking such variables over time and making comparisons among vendors enables purchasing management to negotiate with vendors based on factual evidence of performance.

DISCUSSION QUESTIONS

1. What are the factors involved in acquiring equipment and supplies that managers should attend to in order to minimize the total cost of these acquisitions?
2. What are measurements that can help managers control the cost of supplying a health care delivery organization?

BALANCED SCORECARDS

Comparing performance measures to those of other organizations can give management information as to which activities can be done more efficiently and thus justify management attention even when the organization's own standards are being met. Benchmark comparisons can also serve as inputs to motivation schemes. As such, they can be part of the processes used to set salaries and bonuses or used in determining promotions.

As important, they can indicate problems that are evolving prior to the problems affecting financial results. For instance, discovering an increase in medication errors might indicate training or ordering deficiencies before the occurrence of an incident that could affect the reputation of the organization or lead to expensive litigation. Such performance measurement means that management reports need to include the measure on a spectrum of performance indicators much broader than the standard periodic financial, dollar-denominated reports. Reports that give managers a summary of recent financial performance and report on nonfinancial indicators of future success or failure are referred to *balanced scorecards*. The need to construct and use balanced scorecards is finding increased emphasis in health care delivery. Balanced scorecards are discussed further in the next chapter.

Key Points

- Management should evaluate its organization from the perspective of its customers, internal operations, learning and growth, suppliers, and finances.
- Measures of financial performance can be constructed from information in the financial statements.
- Ratios of financial performance data relative to financial position data are especially informative.
- Measures constructed from financial statement data are historical and do not necessarily indicate future performance and position. Also, they do not indicate why good operational performance does not result from its activities.
- Patients, physicians, and payers can all be considered customers of health care delivery organizations.
- Patients primarily look for the services they need, access to these services, and high quality of care when selecting a care facility. Price is a secondary consideration for most potential patients because most payment is made by third parties.
- Physicians have what is essentially a barter arrangement with hospitals and clinics. They sell admissions and are paid by having facilities in which to do their work.
- The cost of filling a physician's orders should not exceed the revenue from treating the physician's patients. This means that patient costs should be categorized by physician and payer.
- The unused capacity of fixed-cost assets demanded by physicians is a potential source of excessive hospital and clinic expenses.
- Management must understand the levels of skills needed across the array of activities that must take place within the organization and ensure that each activity is adequately staffed. It should also ensure that excess expenses are not incurred by using overskilled labor.
- Prices for care delivery are largely set by third-party payers. The market power of the payers derives from overcapacity of the sellers.
- Selling and administrative costs should be

tracked to individual payers to assure that some payers do not cause more costs than their revenues warrant.
- Control of internal procedures demands monitoring some measures that are not financial.
- Control of costs and other success factors requires standards. There are both internal and external sources of standards for these measures.
- Standards derived from existing best practice do not necessarily represent best

possible practice. Improvement is usually possible, especially when technology is changing.
- Factors other than price are significant to the cost of acquiring equipment and supplies. Measures should be constructed for performance related to logistics costs.
- Measures exist or can be constructed to monitor performance from any of the perspectives from which a health care organization should be viewed.

REFERENCES

[1] Keeney, R. L. and Howard Raiffa. *Decisions with Multiple Objectives: Preferences and Value Trade-offs* (New York: John Wiley & Sons, 1976), Chapter 2.

[2] Kaplan, R. S. and D.P. Norton. *The Balanced Score Card: Translating Strategy into Action* (Boston: Harvard Business School Press, 1996), Chapter 2.

[3] Eastaugh, S. R. "Hospital Costs and Specialization: Benefits of Trimming Product Lines," *Journal of Health Care Finance* 28, 1 (2001): 61–71.

[4] Belkaoui, A. R. *Accounting Theory* (Fort Worth, TX: The Dryden Press, 1993), p. 392.

REPORTING PERFORMANCE MEASURES

INTRODUCTION

This appendix contains examples of quantitative and qualitative health care performance measures. We describe a selection of various measures; most health care performance reports are quantitative; thus, they contain information that can be objectively measured. The examples in this appendix include both quantitative and qualitative measures and are representative of reports prepared by hospitals, by governmental agencies, and by commercial publishers for use as guides.

PHYSICIAN PERFORMANCE REPORTS PREPARED BY HOSPITALS Figure 15A-1, entitled "Hospital's Physician Performance Report—Quantity of Services Provided by Each Clinician," is a count-and-amount type of report. It contains the physician case workload for each physician involved in the service.

Figure 15A-2, entitled "Hospital's Physician Performance Report—Laboratory Testing Ordered by Each Clinician for Each Type of Service," contains the resource usage attributed to each physician for a particular period of time. Thus, each physician's resource utilization of pharmaceuticals, supplies, radiography, laboratory tests, and so forth can be compared against each other and against an overall total.

COMPARATIVE FACILITY PERFORMANCE REPORTS ISSUED BY GOVERNMENTAL AGENCIES Figure 15A-3, entitled "Governmental Facility Performance Report—Hospital Comparative Report," contains information about individual hospitals along with outcomes. The hospital information includes total discharges plus observed and expected average charges. The outcomes include both observed and expected average length of stay (LOS) and mortality rates. Note that the information is aggregated for each hospital; thus, the mortality rates, for example, are across all types of illnesses.

Figure 15A-1 **Hospital's Physician Performance Report—Quantity of Services Provided by Each Clinician**

Physician Case Workload

	Total	DRG 193	DRG 209	Other DRGs
Quantity for all providers	60	8	16	36
Abrams, Dr. William		2	7	0
Jones, Dr. Sherry		6	9	0
Smith, Dr. John L.		0	0	0
Thomas, Dr. Enid		0	0	0

Figure 15A-4, entitled "Governmental Facility Performance Report—Lung Infections, Complicated," also contains information about individual hospitals along with outcomes. The report contains total cases (equivalent to total discharges) and average charges. The report also contains outcomes as to LOS and mortality ratings. In this case, the report includes additional outcomes: the percentage of readmissions for any reason and the percentage of readmissions for complication or infection. Note also that there is a dashboard-type scoring for the mortality rating. The key gives details on the scoring.

Figure 15A-2 **Hospital's Physician Performance Report—Laboratory Testing Ordered by Each Clinician for Each Type of Service**

Physician Laboratory Testing

	Total	DRG 193	DRG 209	Other DRGs
Quantity for all providers	991	274	414	103
Abrams, Dr. William		65	161	0
Jones, Dr. Sherry		209	253	0
Smith, Dr. John L.		0	0	0
Thomas, Dr. Enid		0	0	0
Per case average		34	26	0
Comparison to mean*				
Abrams, Dr. William	0.8811	32.5	161	0
Jones, Dr. Sherry	1.05819	34.83	28.11	0
Smith, Dr. John L.	0.97701	0	0	0
Thomas, Dr. Enid	1.11538	0	0	0
Cases unaccounted by provider	1.25	0	0	0

* Designated physician's number of tests ordered as a fraction of the mean of test ordered per physi-

Figure 15A-3   **Governmental Facility Performance Report—Hospital Comparative Report**

		Average Charges		Average LOS		Mortality Rate	
Hospital	Total Discharges	Observed	Expected	Observed	Expected	Observed (%)	Expected (%)
A	1,061	8,000	8,700	4.26	4.64	2.73	3.51
B	870	10,300	9,600	4.35	4.63	3.22	2.92
C	1,663	9,300	9,700	4.00	5.00	3.61	4.17
D	593	10,900	9,300	4.91	4.76	3.20	4.27

FACILITY PROFILES PUBLISHED AS GUIDES BY COMMERCIAL ENTITIES   Figure 15A-5, entitled "Facility Profiles Published as Guides by Commercial Entities," contains operational, financial, and clinical measures (designated as Part I, Part II, and Part III). The example contains three hospitals, two of which are located in urban areas and one of which is located in a rural area. Operational measures include each hospital's occupancy rate, average overall LOS, and case mix index. The case mix index is a relative weight that indicates the severity of illness in the patients within this hospital over a given period of time (usually a year). The percentage of Medicare discharges and the percentage of Medicaid discharges are also included in the operational Part I.

Figure 15A-4   **Governmental Facility Performance Report—Lung Infections, Complicated**

Hospital	Total Cases	Mortality Rating*	LOS	Readmission % for Any Reason	Readmission % for Complication or Infection	Average Charge (in $)
U	187	⊙	7.2	38.4	12.9	26,893
V	139	⊙	7.2	20.2	3.7	11,766
W	20	●	7.5	35.4	36.4	23,159
X	61	⊙	6.6	15.8	6.0	10,017
Y	122	○	7.5	24.4	7.4	24,849
Z	68	⊙	9.9	37.3	18.3	53,655
Statewide	11,710		7.9	25.4	8.2	20,758

Note: The mortality, length of stay (LOS), and readmission figures account for varying illness levels among patients.

*Key
● = Significantly higher than expected
⊙ = Not significantly different than expected
○ = Significantly lower than expected

Source: Reprinted from the *2001 PHC4 Hospital Performance Report*, published by the State of Pennsylvania.

Figure 15A-5 **Facility Profiles Published as Guides by Commercial Entities**

Part I: Operational

Hospital	Occupancy Rate (%)	Average LOS	Case Mix Index	Medicare (%)	Medicaid (%)
Urban 1	76.6	4.3	1.3965	26	4
Urban 2	61.3	4.4	1.3421	32	29
Rural	36.3	3.5	1.1280	57	12

Part II: Financial

Hospital	Outpatient Revenue (%)	Operating Revenue*	Days in Accounts Receivable	Average Pay Period
Urban 1	24	190.6	57.3	113.9
Urban 2	33	57.4	82.1	105.9
Rural	54	54.0	65.4	68.8

* Listed in millions of dollars

Part III: Clinical (Top 5 DRGS)

Hospital		DRG 1 Average LOS	DRG 2 Average LOS	DRG 3 Average LOS	DRG 4 Average LOS	DRG 5 Average LOS
Urban 1	DRG	127	089	088	462	014
	LOS	(6.0)	(6.0)	(5.6)	(8.3)	(7.2)
Urban 2	DRG	127	079	014	089	416
	LOS	(4.7)	(7.3)	(6.5)	(5.5)	(7.5)
Rural	DRG	127	089	088	140	182
	LOS	(4.3)	(5.0)	(4.1)	(2.5)	(3.4)

DRG Key

127 = Heart failure and shock

089 = Simple pneumonia and pleurisy, age greater than 17 w/complications

088 = Chronic obstructive pulmonary disease

462 = Rehabilitation; 014 = intracranial hemorrhage and stroke w/ infarction

416 = Septicemia, age greater than 17

140 = Angina pectoris

182 = Esophagitis, gastroenteritis and miscellaneous digestive disorders, age greater than 17 w/complications

The financial measures include each hospital's outpatient revenue percentage of revenue and its overall operating revenue (listed in millions of dollars). The traditional performance measures of number of days in accounts receivable and number of days in accounts payable ("average pay period") are also included in the financial Part II.

The clinical measures include each hospital's top five DRGs, along with the average LOS for each of the five DRGs. A key that describes each DRG appears with the clinical Part III.

Qualitative Measures

Qualitative performance reports contain information that must be measured in a subjective manner. The most common qualitative measure used in health care facilities is the customer satisfaction survey. The survey can be administered by telephone or in written form such as the examples contained in this appendix.

EMERGENCY ROOM CUSTOMER SATISFACTION SURVEY Figure 15A-6, entitled "Customer Satisfaction Survey—Emergency Room," is a simple easy-to-complete form. A survey such as this one is sometimes given to the patient during the check-out process.

INPATIENT CUSTOMER SATISFACTION SURVEY Figure 15A-7, entitled "Customer Satisfaction Survey—Inpatient," is a somewhat longer survey form. A form such as this is sometimes mailed to the patient after discharge. Surveys that are mailed have a lower response rate than the one described in the preceding paragraph that can be collected on the spot.

Figure 15A-6 **Customer Satisfaction Survey—Emergency Room**

Please check one:

	Excellent	Good	Average	Poor
What was your general impression:				
of our emergency room service	☐	☐	☐	☐
of our professional staff				
prompt	☐	☐	☐	☐
courteous	☐	☐	☐	☐
concerned	☐	☐	☐	☐
of how you were informed of your progress				
of care	☐	☐	☐	☐
of how discharge instructions were				
explained ☐ ☐ ☐	☐			

	Yes	No
Do your comments reflect treatment given		
by our:		
doctors	☐	☐
nurses	☐	☐
clerical staff	☐	☐
x-ray technician	☐	☐
other _____	☐	☐

(specify)

Other comments?

_____

_____

_____

_____

_____

Figure 15A-7   **Customer Satisfaction Survey—Inpatient**

Patient Questionnaire

Admitting
Were you treated courteously and promptly by the admitting staff?   ___Yes ___No

Your Room
Was your room satisfactory in terms of:

Housekeeping	___Yes ___No
Lighting	___Yes ___No
Temperature	___Yes ___No

Your Care
Was your nursing care:
   Excellent ___ Good ___ Fair ___ Poor ___
Did you receive adequate information about medical procedures? ___Yes ___No

Visiting
Were visiting hours:
 Too short ___ About right ___ Too long ___
Were your visitors directed to you without confusion or delay? ___Yes ___No

Food
Considering your dietary needs, was your food:
   Excellent ___ Good ___ Fair ___ Poor ___

Summary
Overall, how would you rate the quality of care you received at our hospital?
   Excellent ___ Good ___ Fair ___ Poor ___

After studying this chapter, students should be able to:

1. Identify three general categories of decisions.

2. Explain the differences between periodic performance reports and ad hoc reports.

3. Explain the philosophy and content of balanced scorecards.

4. Explain the relationships among organization charts, hierarchies of objectives, strategies, and balanced scorecards.

5. Explain the uses of balanced scorecards.

6. Explain the criteria and methods for selecting content for specific reports.

7. Explain the advantages and appropriate use of pie, column, and line charts in reports.

INTRODUCTION

Early in this book, we emphasized that the purpose of management accounting was to measure and present to managers information they need in order to perform their jobs. In performing their jobs, they must continually make decisions. When making decisions, manager's use thought processes, which were referred to as decision models. These models consider the relationships among factors that bear on the problem demanding a solution; these factors are called variables. In most situations, the decision maker needs measurements on these variables in order to apply the appropriate decision model. These decisions fall into three general categories:

1. Decisions that involve identifying and correcting current problems reflected in the organization's position and performance. Reporting cost variances to spot activities whose costs appear to be out of control is an example of information supporting this type of decision.

2. Decisions that involve identifying and correcting situations that may cause poor performance in the future. An example of information supporting such a decision is finding causes of low customer satisfaction.

3. Decisions that involve choosing among action alternatives. The results of capital budgeting analyses provide information supporting this class of decisions.

In all of these situations, the appropriate measures are those that fit the decision model used for the situation being addressed. Reports to support these three general categories of decisions can be divided into two basic types:

1. The first type is reports on historic performance and current position. These report are the results of the measurement step in the control process and support the first two decision categories just mentioned. These are generally referred to as *periodic performance reports*.
2. The second type is reports of information needed to construct alternative actions and choose among them. These are generally generated on request from a specific manager and are referred to as *ad hoc reports*.

PERIODIC PERFORMANCE REPORTS

Performance reporting assumes the organization has previously established its mission and the strategies it will follow to accomplish the mission. It also assumes that, based on the organization's mission and strategy, objectives have been established for activities at all management levels and across all activity centers. The basic purpose of the reports is to see if the objectives are being met, to identify reasons why objectives have not been met, and to track success or failure to reach specific objectives to those responsible for them.

Balanced Scorecards

Traditionally, management accounting reports have concentrated on measures that reflect financial performance. This has been encouraged because, as mentioned earlier, organization viability and financial viability are virtually synonymous. So far, this book has concentrated on performance with reference to resource use and costs. There is increasing awareness of the importance of the need to track nonfinancial measures if managers are to understand the causes of poor financial performance within their competitive environment.[1] Periodic reports that attempt to give a comprehensive view of the level of performance and specific weaknesses in performance are called *balanced scorecards* (BSCs). The specific content of a specific BSC depends on the level of the manager it supports, the time interval of the performance, or the time at which the position is being reported. BSCs necessitate careful examination of the objectives that were established during the organization's planning process.

OBJECTIVE HIERARCHIES   Keeney and Raiffa contend that after establishing the mission, management must decide what objectives lead to its being accomplished. These objectives can flow from responses to a series of questions. The first could be: "If we are going to accomplish the mission, what must happen?" Each response to this question describes an objective that must be reached and implies a set of activities needed to reach it. These can be referred to as *first-level objectives*. The next set of questions is of the form, "In order to reach each first-level objective, what must happen?" For each of the first-level objectives a set of subobjectives is specified. Continuing this procedure lays out a hierarchy of objectives.[2] Figure 16-1 is a schematic of such a hierarchy. As lower level objective are specified, they become more narrow and limited in scope. Eventually the analysts will reach a point that further specification of component objectives is of little value. This stopping point is a matter of manager and analyst judgment.

The hierarchy depicts the linking of the organization's mission to its strategy through the specific chain of objectives that the strategy dictates. Kaplan and Norton suggest that high-level objectives be established from the perspectives discussed in Chapter 15.[3]

Inspection of Figure 16-1 shows that if the objectives at the bottom of each hierarchical chain are reached, the mission is accomplished. For instance, in Figure 16-1, to reach objective *B*, objectives *c, d, e,* and *f* must be reached. But to reach objective *d*, objectives *5, 6,* and *7* must be reached. Similarly, to reach objective *5*, objectives *bb, cc,* and *dd* must be reached. This analysis of objective *B* can be completed by looking at objectives *c, d, e,* and *f* in the same way. Working from the bottom up, we can see that when objectives *c, bb, cc, 1a, 2b, 6, 7, e, 8, ee,* and *ff* (the

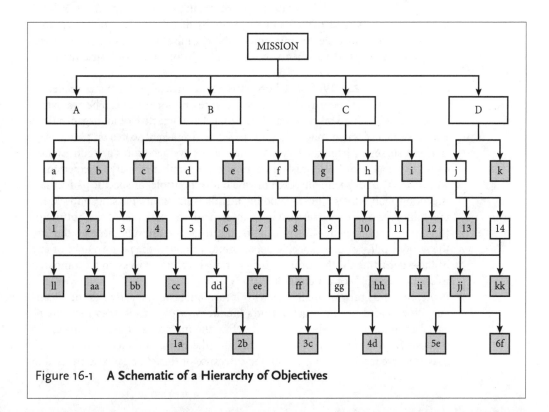

Figure 16-1   **A Schematic of a Hierarchy of Objectives**

shaded objectives supporting objective B) are achieved, objective *B* has been achieved.

OBJECTIVES AND CONTROL   Performance goals can be set for every objective in the hierarchy. For control purposes, however, if the goals are reached for the lowest level objective in each branch of the hierarchy, the organization is effectively implementing its strategy. This means that control can be simplified by paying routine attention to only those objectives. We speak of balanced scorecards because many of these goals may not be measured in financial terms. *Balance* refers to a balance of financial and nonfinancial measures. For instance, an objective may be to reduce returns to surgery to less than a specified number; the control measure here would be *returns to surgery*, not an amount of money.

It is important to realize that the hierarchy of objectives is not an organization chart. An organization's departments are usually organized around common technology and skills. This is especially true where the salable product is a patient's discharge or fulfillment of a capitated care contract, as opposed to a set of line items. Hierarchies of objective are the result of the analysis of the sequences of objectives that must be reached in order to accomplish the mission under a given strategy. This creates a dual set of relationships in our performance evaluation process. The objective hierarchy depicts the relationship of objectives and activities to the organization's mission and strategies. The organization chart depicts the structure of responsibilities of people managing groups of resources. A linking of these two sets of relationships is made by distributing the objectives that must be reached in order to implement the organization's strategy among the groups of resources (departments or centers) in the organization's structure.

REPORT CARD USES   With stated objectives, measures of performance related to them, and goals (or standards) for those measures, performance can be evaluated. Assume that high patient satisfaction is a high-level objective of an organization. Executive management may only want to see an average of scores on patient satisfaction surveys. They may take no action if the average scores are consistently above the goal. However, satisfaction rests on a number of patient experiences with a variety of departments, each of which is responsible for specific patient satisfaction subobjectives. These would include the admissions, nursing, housekeeping, billing, and other centers having contact with the patients. At the bottom of the hierarchy of objectives affecting patient satisfaction are subobjectives that are the responsibility of these specific department. To review the performance of any of these departments, the measurements on their subobjectives can be compared to established goals or benchmarks.

Report cards provide managers with information on the activities they manage. When based on the organization's hierarchy of objectives, they focus managers' attention on the objectives that define the mission and the organization's strategy for accomplishing it. They measure the degree of success with which managers are implementing the strategy. Because of this, they can also be used to appraise the performance of managers and departments. Because each report shows measures related to a set of objectives, a weighting system can be used to produce an overall performance score. Such a score can be used as the basis for awarding bonuses or other motivating rewards. However, for awards to motivate high-level performance, managers and workers must believe that the scores on which they are based indicate the level of their performance. To be effective, the scores must indicate the degree to which the organization's strategy is being implemented. If it is true that "what gets measured and rewarded gets attention," a BSC based on the hierarchy of organization objectives should be a powerful control tool. It should focuses managers' attention on the organization's strategies for accomplishing its mission.

The BSC can also promote improved coordination. For instance, suppose that an objective at the level of the director of clinical care has a low rate of returns to surgery and some of its subobjectives are the responsibility of the surgery department, while others are the responsibility of nursing services. The poor score on *returns to surgery* should automatically stimulate investigation within the directorate to see what subobjectives are not being met and if coordination among them is a problem. This cross-department reaction to the three scorecards involved can be a strong enabler of quality improvement.

Although not a use of the scorecards themselves, the need to relate effective scorecards to a hierarchy of objectives forces management to precisely articulate the organization's mission, the objectives necessary to reach the mission, and the relationships among these objectives and the departmental structure of the organization. Such reviews can spot unnecessary activities and inappropriate organization structure.

DISCUSSION QUESTIONS

1. What are the differences between periodic performance reports and ad hoc reports?
2. Why must the mission, strategy, and objectives of an organization be established before performance reports are designed?
3. What are the differences between BSCs and traditional management performance reports?
4. Why can we say that if the lowest level objectives in each branch of an objective hierarchy are met, the mission, as planned, is accomplished?
5. What is the relationship between attributes of objectives and the control function?
6. What are the differences between a chart of the hierarchy of objectives and an organization chart? What does each tell us? What is the relationship between them?
7. Explain the uses of a BSC.
8. Why must subordinate managers agree with executive managers on the appropriate content of BSCs for their activities?

Executive Management

Executive managers are interested in the overall, general performance of their organization. They are concerned with whether the organization has an appropriate mission and is using the best strategies to achieve it. These can be called executives' *outside* interests. Traditional financial statements partially meet the requirements of executive performance reporting on outside interests. They summarize the overall performance of the organization using a common numeric, which is money. Additionally, executives are interested in the degree to which success is being achieved from the perspectives of customers and suppliers, which are also outside interests.

Executive management must also be interested in the performance of operations and learning and growth within the organization. These are *internal* interests. They want information about the performance of first-level objectives and some key subobjectives. Unfortunately, financial measures are limited in their ability to measure the performance of centers within the organization. Where revenue cannot accurately be assigned among internal centers, financial statements can not reflect the profitability of those centers. Money-denominated measures related to these centers are restricted to cost analysis. Financial statements as performance reports do not include nonfinancial measures that can often indicate weaknesses in activities leading to key objectives. These weaknesses might not show up in financial statements until later, after considerable damage has been done. As an example, managers want to know about low patient satisfaction before it causes a reduction in admissions that could eliminate profits.

Executive managers, however, are not routinely interested in following the activities involved in meeting low-level objectives. Failure in reaching these objectives can be reflected in aggregate measures of success that appear on the executive's scorecard. For example, a measure of overall patient satisfaction computed from patient surveys is adequate for an executive report card. When this measure indicates low patient satisfaction, executive managers can ask for explanations from those with responsibility for the failed objectives involved. They can also drill through measures of the components of patient satisfaction shown in the scorecards of those responsible for the subobjectives in question. In reality, such lower level analysis should be a joint effort of executive management and the operating managers responsible for activities related to the unmet objectives.

Operations Managers

Managers of production and staff operations are interested in the activities assigned to them. They are, therefore, interested in performances related to the objectives of those activities. They would like a scorecard that gives them information on the degree to which those lower level objectives are being met.

The keys to creating an effective scorecard for a given center are to:

- Pick important objectives from the objective hierarchy for which the center is responsible. The center's personnel must acknowledge that these objectives relate to their performance and the organization's strategy for mission accomplishment.
- Determine valid measures that accurately reflect the degree to which these objectives are being met. The validity and accuracy of the measures must also be agreed on by the center's personnel and higher management if they are to motivate effort toward the objectives. Avoid redundant measures, measures that do not relate to mission-oriented objectives, and measures related to objectives that are not the responsibility of the center or manager whose performance is being reported on the scorecard.

Report Complexity

The purpose of performance reports is to give managers indicators of whether or not their organization strategy is being effectively and efficiently implemented. Performance reports should, therefore, be complex enough to provide that information without presenting content that is not needed. The key to doing this is to present a summary measure on the objectives for which the recipient is responsible. The objectives appropriate for a given manager's report are indicated in the objective hierarchy. The idea is to have routine performance reports that are adequately comprehensive but as concise as possible. Adequately comprehensive means that, if any objective in the hierarchy branch within the manager's responsibility is not being met, the failure is indicated by an item in that manager's report.

Report Frequency

Because operating managers are concerned with daily activities, they want more frequent performance reports on some objectives than would higher level managers. Increased frequency decreases the lag time between detecting a weakness and responding to it. For example, the chief of nursing may want census data three times a day or even in real time to help manage coordination of ward activity, bed space, and admissions. Executive managers may want to see summaries of this information only weekly or monthly. The point is that report cards may be formulated for different managers to receive performance information on various sets of objectives at varying intervals. Decisions about the content and frequency of reports to specific manager should be up to the manager. Reports that are not requested are usually not used.

Management Accountants and Performance Report Cards

From this discussion, it is obvious that performance reporting in today's health care organizations should entail more than periodic reporting of summary financial figures, product costs, and cost and revenue variances. Expanding from the traditional financial reports to a BSC requires a great deal of management action. Niven presents a seven-step process for the development of BSCs that involves:[4]

- Forming a BSC team
- Confirming the mission and strategies of the organization and assuring everyone in the organization understands them
- Conducting a series of management interviews and group sessions to define key objectives, isolate appropriate measure for each of them, and set target values or goals for each measure
- Communicating the measures and goals to all involved and getting feedback on their relationship to the mission and strategy, their validity and accuracy, and their fairness
- Developing a mechanism to maintain the validity of the scorecards as strategies are revised

The measurement and information implications of the last three items put the BSC system in the management accounting arena. Management accountants are suited to serve as the link between the system and the managers it supports. To do this well, management accountants must thoroughly understand the mission, strategy, and goals of the organization and its hierarchy of key objectives. These requirements expand the knowledge base of many management accounting centers beyond that which they currently have.

The last two of these items involve skills usually located in an information systems (IS) department, along with the decision analysis and measurement skill of management accountants. Because IS departments tend to focus on the configuration of computer hardware and software along with electronic communication links more than on information content, the demand for coordination between these two groups of staff specialists is increasing.

APPROPRIATE PERIODIC REPORT INFORMATION

Information appropriate for a specific report is that which is relevant to the purpose of the report. It must provide understanding of the level of accomplishment of the objectives that are the responsibility of the manager or department of concern. In reviewing existing reports, it is critical to ask why the report was created in the first place. What information was it intended to provide, to whom, and why did they need it? Who requested the report? Who is now receiving it? For what purpose do they use it—or do they use it at all? The search for answers to these questions may well lead to the elimination of some reports and the improvement of others.

Performance reports using a balanced scorecard approach are sometimes referred to as *dashboards*. The analogy comes from the attempt to present a small number of financial and nonfinancial measures that quickly indicate the degree of progress in implementing the organization's strategy. Reports should contain enough indicators to assure that a problem in strategy implementation is detected but yet not bog the reader down in detail when more detail is unnecessary. Cleverly suggests that reported variables be those that are most important to success, reflect critical drivers influencing goal attainment, are the most relevant measures of those drivers, and have relevant benchmarking data available. As an example, he suggests that a dashboard reflecting organization performance from the financial perspective contain return on equity, economic value added, a financial strength index, and total margin.[5] If any of these measures indicate a problem, executive managers can look at measures on components of the indicator reflecting a problem.

To be of value, the variables reported must be *valid;* that is, they must indicate differing levels of the concept that is being measured. In the mid-1980s, Health Care Financing Administration required that hospitals report their mortality rates. Reporting mortality rate was intended to give potential patients a measure of the concept of *quality of care* for individual hospitals. However, this variable, by itself, is simply not a valid measure of the quality of care. Mortality rates are a function of other variables as well. The most obvious of these are the mix of patients' diseases and the severity of their conditions on admission. Hospitals providing superior care to very sick or extremely injured patients with high expectations of dying could have much higher mortality rates than other hospitals.

Additionally, the measures on variables that are appropriate must be *accurate.* Previous chapters have discussed the need to improve the accuracy of cost measures, especially for comparison of the costs among different cost targets. Obviously inaccurate measures are of no help in comparing different entities on any dimension.

DISCUSSION QUESTIONS

1. Why is the detail in reports for lower level managers greater than that for executive managers?
2. What are senior managers' reaction alternatives when a performance report shows poor results?
3. What are the basic steps in structuring a BSC? Why is each important?
4. Why is it necessary for management accountants and information system technologists to collaborate extensively?

Nonroutine Decision Support

Unlike performance reporting, nonroutine reports are usually not based on continued measurement of performance indicators relevant to a defined set of objectives. Management accounting to support these ad hoc decisions frequently demands measurements that are not made continually. Reporting requirements for these decisions are defined by the choice models used to make them. In supporting these decisions, management accountants face a serious complicating issue.

Understanding Decision Models

The work of management accountants can be complicated because decision makers often have a difficult time articulating their decision models. Management accountants and information systems personnel frequently complain that after preparing and delivering reports containing the information operating managers said they wanted, the managers complain that it is not what they need. The more the management accountant is familiar with the managers' problems and decision models, the less likely it is that this will occur. However, gaining this understanding is not easy. Davenport contends that an effective approach should make the people who need and use information responsible for the information content of the reports they use.[6] Failure to do this can lead to formalizing models that do not consider all the important variables or to creating models that are overly complicated and require more data collection and processing than is necessary. For management accountants to gain an adequate level of familiarity with managers' decision models may take a considerable amount of time and effort.

Established Models

Generic models for the solution of some sorts of common, though not routine, problems are being widely used. The net present value approach to analyzing capital asset purchases, discussed in Chapter 14, is an example of such a model. Isolating the information needed by the model requires coordination with the decision maker and those who will be involved with the new asset. This coordination must ensure that all the revenue sources and asset needs have been identified. Then accountants must work with purchasing, personnel, marketing, maintenance, and other specialists to obtain accurate predictions of the cash inflows and outflows that will occur in the periods of the asset's life. This is not a trivial task in a period of uncertain asset operating lives and resource prices. This task can be made easier when the organization knows that it will acquire certain types of equipment periodically. It can then maintain current information on prices, quality, and support capabilities of potential vendors. This information can reduce data search time when specific analyses are needed. Measures on the risk of flows not being at their expected values should also be included. Procedures for doing this risk analysis are beyond the scope of this book; they are a standard topic in financial management texts.

Decisions Without Precedence

Accounting support for decisions for which there is little or no precedence demands close cooperation between the decision maker and the accountants attempting to provide decision support. In these situations, management accountants become coordinators; they must work with the decision maker to determine what variables are being used in the decision model. Then they must work with the variety of specialists who are best able to measure these variables.

Ad Hoc Reporting Information

Ad hoc reports are usually prepared in response to a manager's request for a specific set of measures on specific phenomena. The information support effort necessary to support ad hoc decisions depends on the degree of specificity of the decision. The capital budgeting decisions discussed in Chapter 14 are generally well specified. A well-understood model is used, and this model indicates the cash flows that must be measured. The decision to merge with another organization could be placed at the opposite end of the specificity spectrum. Though both use a present value analysis, the marginal cash flow data needed for decisions about mergers depends heavily on the nature of the current products, cost structure, organization culture, market positions, and the financial position of both organizations. Assembling appropriate measures of these variables requires data collection from many more sources. Additionally, this collection must be based on much more detailed understanding of the process used in making the decision than is needed in a capital budgeting decision.

The capital budgeting analysis is usually reported by presenting the complete present value computation matrix with an explanation of assumptions made. Frequently, the report also contains analyses of the situation's sensitivity to changes in key variables. The report is often prepared by management accountants after they have coordinated data collection efforts by many staff specialists. Reporting information in support of the more complex merger decision generally requires preliminary reporting of information relevant to the components of the decision just mentioned prepared by experts in each area. For instance, financial managers will be asked to make a judgment as to the effect of a merger with a particular organization on the credit rating and borrowing capacity of the new entity. Managers of administrative activities will be asked to project the total administrative savings available from consolidating organization-sustaining activities. Estimates of reductions in the costs of production by combining some production activities at a single location will be requested from production managers. This information can be presented in tabular of graphic format. A difference is that integrating it into a specification of alternatives and criteria for comparisons among alternatives requires a sequence of exchanges between the information sources and executive management. These are necessary in order to understand and articulate the interactions among these factors and the best attributes with which to judge potential advantages from a merger. Reports that prepare executive management to initiate such interaction usually require prose explanation as well as quantitative measures.

DISCUSSION QUESTIONS

1. What is the purpose of reviewing the content of current periodic reports? What questions should be asked in the review process? Why?
2. What does the term dashboard mean with respect to management reporting?
3. What criteria should be used in selecting dashboard-reporting measures?
4. What is meant by the terms validity and accuracy?
5. Why is identifying appropriate information for reports supporting ad hoc decisions frequently more complex than for periodic reports?

CONTENT FORMATS

Some reports required by outside users have required formats, such as the financial reports required by the Securities and Exchange Commission (SEC) and the Financial Accounting Standards Board (FASB), cost reports required by CMS for Medicare and Medicaid remuneration, and reports required by state regulatory agencies. Health care organizations have little discretion in the formatting of these types of reports. Reports for internal use can, however, be designed as the organization believes is most effective for their purpose. Once the content of a report is set, the design objective is to make the content as clear as possible. Some ways to do this are to:

- Use graphics versus tables or prose to present basic relationships.
- On routine performance reports, use a consistent format.
- Use terms that are well defined and understood throughout the organization.
- When using tables and charts, label and footnote them so that they can stand alone, without references to the text of the report.
- Add comments graphical presentations when they help in understanding the relationship among variables.

Graphic Presentation

If a picture is worth a thousand words, it is probably worth ten thousand numbers. Information that is presented in tables of numbers must be reprocessed in the reader's mind if it is to provide an understanding of relative values. Graphic presentations can eliminate much of this reprocessing. Table 16-1 shows information on the cost of DRG 089 patients categorized according to their attending physician. The following discussion will show how comparisons made from this information can be presented to managers more clearly. The three types of graphic presentations most commonly used in internal reporting are pie charts, column charts, and line charts.

PIE CHARTS   Pie charts present the distribution of the component parts of a phenomenon. In the example, Figure 16-2 shows the portion of DRG 089 cases attended by specific physicians. It tells what physicians are treating these cases and compares the share of these cases handled by each.

Table 16-1   DRG 089: Simple Pneumonia and Pleurisy Greater than Age 17 Quarter ending 12/31/2003

Physician Identification	MD 1	MD 2	MD 3	MD 4	MD 5	Average
Number of cases						
Medicare	23	47	5	14	25	
Other	0	15	7	0	0	
Total cases	23	62	12	14	25	
Hospital ALOS	7.2	9.8	14.7	10.7	13.4	
Medicare ALOS						
Other ALOS						
Expected Medicare Revenue	$4,592.00	$4,592.00	$4,592.00	$4,592.00	$4,592.00	$4,592.00
Room & board costs						
Med/surg ALOS	6.6	9.3	13	10.7	13.4	
Med/Surg cost	$1,802.00	$2,505.00	$3,782.00	$2,712.00	$3,575.00	$2,710.00
ICCU ALOS	0.6	0.5	1.5	0	0	0.5
ICCU cost	$346.00	$288.00	$865.00	$0.00	$0.00	$268.00
Ancillary costs						
OR	$0.00	$0.00	$0.00	$0.00	$136.00	$24.00
PACU	$0.00	$0.00	$0.00	$0.00	$2.00	$1.00
Anesthesia	$0.00	$0.00	$0.00	$0.00	$4.00	$1.00
ER	$345.00	$137.00	$373.00	$0.00	$108.00	$174.00
Ambulance	$31.00	$60.00	$152.00	$10.00	$31.00	$52.00
Lab	$260.00	$299.00	$601.00	$352.00	$263.00	$318.00
Pathology	$0.00	$0.00	$0.00	$0.00	$6.00	$2.00
EKG	$84.00	$53.00	$84.00	$56.00	$50.00	$61.00
Cardiac rehab	$0.00	$0.00	$0.00	$16.00	$50.00	$12.00

Continued

Table 16-1 **(Continued)**

Physician Identification	MD 1	MD 2	MD 3	MD 4	MD 5	Average
Radiology	$141.00	$140.00	$219.00	$335.00	$227.00	$183.00
Echocardiology	$58.00	$73.00	$146.00	$97.00	$58.00	$77.00
CAT scan	$20.00	$27.00	$0.00	$69.00	$101.00	$41.00
Pulmonary	$349.00	$253.00	$630.00	$283.00	$420.00	$336.00
Physical therapy	$24.00	$48.00	$82.00	$75.00	$0.00	$41.00
Central supply	$32.00	$63.00	$43.00	$74.00	$43.00	$54.00
Pharmacy	$524.00	$608.00	$843.00	$692.00	$1,056.00	$703.00
Total ancillary cost	$1,868.00	$1,761.00	$3,173.00	$2,059.00	$2,565.00	$2,080.00
Average ancillary cost per day	$256.00	$181.00	$219.00	$193.00	$191.00	$198.00
Total cost	$4,016.00	$4,554.00	$7,820.00	$4,771.00	$6,140.00	$5,058.00
Net income (loss) per case— DRG 089	$576.00	$38.00	−$3,228.00	−$179.00	−$1,548.00	−$466.00
Average cost for DRG 089— all physicians	$5,058.00	$5,058.00	$5,058.00	$5,058.00	$5,058.00	$5,058.00
Average cost per day—DRG 089	$588.00	$476.00	$539.00	$447.00	$458.00	$482.00
Average cost over all DRGs attended	$4,660.00	$4,555.00	$8,850.00	$4,825.00	$5,770.00	$5,265.00
Average cost across all physicians	$5,265.00	$5,265.00	$5,265.00	$5,265.00		

COLUMN CHARTS Column charts present the frequency or amount of a variable (or variables) attributed to various entities. Figure 16-3 shows the average medical/surgical, ICCU, and ancillary cost of each physician's patients, along with their totals. Column charts rapidly give an understanding of the relative amounts of variables associated with various entities. When column charts are rotated 90 degrees, with the entities named along the vertical axis, they are called *bar charts*.

LINE CHARTS Information presented in column charts can also be shown on a line chart. Here, a line connects the value associated with each entity. These charts can be made a bit more informative when the average among the entities is also shown as a horizontal line. Figure 16-4 is an example.

When trends in variables are of interest, the x-axis can show chronological time and the value of a variable over time can be shown on the y-axis. The line then presents the amount and change of the variable over time. Figure 16-5 is an example of such a trend line.

In many situations, it is understood that a variable will change with time, but the change is to be kept within limits around a desired level. In these cases, a trend line can be maintained using measures made as close to the time of reporting as possible. The chart can also show horizontal lines at the level of the upper and lower acceptable limits of variation from the desired

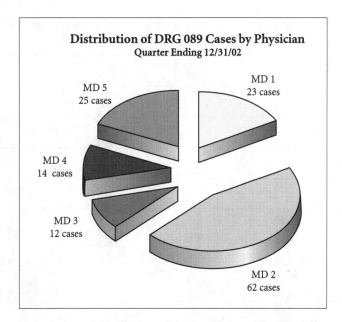

Distribution of DRG 089 Cases by Physician
Quarter Ending 12/31/02

MD 5
25 cases

MD 1
23 cases

MD 4
14 cases

MD 3
12 cases

MD 2
62 cases

Figure 16-2   **Distribution of DRG 089 Cases by Physician**

value. Such line charts are called *control charts*. They indicate at a glance when the variable is trending toward unacceptable values.

SUMMARY SYMBOLS   It may be simpler to reduce tabular numbers to symbols representing the relative quality of key measures reported. For instance, Cleverly presents the dashboard report on financial performance mentioned by noting where subject hospital's performance falls in a quartile distribution of benchmark information from similar hospitals. The hospital's relative performance is shown on the dashboard by a set of stars.[7] For instance, performance in the second quartile is shown by two stars. Pink and associates divide measures on dashboard-performance factors into three categories: average, above average, and below average. They report each factor's performance using an open circle for below average, a half-shaded circle for average, and a fully shaded circle for above-average performance.[8]

GRAPHIC CHOICES

The choice of graphics should be appropriate to the intended use. Tufte, in his discussion of the visual display of quantitative information, sets out the following principles of graphical excellence:[9]

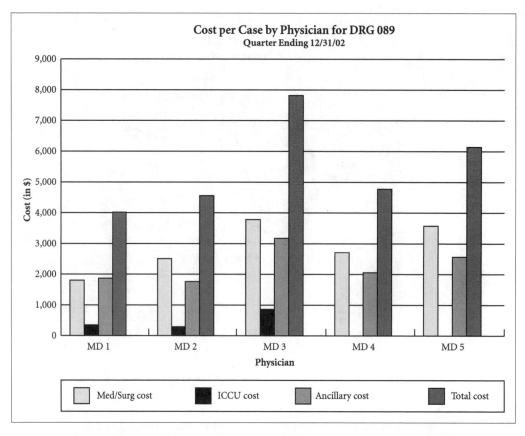

Figure 16-3   **Cost per Case by Physician for DRG 089**

- Graphical excellence is the well-designed presentation of interesting data—a matter of substance, of statistics, and of design.
- Graphical excellence consists of complex ideas communicated with clarity, precision, and efficiency.

Too often, analysts do not design a graphic to its use, but instead rely on two or three formats that are used over and over. Tufte went on to give three additional principles of graphical excellence:[10]

1. Graphical excellence is that which gives to the viewer the greatest number of ideas in the shortest time with the least ink in the smallest space.
2. Graphical excellence is nearly always multivariate.

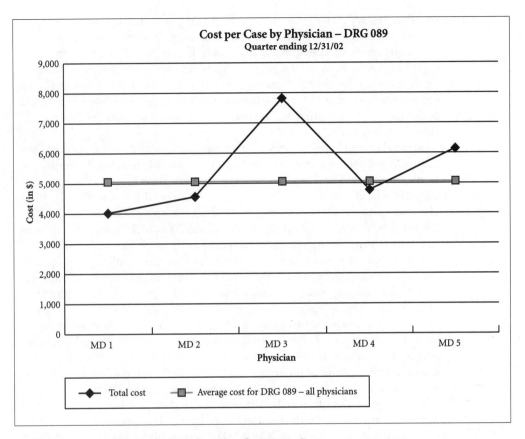

Figure 16-4 **Cost per Case by Physician for DRG 089**

3. Graphical excellence requires telling the truth about the data.

It should go without saying that telling the truth about the data is the foundation of all management accounting reports.

REPORT DISTRIBUTION

Table 16-1 (see p. 373) contains information about the cost of DRG 089 cases under the care of different attending physicians. Although the table contains a great deal of information, it is not easily interpretable. The hospital's chief of medicine will not want to take the time to review the large quantity of numbers it contains. The key item of information she would want from this table is the average cost of care for these patients. A second item would be information about any physicians who are causing overly high costs. It may be that a figure similar to Figure 16-4 that shows the average case costs across all cases for each attending physician is all the executive management would want. If that chart indicated some physicians were well above the hospital's average, executive management could query the appropriate section heads or drill down to more detailed presentations by themselves.

Medical section heads might want to begin with a more detailed analysis. They may want to establish a cost-over-average percentage. More detailed information would be requested on any physicians over the cut-off percentage. The appropriate section head may want to look at information on the cost profiles of these physicians for each DRG they treat. Figure 16-3 is such a graph for MD 3's DRG 089 patients. This figure clearly shows that, in this DRG, MD 3 causes far more ancillary costs than other physicians and significantly more medical/surgical ward cost than three of the four other physicians. To look more closely at the specific ancillary services used, a presentation like Figure 16-5 is revealing. It indicates that MD 3 used radically more pharmacy and somewhat more pulmonary services than the other physicians.

The section heads may also want to check trend lines such as those in Figure 16-6 to see if the quarter of the report is typical of individual physician's performance or if trends exist in the control of costs. Figure 16-6 indicates that MD 1 has demonstrated a history of improved cost control. MD 2 has also controlled costs; he seems to have reached a steady level at somewhat over $4,500 per case. MD 4 has also lowered costs, but leveled off at around $4,800 per case. Similarly, MD 5 had leveled at about $5,200 but had an atypically high last quarter. The significant bit of information in the chart is that MD 3 creates high costs and has done so consistently over the past six quarters. This information should prompt an investigation as to the legitimacy of these costs, and if not appropriate, how to reduce them.

Physicians should also be presented information like that in Figure 16-6. In order to get those who cause costs to change their behavior, they must see evidence that dictates a need for change. The concept of balance in the types of variables reported can be illustrated here. MD 3 might contend he orders more costly hospital services because his patients are sicker or represent more complex cases than those of other physicians. If this is not true, that fact can be communicated by inserting scores on each physician's average patient severity at admission into the figure. The reports of relative costs among physicians are really not complete until information on differences in related causal variables are included. Realize that Figure 16-7 presents exactly the same information as Figure 16-6. Intuitively, both present their content more clearly and more easily interpreted than does a table containing the numbers presented graphically. The choice of which graphical presentation to use should rest with the person using the report.

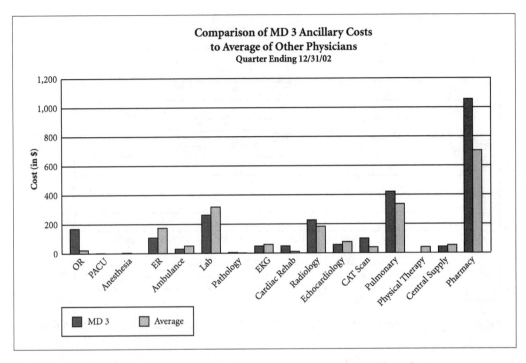

Figure 16-5   **Comparison of MD 3 Ancillary Costs to Average of Other Physicians**

DISCUSSION QUESTIONS

1. Why are graphical information presentations often superior to reporting information in matrixes of measurement results?
2. What are appropriate uses of pie charts, line charts, and summary symbols?
3. What should be the difference in the content of periodic reports to executive managers as opposed to operating managers?
4. Who should decide on the content of periodic reports for executive managers? For operating managers? Why?
5. What is the purpose of producing periodic reports of management information for attending physicians?

KEY POINTS

■ Periodic performance reports assume that the organization has established its mission, strategies for accomplishing the mission, and periodic goals for the objectives that must be reached in order to accomplish the mission.

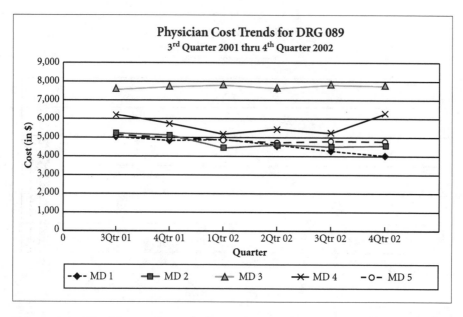

Figure 16-6 **Physician Cost Trends for DRG 089 3rd Quarter 2001 thru 4th Quarter 2002**

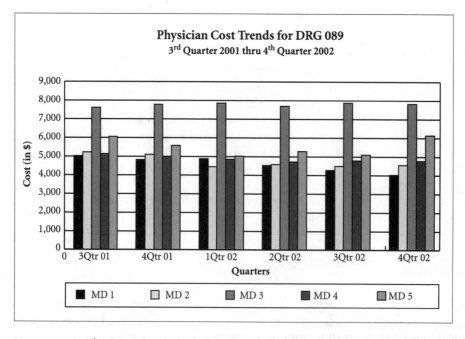

Figure 16-7 **Physician Cost Trends for DRG 089 3rd Quarter 2001 thru 4th Quarter 2002**

- Periodic reports are to indicate the level of success in reaching or maintaining the stated objectives.
- Balanced scorecards are periodic performance reports on key nonfinancial as well as financial objectives. They use nonfinancial as well as financial measures.
- An objective hierarchy shows the sequence of objectives that must be reached.
- If the lowest level objectives in each branch of the hierarchy are reached, the mission is being accomplished.
- Objective hierarchies are not organization charts.
- Objective hierarchies depict the linking of an organization's activities to its strategies.
- The content of report cards should be determined by the user of the report.
- Report cards for operations managers will contain more detailed measures than do those for executive managers.
- Report card measures for middle and higher level managers can indicate the effectiveness of coordination among activity centers.
- Many reports for operations managers will be prepared more frequently than those for executive managers.
- Report card scores can be used as the basis for motivational rewards for employees.
- To be effective as motivators, reported measures must be considered valid and accurate by employees.
- To design a report card system, management should:

    Form and BSC team

    Confirm the organization's mission and strategies and ensure the personnel's understanding of them

    Communicate measures and goals report recipients

    React to feedback from report and recipients.

    Develop methods for keeping objectives, measures, and goals up to date.
- Ad hoc reports are reports that are not required at set intervals of time.
- The content of ad hoc reports is dependent on the model used for the specific decision being supported.
- Articulating models used by decision makers can be extremely difficult when established models have not been accepted and previously used. It demands mutual confidence and understanding between the decision maker and the information specialists.
- Formats for internal reports should be jointly designed by the recipient and management accountants.
- Graphical presentation of key relationships is usually more beneficial than matrixes of figures. Their effectiveness increases for reports to higher level managers with more general responsibilities.
- The common types of graphical presentation are pie, column, and line charts. These are easily prepared from data matrixes using common graphics software.
- Reports should be distributed only to decision makers who use their content. As a corollary, a report to a specific user should not contain information the recipient does not use.

REFERENCES

[1] Niven, P. R. *Balanced Scorecard Step-by- Step: Maximizing Performance and Maintaining Results* (New York: John Wiley & Sons, 2002), pp. 6–8.

[2] Keeney, R. L. and Howard Raiffa. *Decisions with Multiple Objectives: Preferences and Value Trade-offs* (New York: John Wiley & Sons, 1973), pp. 41–45.

[3] Kaplan, R. S. and D. P. Norton. *The Balanced Scorecard: Translating Strategy into Action* (Boston: Harvard Business School Press, 1996), pp. 21–29.

[4] Niven, P. R. *Balanced Scorecard Step-by- Step: Maximizing Performance and Maintaining Results* (New York: John Wiley & Sons, 2002), pp. 61–65.

[5] Cleverly, W. O. "Financial Dashboard Reporting for the Hospital Industry," *Journal of Health Care Finance* 27, 3 (2002): 33, 35.

[6] Davenport, T. H. *Information Ecology: Mastering the Information and Knowledge Environment* (New York: Oxford University Press. 1997), p. 11.

[7] Cleverly, W. O. "Financial Dashboard Reporting for the Hospital Industry," *Journal of Health Care Finance* 27, 3 (2002): 34.

[8] Pink, G. H. and I. McKillop, E. G. Schrae, C. Aroya, C. Montgomery, G. R. Boker. "Creating a Balanced Scorecard for a Hospital System," *Journal of Health Care Finance* (2001). Vol 27 No 3 pp 1–20.

[9] Tufte, E. R. *The Visual Display of Quantitative Information* (Cheshire, CT: Graphics Press, 1983), p. 51.

[10] Ibid.

CHAPTER 17

SUMMARY AND A LOOK TO THE FUTURE

SUMMARY

This book has stressed the importance of generating the information that managers need in order to make necessary decisions. Because these decisions are made at the margin of ongoing operations, information activities should support choices among possible alternatives for future operations by providing accurate estimates for use in both operational and financial choice models. As pointed out earlier, one manages the future, not the past. However, to do that well, one must generally understand the past and adjust for a changed future. Activity-based management involves attempting to understand the component activities within an organization's total operations. If this is done, a new operation can be analyzed by thinking of it as an aggregate of such components. To understand the cost of any activity or output, the costs of the resources it uses must be known. These include the cost of resources that flow into it and the cost of previous activities that must be accomplished to enable its production. To make choices among alternatives actions, the relative costs and benefit of their results should be known.

Activity-based costing (ABC) does two basic things. First, it eliminates much of the overaveraging which, in traditional costing approaches, distorts the relative cost of different outputs. Second, it considers all the activities necessary to earn specific revenues, so that the total financial effects of specific transactions can be understood.

Knowing the amount of direct costs used in any department, activity, or product is relatively easy because, by definition, they are directly traceable to the cost target. ABC involves the appropriate assignment of overhead costs to the targets that cause them to be incurred. Some overhead activities are in response to a countable activity by the cost target. For instance, the cost of payroll activities is caused by other activities requesting that their employees be paid. The requests to pay individuals necessitate the actions of the payroll activities and the costs they incur. This is an example of an activity driver. When a causative activity of the users of overhead cannot be identified, analysts try to identify a resource whose consumption by the users is associated with the amount of the overhead activity performed. These are called resource drivers. An example is finding that equipment repair costs correlate highly with the amount of time the equipment is run.

ABC emphasis is on activities, rather than departments, for two reasons. First, costs are caused by the use of resources in performing activities, not simply by the existence of departments. Department costs cannot be controlled unless the use of resources by the department is understood. Activity analysis creates this understanding. Second, several overhead activities may be performed within a single department. These may have separable costs, different drivers, and be used to varying extents by different users. Not recognizing these differences and simply assigning the department's cost using a single allocation variable overaverages the cost among the users. The cost of some is stated too high while that of others is understated.

The flows of selling and administrative activities conducted by an organization are also analyzed because their costs are no less significant to financial performance than production costs. Doing business with different suppliers and different customers can incur varying levels of cost. Analysis of the activities involved in dealing with various vendors and customers can identify those who can be dealt with efficiently and those with whom it is unnecessarily expensive to do business. For instance, some vendors may necessitate more coordination to assure specifications are met, more order tracing, more inspection when purchases are received, more management of just-in-time support, and other activities. It is important to know what these activities cost when selecting vendors and computing the total cost in inputs.

The Health Care Environment

Financial pressure is exerted on health care deliverers from several elements within their environment. Three are of particularly important: (1) the market power of third-party payers, (2) the pervasiveness of excess capacity in the industry, and (3) the rapid rate of technological innovation.

Power of Third-Party Payers

Most payment for health care services is made by third parties: managed care organizations, casualty insurance companies, self-insured employers, or government agencies. Because these payers can affect where the large groups of potential patients they cover will seek care, they have great market power. In order to reduce their own costs, these payers use their market power to reduce the prices they pay care providers. In negotiating prices with these payers in today's buyers' market, care deliverers must be able to substantiate the costs they incur to produce each service.

Because payers can contract with different care providers for varying services, providers must understand the relative cost of their various services. To the extent that a service is undercosted, it will probably be underpriced. In this case, its profitability will be less than the accounting system indicates. In extreme cases, the service could actually be unprofitable, though the accounting system indicates it is a profit producer. The accounting error leads to pricing the product lower than the competition, very likely producing high sales volume. This causes both overstating profits and diverting resources from other, high-profit services. For services that are overcosted, unit profitability will actually be higher than accounting data indicates, but sales of services will be low because of their relatively high price. The care deliverer loses sales volume in its more profitable service or product. These situations are magnified by the fact that payers will steer their patients or members to the provider with the lowest prices on the specific services needed by each patient or member. This is why the reduction of overaveraged cost gained though ABC is valuable. It can prevent providers from entering contracts to provide large quantities of services that will not be remunerated adequately.

Overcapacity

Kaplan and Cooper claim that ". . . measuring and managing used and unused capacity is the central focus of activity-based costing."[1] In producing services, the vast majority of costs are fixed: facilities, equipment, and salaried labor. Compared to manufacturing, the quantity of materials is low. This means that the cost per unit of service is primarily dependent on the degree to which fixed costs are spread over the maximum possible volume of services; that is, the extent to which utilization is near capacity. The analysis of the use of fixed-cost resources in any activity coupled with understanding how the driver of the activity allows managers to know how much of their capacity is being used. Reporting capacity variances keeps managers aware of continuing unused capacity. ABC analysis will also inform managers of the amount of output increase needed to increase utilization to capacity.

The capacity issue is, of course, related to price negotiation in that the lowest profitable price can be offered only if production of services is at effective capacity. A critical condition exists when there is overcapacity throughout a service area. When payers are aware of this, they can offer prices that do not enable long-term financial viability but furnish a financial contribution. If a care deliverer refuses such a price, the payer can direct (or threaten to direct) its patients or members to another provider. The provider must decide if the short-term contribution justifies the long-run financial damage caused by accepting a price below the full cost of producing services. As the health care industry brings its resources into line with demand, this ability for payers to play one provider against others will decline.

The most financially productive way for a care provider to correct an unused capacity situation is to increase the volume of its sales of services. However, this is the case only if the sales price of the services is above the variable cost (there is a positive unit contribution) or the decrease in fixed cost per unit is more than an existing negative unit contribution. Managers will not know if this is the case unless they have accurate measures of the variable costs for each service they sell.

Motivation for Efficiency

To increase sales, potential patients must believe that the providers' services are at an acceptable level of quality, though attaining the goal of providing the highest quality at the lowest cost is wishful thinking. In most industries, providing less than the best quality available (however "the best" might be perceived by potential patients) must be coupled with lower prices. However, in health care, because the great majority of patients' bills are paid indirectly through an insurance or government system, when they receive services, they tend to expect the very best care. They feel that they or their employer have already paid for the best quality available in advance, through their insurance program. At the same time, the population in the aggregate is demanding lower health care costs. To respond to this demand, information about the relationship of the quality of the outcomes of care to the cost of the care must be available. Unless potential payers know the cost they incur by receiving more, or more expensive, care than acceptable outcomes demand, there will be little motivation for patients to attempt to reduce the quantity or complexity of the care they request. For this to happen, providers must price care in proportion to its cost and control cost by choosing the lowest cost alternatives that will produce an acceptable outcome.

Because of today's overaveraging costing procedures, the lack of attention to the ease of access versus capacity utilization trade-offs, and the use of CCRs to establish individual service/product costs prevent the necessary cost information from existing. The need for cost benefit awareness also demands quality of care, or outcomes, measurement. The association of outcomes information with cost information allows managers and clinicians to structure efficient care delivery systems for achieving the types of outcomes desired by patients, payers, and communities, given the opportunity costs involved.

The need for managers to understand and react to the wide variety of variables that define and track costs and outcomes resulting from performance results in the need for what is now called balanced scorecards. A great need exists to integrate the measurement of this variety of variable used in an array of models that support decisions regarding the benefits and costs of health care activities. We believe this will cause the work of management accountants to be more closely linked to that of industrial engineers and information technologists than to the work of financial accountants. Additionally, we believe that the application of behavioral studies we have referred to as information ecology will be recognized as a crucial part of the information-support activities that support managers' decision demands.

A Look to the Future

Providers will need to better manage their contracts with third-party payers if they are to keep their doors open. To do so, the provider needs reliable timely information. The overcapacity issue will drag a provider down, but to avoid negative margin contribution caused by overcapacity, the provider needs accurate measures of fixed and variable costs.

The future of technological tools may help to save the day. Today, health care providers can be grouped into those who possess sophisticated computer technology and use it (the "haves") and those who, for one reason or another, do not (the "have-nots"). At present, the "haves" are in the minority and the "have-nots" are in the majority. As technology evolves, its ease of use increases as its capital cost decreases. This is good news for providers, who desperately need appropriate computer capability to process necessary information.

In summary, the provider must achieve a motivation for efficiency as a weapon of survival. However, cost benefit awareness and a knowledge of the rewards of efficiency hinge upon having cost information available for decision making.

Do we detect a theme? Yes, we do: The future will belong to those who initiate, support, and use costing and accounting systems for managerial decision making.

Reference

[1] Kaplan, R. S. and R. Cooper. *Cost and Effect: Using Integrated Cost Systems to Drive Profitability and Performance.* (Boston: Harvard Business School Press, 1998), p. 122.

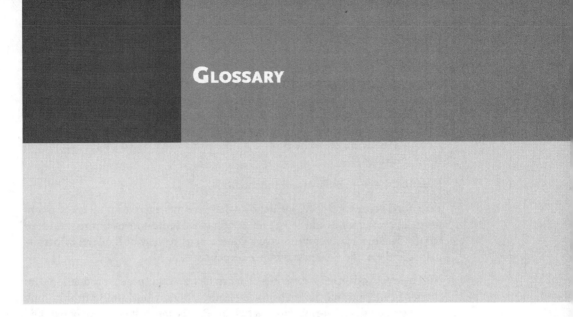

GLOSSARY

Underlined terms can be found elsewhere in the glossary.

Absorption cost—The full cost of all items produced; thus, the fixed production cost is absorbed into the cost of the finished goods. (See also *Full cost of manufacturing.*)

Accounting—The process of identifying, measuring, and communicating economic information to permit informed judgments and decisions by users of the information.

Accrual basis—In the accrual basis of accounting, revenues are recorded when they are earned (that is, when the service, drug, or medical supply item is provided), and expenses are recorded when they are incurred. (See also *Cash basis.*)

Activity—Work performed within an organization. An aggregation of actions performed within an organization that is useful for purposes of activity-based costing.

Activity center—A center within a service or a product center where an activity is performed whose cost can be separated from other activities and traced or allocated to a subsequent overhead center or product. Activity centers are the locations at which costs are incurred. (*See* Exhibit 6-1 for a listing of other structural unit types.)

Activity driver—A specific variable that defines demand for each cost target's use of a separable activity.

Ad hoc reports—Reports of information needed to construct alternative actions and choose among them. Generally generated on request from a specific manager.

Allocating/allocation—An apportionment or distribution. A process of assigning cost to an activity or cost object when a direct measure does not exist or when the cost benefit of measurement cannot be justified.

Arithmetic average—The sum of all the measures divided by the number of items measured.

Balance sheet—*See* Financial statements.

Balanced scorecard (BSC)—Reports that give managers a summary of recent financial performance and report on nonfinancial indicators of future success or failure. The reports attempt to give a comprehensive view of the level of performance and specific weaknesses in performance.

Batch-level activities—Activities that can be traced to specific production runs of specific outputs but cannot be traced farther to individual units of the output. (See also *Organization-sustaining activities*, *Production-sustaining activities*, and *Unit-level activities*.)

Batch costs—The costs of batch-level activities. Also known as *Setup costs*.

Billable line items—Items such as drugs, surgical procedures, and so forth, each of which appears on a separate line on the patient's bill.

Bottom-up analysis—Costing that starts with the cost object and works upward through all the activities necessary to achieve it. (See also *Top-down analysis*.)

Breakeven analysis—Analysis to discover that quantity of output where the total revenue and the total cost will be equal and where the operating income is therefore zero.

Budgets

    capital budget—A budget containing figures that require capital investments; thus, a capital budget concerns fixed assets that are long-term additions to the business.

    cash budget—Adjusts the figures in a pro forma income statement to reflect cash flows during shorter, imbedded periods. The purpose is to indicate if available cash will be adequate to meet short-term cash needs.

    cost budget—A statement of the anticipated cost of implementing or operating a plan over a set upcoming period; thus, the dollar-denominated restatement of plans. Cost budgets generally reflect expected revenues and expenses for a coming accounting period.

    extended budget—Covers an accounting period or periods that falls after the upcoming operating period. Also called an *Intermediate budget*.

flexible budget—Assumes a range of activity; thus, budgeted amounts for an operating period are flexible with respect to the level of output of the period. (See also *Static budget.*)

intermediate budget—*See* Extended budget. The term intermediate refers to the budgets in between the operating budget and the strategic budget.

long-term budget—*See* strategic budget.

operating budget—Generally covers a 1-year period of time, which corresponds to the standard financial reporting cycle.

program budget—Covers the expected amount and timing of costs over the life of a project; therefore, often multiperiod. May cover the costs and timing of a specific service.

rolling budget—Generally a series of budgets covering periods further and further into the future; the further into the future, the less detail is contained in the budget for that period.

static budget—Assumes one level of activity; thus, actual results are always compared to budget costs at the original activity level. (See also *Flexible budget.*)

strategic budget—Covers a long period of time for which management believes a given strategy will be used. Also known as a *Long-term budget.*

zero-based budget—Starts from zero; that is, each activity and its resource demand are analyzed using new measurements on all the variables involved.

Calendar year—A 12-month period that always begins on the first of January and ends on the last day of December; thus, it follows the calendar. (See also *Fiscal year.*)

Capacity variance—*See* Variances.

Capital budget—*See* Budgets.

Capitation—When the care provider is paid a flat fee to provide a client whatever services are necessary (as prescribed in a contract with the payer) over a defined period of time.

Cash basis—In the cash basis of accounting, revenues are not recorded until the cash payment is received and expenses are not recorded until they are paid for in cash. (See also *Accrual basis.*)

Cash budget—*See* Budgets.

Center—A term used to designate either departments or parts of departments. (*See* Exhibit 6-1 for a listing of other structural unit types.)

Charge—What an organization bills its payers for a product sold.

Charge master—A computerized listing of uniform billed charges; thus, the master list of charges.

Competition imperative—Assuming two key assumptions are operating, competition among producers attempting to sell to well-informed customers controls prices and promotes improvements in both products and services.

Complete observer—An observer that is removed from the activities and not noticed by those involved in them.

Cost-behavior analysis—Used to separate mixed costs into their fixed and variable components.

Cost-behavior pattern—The pattern of which costs are fixed and which costs are variable.

Cost budget—*See* Budgets.

Cost center—A unit within an organization to which costs can be traced or allocated but revenue cannot. (*See* Exhibit 6-1 for a listing of other structural unit types.)

Cost-to-charge ratio (CCR)—At the end of a period, the total costs in the profit center's cost pool are divided by the total revenues received form the center's sales. The CCR is a used as a cost-finding ratio. Also known as the *Ratio of cost to charges* or RCC.

Cost of goods sold—Expenses associated with the sale of acquiring goods.

Cost object—A general designation for the item whose cost management would like to understand. Also known as *Cost target*.

Current procedural terminology (CPT) codes—A listing of descriptive terms and unique numeric identifying codes for reporting medical services and procedures developed by the American Medical Association. Used to designate services and procedures on claim forms and bills.

Current ratio—*See* Financial measures: Ratios.

Dashboard—An abbreviated performance report using a balanced scorecard (BSC) approach.

Debt-to-assets ratio—*See* Financial measures: Ratios.

Debt-to-equity ratio—*See* Financial measures: Ratios.

Decision analysis—A method of analysis composed of processes in which an individual decision maker contemplates a choice of action.

Decision maker model—An approach to generating information that analyzes specific types of decision processes to understand how the decision is made, what variables are considered, and how measures on these variables can be aggregated to support each specific type of decision.

Decision model—An approach to generating information that uses predetermined, normative methods to identify variables and measure them.

Department—A group of people and resources formally differentiated by the organization and having a single individual responsible to the organization for its performance. Also, a unit shown on the formal organization chart of an organization. (*See* Exhibit 6-1 for a listing of structural unit types.)

Diagnosis-related group (DRG)—A category of patients. This category contains patients whose resource consumption, on statistical average, is equivalent.

Direct cost—Unit-level resources that can be traced to each unit of each product made; also, costs that can be physically traced to units of each product.

Direct labor—One category of direct cost; that is, labor that can be physically traced to units of each product.

Direct labor variance—*See* Variances.

Direct material—Another category of direct cost; that is, materials that can be physically traced to units of each product.

Discretionary costs—Costs, which, if incurred, will not affect the operation of the organization within the current accounting period.

Driver—The variable or phenomenon that causes a cost to be incurred.

Economic value added (EVA)—*See* Financial measures other than ratios.

Efficiency variance—*See* Variances.

Expense—The costs necessary to earn revenue. Expenses are the cost of doing business.

Extended budget—*See* Budgets.

Fee for service—A type of payment system whereby the provider is paid separately for each item of service it delivers in the care of a patient. The amount is determined by the cost of the resources used to produce the services.

Financial measures: Ratios

    current ratio—The ratio of current assets to current liabilities that indicates the ability to pay short-term liabilities as they come due.

    debt-to-assets ratio—A comparison of debt to the book value of total assets.

    debt-to-equity ratio—A comparison of long-term capital from creditors to that from providers of equity.

    quick ratio—Current assets less inventories divided by current liabilities;

indicating the ability to pay short-term liabilities if inventories are not turned into cash.

Financial measures other than ratios

economic value added (EVA)—Operating profit less the total cost of capital.

market value added (MVA)—The market value of equity less its book value.

return on assets (ROA)—Profit as a percentage of the assets used to produce it.

return on investment (ROI)—Profit as a percentage of the equity furnished by investors.

Financial statements

balance sheet—Provides measures of financial position at a point in time. Also known as the statement of financial position.

income statement—Provides the primary measure of financial performance from an operations standpoint. Also known as the operating statement.

statement of cash flow—Provides the measure of how the organization's resources were used by summarizing the causes of cash inflows and cash outflows.

statement of changes in equity—Provides a picture of changes in the equity (or the fund balance) of the organization. This information can also appear at the bottom of the income statement instead of appearing as a stand-alone statement.

Fiscal year—A 12-month period that begins on the first of a month other than January and ends on the last day of a month other than December. (See also *Calendar year*.)

Fixed costs—Cost elements of an activity that do not vary with changes in the volume of the driver.

Fixed production overhead—Costs that must be paid whether or not the organization produces anything.

Flexible budget—*See* Budgets.

Full cost of manufacturing—All costs of manufacturing an item, including variable costs and a fair share of fixed production overhead costs, are included in the finished goods inventory value.

Generally accepted accounting principles (GAAP)—The authoritative basis of accounting theory and practice. GAAP should always be used in financial statements intended for external users.

General service center—Term used I Medicare cost finding for departments such as housekeeping that perform services for almost all other departments.

Goals, organizational—Thresholds on measures that indicate whether organizational objectives are being reached.

Incremental cost—The additional cost brought on by a change in operations or the additional cost resulting from an operating decision. Also known as *Marginal cost*.

Income statement—*See* Financial statements.

Indirect cost—Costs that cannot be physically traced to units of each product, or if they can, the cost of tracing is more than the value of the information; also, a cost that must be allocated because it cannot be directly traced to the activity being costed.

Information ecology—An additional dimension of information systems that involves understanding the culture, behavior, and work processes and politics of the organization.

Information tech—An environment comprising the computer and electronic communication system.

Intermediate activities—The basic building blocks for estimating the cost of meeting the demands of any payment system or the product for which it pays.

Intermediate budget—*See* Budgets.

Intermediate product center—A center that produces a product that is a direct input to a subsequent product. (This is a special case of a product center.) (*See* Exhibit 6-1 for a listing of other structural unit types.)

Intermediate products—The output of a center, that contributes to the final product.

International Classification of Diseases, 9th revision (ICD-9)—A statistical classification system that arranges diseases and injuries into diagnostic groups according to established criteria.

Job costing system—A costing approach that responds to separate orders for quantities of a specific item. Items are not produced continuously, as on an assembly line. Instead, batches of items are produced. Each item produced in a job is identical. The cost of the job is the total of direct labor and direct materials that flow into the job plus the variable overhead assigned to the job and an allocated share of the producing organization's fixed overhead. The cost of a single unit of the item produced in a job is the cost of the job divided by the number of units the job produced.

Job shop—The production center that performs direct production activities using job costing system. The order to be filled is called a job.

Joint cost—A resource that must be purchased in order to produce any one or all of a number of products.

Learning curve—A mathematical model of the decrease in cost that occurs with experience.

Long-term budget—*See* Strategic budget under Budgets.

Major diagnostic category (MDC)—Broad categories of similar patient types that serve as an umbrella classification system for diagnosis-related groups (DRGs). MDCs are the overall clinically related categories that classify diseases and disorders of the body.

Managed care organization (MCO)—Those organizations that assume the casualty insurance function and attempt to influence some control over provider behavior and payments to providers.

Management control—The process by which managers influence other members of the organization to implement the organization's strategy.

Marginal cost—The additional cost brought on by a change in operations or the additional cost resulting from an operating decision. Also known as *Incremental costs*.

Marginal revenue—The additional revenue gained by a change in operations or the additional cost resulting from an operating decision. Also known as *Incremental revenue*.

Market price—The price that the seller could get if the seller sold the product outside the organization.

Market value added (MVA)—*See* Financial measures other than ratios.

Material variance—*See* Variances.

Mean—The sum of all measures divided by the number of items measured. Also called the *Arithmetic average* or the expected value.

Median—The quantity at which half the observations have a higher value and half have a lower value.

Mission (organizational)—Articulates why the organization should exist; it states the societal needs the organization intends to satisfy. Meeting an organization's general, overreaching objective is often referred to as the organization's mission.

Mixed costs—Cost elements that have both a fixed and a variable component.

Mode—The value that exists most often in the group of measurements being analyzed.

Objectives, organizational—Specific intermediate accomplishments that must happen if the organizational mission is to be achieved. (See also *Goals, organizational.*)

Operational costing system—A system that possesses characteristics of both the job cost and process cost systems; a hybrid system often used in some health care organizations.

Organization-sustaining activities—Activities that are necessary to keep the organization functioning. (See also *Batch-level activities, Production-sustaining activities,* and *Unit-level activities.*)

Overhead variance—*See* Variances.

Perfect knowledge assumption—An assumption that allows buyers to make appropriate choices in spending limited funds among alternative products.

Period costs—Costs not traced to specific products, but instead considered costs of the period in which they are incurred rather than the period in which the item manufactured is sold.

Periodic performance reports—Reports on historic performance and current position.

Price variance—*See* Variances.

Process costing system—In process costing, the costs of a steady flow of allocated and traced resources are measured for a production period. The quantity of the product output during the period is counted. The total resource cost is divided by the total quantities of output to arrive at a cost per unit of output.

Product center—A unit of the organization that produces a countable product that can be traced as a direct input to a subsequent product as opposed to flowing to an overhead pool, or a center that produces a product that is sold. (*See* Exhibit 6-1 for a listing of other structural unit types.) This term is also used in the traditional sense for centers whose output is a saleable product.

Product center overhead—Can be traced to its product center but not to specific products. (See also *Product overhead.*)

Product overhead—Can be traced to specific products but not to units of the products. (See also *Product center overhead.*)

Production costs—Cost incurred to produce an output for sale.

Production-sustaining activities—Activities that can be traced to specific outputs but cannot be traced farther to specific units of the output. (See also *Batch-level activities, Organization-sustaining activities,* and *Unit-level activities.*)

Profit center—A unit within an organization such as a department to which both costs and revenue can be traced; a unit that generates revenues as well as cost. (*See* Exhibit 6-1 for a listing of other structural unit types.) Also called a *Revenue center.*

Program budgets—*See* Budgets.

Prospective payment—Under this payment system, set prices for specific outputs are established ahead of the time care is delivered. The set price is the payment regardless of the amount of resources used to produce the output.

Pseudoprofit center—A unit within an organization to which costs can be traced but revenue must be attributed through the use of transfer prices. (*See* Exhibit 6-1 for a listing of other structural unit types.)

Quantity variance—*See* Variances.

Quick ratio—*See* Financial measures: Ratios.

Ratios—*See* Financial measures: ratios.

Ratio of cost to charges (RCC)—Another term for the cost-to-charge ratio. The RCC is used as a cost-finding ratio.

Regression analysis—A linear model with which to predict Y if one knows X.

Relative value unit (RVU)—The basic measurements (units) in the resource-based relative value scale. Units weight services according to the level of work effort or to their relative cost.

Relevant costs—Those costs considered for a decision at the margin. (See also *Marginal costs.*)

Relevant range—A segment of activity within which cost-behavior assumptions are valid.

Report cards—Reports that provide managers with information on the activities they manage.

Resource driver—A variable that can logically be thought to cause changes in an overhead input in question. Also known as a driver of untraceable costs.

Responsibility accounting—Accounting to support and evaluate control by selected managers at designated centers in the organization.

Return on assets (ROA)—*See* Financial measures other than ratios.

Return on investment (ROI)—*See* Financial measures other than ratios.

Revenue center—A unit within an organization such as a department whose output is sold to buyers outside the organization. So called because prices paid for the outputs are revenue to the organization. Sometimes called a *Profit center*.

Revenues—The amount earned by an organization when the organization is going about its business. In the case of a health care organization, most revenues are earned from delivering services.

Rolling budget—*See* Budgets.

Rules of thumb—Rules that are easy to apply but are overly simple, thus producing solutions that are far from optimal.

Separable activities—Activities that use direct-to-activity resources that are not shared with other departments or centers; thus they are separable.

Service center—A unit in an organization whose output is not sold to external customers but produces organization- and production-sustaining activities for other units of the organization. (*See* Exhibit 6-1 for a listing of other structural unit types.)

Setup costs—*See* Batch costs.

Simple moving average—An average cost over a set of recent periods, used to forecast the next period, that weights all period equally. (See also *Weighted moving average*.)

Spending variance—*See* Variances.

Staffing—The process of selecting specific people to fill positions within the organization.

Standard cost—The cost that the organization should suffer to produce the product; or, the amount a cost ought to be. The classic definition of standard cost is the per-unit cost of an output at a good—or best—level of performance.

Standard deviation—The square root of the variance; the statistic most used to describe variability.

Standard error—The standard deviation of a distribution of sample means is the standard deviation of the population from which the samples were taken divided by the square root of the sample size. Also called standard error of the means.

Statement of cash flow—*See* Financial statements.

Statement of changes in equity—*See* Financial statements.

Static budget—*See* Budgets.

Step-down cost allocation—A method of cost allocation that allocates general services, or overhead, departments one by one to departments that use the services.

Strategic budget—*See* Budgets.

Strategic planning—Deciding on the organization's mission and the strategies for attaining it.

Strategies—General approaches to accomplishing organizational missions.

Strategy (organizational)—The general approach the organization plans to take in order to accomplish its mission. (See also *Mission.*)

Sunk cost—A special type of fixed cost; a cost that has already been incurred and thus, will not be affected by future actions. This cost cannot be recovered; it is sunk.

Task—A subset of an activity. One activity is made up of a series of tasks.

Task control—The process of assuring that specific tasks are carried out effectively and efficiently.

Top-down analysis—Costing that starts with overhead activities and allocates accumulations of cost down toward products. (See also *Bottom-up analysis.*)

Traceable—The resource causing a cost can be visually or physically traced to the cost object in question.

Unit-level activities—Activities performed for each unit of output that can be considered direct costs of each unit; e.g., a single unit of production. (See also *Batch-level activities, Organization-sustaining activities*, and *Production-sustaining activities.*)

Usage variance—*See* Variances.

Variable cost—Cost that changes in total in proportion to changes in a cost driver.

Variances

Variable production overhead—Indirect costs whose total during an accounting period increases as output increases.

    capacity variance—A subset of overhead analysis that focuses on whether fixed-cost resources are used at their capacity.

    direct labor variance—A subset of variance analysis focused on direct labor; utilizes volume, efficiency, and price variances related to labor. The direct labor price variance is also known as the *Wage rate variance.*

    efficiency variance—Actual costs are different from planned costs because more of the variable cost resource has actually been used than the amount that was planned. Also called *Usage* or *Quantity variances.*

material variance—A subset of variance analysis focused on materials; utilizes volume, efficiency, and price variances related to materials.

overhead variance—A subset of variance analysis focused on overhead; utilizes volume, efficiency, and spending, variances related to overhead. The three types of variances may also be divided into subtypes of fixed overhead variance and variable overhead variance. A fourth type of overhead variance known as *Capacity variance* may also be utilized.

price variance—Actual costs are different from planned costs because prices that were paid for by the variable resources are different from the prices that were planned.

quantity variance—*See* Efficiency variance.

spending variance—*See* Overhead variance.

usage variance—*See* Efficiency variance.

variance—The difference between planned and actual results.

volume variance—Actual costs are different from planned costs because the actual output produced is more or less than the output that was planned.

wage rate variance—The Direct labor variance is also known as the Direct labor price variance.

Vision (organizational)—The place the organization sees for itself at points in the future within the markets it plans to serve.

Volume variance—*See* Variances.

Wage rate variance—*See* Variances.

Weighted moving average—An average cost over a set of recent periods, used to forecast the next period, that weights some periods more heavily than others (rather than weighting all periods equally). (See also *Simple moving average*.)

Zero-based budgets—*See* Budgets.

ACRONYMS

ABC - Activity-based costing

ABM - Activity-based management

AHA - American Hospital Association

AICPA - American Institute of Certified Public Accountants

AMA - American Management Association

APC - Ambulatory payment classification

BSC - Balanced scorecard

CAM-I - Computer Aided Manufacturing International

CCR - Cost-to-charge ratio

CMS - Centers for Medicare and Medicaid Services

CPT - Current procedural terminology

DRG - Diagnosis-related group

EVA - Economic value added

FASB - Financial Accounting Standards Board

GAAP - Generally accepted accounting principles

GASB - Governmental Accounting Standards Board

HCFA - Health Care Financing Administration

ICD-9 - International Classification of Diseases, 9th Revision

MCO - Managed care organization

MDC - Major diagnostic category

MVA - Market value added

RCC - Ratio of cost-to-charges

ROA - Return on assets

ROI - Return on investment

RVU - Relative value unit

SEC - Securities and Exchange Commission

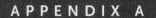

APPENDIX A   A REVIEW OF FINANCIAL ACCOUNTING CONCEPTS

THE CONCEPT OF FINANCIAL ACCOUNTING: INTRODUCTION

Financial accounting is generally intended for external users. This is in contrast to managerial accounting, which is intended for internal users. Financial accounting reports are used by third parties while management accounting reports are used by individuals within the organization. The purpose of financial accounting reports for external use is to communicate the organization's financial status. Because financial accounting is generally for outside users, the principles of accounting and reporting are regulated by a variety of governmental and private sector agencies.

ORGANIZATIONAL STRUCTURE AFFECTS FINANCIAL ACCOUNTING

An organization's type of business and purpose in large part determines what type of financial accounting will be required of the organization.

Organization's Type of Business

Financial accounting originally focused upon the manufacturing industry. A manufacturing type of business creates goods for sale, such as widgets. Financial accounting for manufacturers therefore includes costs of production ("cost of goods sold") along with the cost of distributing and marketing the goods that have been manufactured.

Another type of business is the service industry. The service industry does not create an actual product; instead, it offers services. Therefore, the financial accounting for the service industry disregards measurement of the cost of goods sold and focuses instead on offering services and the costs involved in providing these services. A commercial laundry, the practice of law, and banking are common examples of service industries.

The health care industry is a branch of the service industry, because health care providers offer services. Generally speaking, however, the health care organization offers many types of services, from physical examinations and diagnostic tests to medical and surgical interventions. It also has many more types of payment arrangements for these services. Financial accounting for health care, therefore, has to take these differences into account.

There are also many different types of health care service providers. Exhibit A-1 illustrates types of health care organizations that use financial accounting.

Organization's Purpose

The organization's purpose also determines what type of financial accounting is required. The basic difference is between for-profit and not-for-profit organizations. For-profit, or *proprietary*, organizations are expected to make a profit. Their mission is quite different from not-for-profit organizations, which are expected to have a charitable and/or educational purpose that justifies their nonprofit status.

The wording of the financial reporting varies between and among for-profit and not-for-profit organizations. There is also a difference in the level of

Exhibit A-1 Examples of Health Care Organizations That Use Financial Accounting

1. Health systems
2. Hospitals
3. Skilled nursing facilities
4. Nursing homes
5. Home health agencies
6. Ambulatory surgery centers
7. Clinics
8. Physician practices
9. Laboratories
10. Pharmacies

responsibility between privately held for-profit companies and publicly held for-profit companies. The publicly held companies such as a hospital chain that is traded on the New York Stock Exchange are held to a higher level of reporting and related disclosure responsibilities. Likewise, there is a difference in financial accounting between nongovernmental not-for-profit organizations (a university hospital or a church-owned hospital, for example) and a governmental not-for-profit organization (a county hospital that can receive tax revenues, for example).

THE OVERSEERS OF FINANCIAL ACCOUNTING

Most financial accounting and financial reports in the United States are governed by generally accepted accounting principles, or GAAP. These principles serve as the authoritative basis of accounting theory and practice. Financial statements intended for third-party use should be created in accordance with GAAP. Several bodies that serve as overseers of financial accounting are discussed here.

Financial Accounting Standards Board

The Financial Accounting Standards Board (FASB) is a nonprofit private-sector body; this means the FASB is not an agency of the government. The responsibilities of FASB include researching problem areas, holding public hearings as part of the research process, and determining and publishing appropriate accounting treatments. The published accounting treatments then become additional GAAP for all nongovernmental organizations.

Governmental Accounting Standards Board

The Governmental Accounting Standards Board (GASB) was created to establish GAAP for state and local governments. Governmental units are required to use financial reporting practices that acknowledge the usual governmental divisions and revenue sources. These governmental units include health care organizations such as hospitals that are taxing districts. Because they have taxing power, they are considered to be governmental units.

Securities and Exchange Commission

Organizations that are publicly held fall under the authority of the Securities and Exchange Commission (SEC). Publicly held organizations sell stock to the public and are therefore responsible to their stockholders and to the public. Congress designated the SEC to have final responsibility to specify GAAP for those organizations that trade their stock publicly. The SEC, in turn, delegated part of its power and authority to the FASB.

Public Company Accounting Oversight Board

In 2002, Congress passed a law to create an accounting oversight board in the wake of revelations of accounting scandals such as Enron. This regulatory board must have its actions approved by the SEC. Its responsibility is to oversee that part of the accounting profession that performs audits and financial reporting for publicly held organizations.

American Institute of Certified Public Accountants

The American Institute of Certified Public Accountants (AICPA) is the public accountants' trade organization. The AICPA supports the actions and publications of FASB and also publishes its own guidelines for certified public accountants.

OTHER INFLUENCES ON HEALTH CARE REPORTING

Health care organizations have other agencies that also require special reporting. The arrangement of accounts in the books and records of the organization often reflect these special reporting requirements.

Medicare Cost Reports

The Medicare program is administered by the Centers for Medicare and Medicaid Services (CMS). The federally funded Medicare program was created under Title XVIII of the Social Security Act to assist with covering the costs of health care for the elderly and disabled who qualify. Health care providers who choose to participate in the Medicare program must sign a participation agreement. One of the conditions of participation in this agreement is that the provider must file an annual cost report with CMS. The Medicare cost-reporting requirement has been in place since 1966, and it has profoundly affected the way books and records for health care providers are arranged.

Medicaid Cost Reports

The Medicaid program is administered by the individual states but is overseen by the federal government through the CMS. The Medicaid program was created under Title XIX of the Social Security Act to assist with covering the costs of health care for eligible individuals that generally include low-income women and children plus low-income elderly and the disabled to some extent. The Medicaid program is funded by a combination of state and federal funding, and each state has its own cost-reporting requirement. Although some impact on the way books and records for health care providers are arranged may be attributed to

Medicaid cost reporting, the Medicare program's influence is generally much more pronounced.

Specially Funded Projects Such as Research or Demonstration Projects

Research projects or funding for demonstration projects often require special reporting as a condition of the funding. Although these reports may be submitted separately from the usual financial accounting, they often influence the arrangement of the accounts in the organization's books and records.

American Hospital Association

The American Hospital Association (AHA) is the hospital industry's trade organization. The AHA Health Data and Coding Standards Group gathers hospital data and sets certain standards. For example, this group produces the *Estimated Useful Lives of Depreciable Hospital Assets*. Its influence is evident because this asset useful life information is accepted by the federal government as the "gold standard" for depreciable asset treatment in Medicare cost reporting.

FINANCIAL ACCOUNTING CHARACTERISTICS, CRITERIA, AND ASSUMPTIONS

In order to fully understand the principles of financial accounting, it is necessary to first examine its characteristics, its criteria, and its assumptions. All three are discussed in this section.

Financial Accounting Characteristics

Financial accounting exhibits the following four characteristics:

1. Financial accounting is usually *retrospective;* that is, it looks to the past. Financial accounting generally reports past history such as revenue and expenses for a period that has already occurred.
2. Financial accounting is *restricted* by the requirements to adhere to GAAP.
3. Financial accounting's primary concern is often about adequate *disclosure.*
4. Financial accounting reports are usually in *summary* form; that is, they report in the aggregate and not in detail.

The third and fourth characteristics of financial accounting are in direct contrast to management accounting. Although disclosure to outside third parties is a financial accounting's concern, management accounting wants and needs to get information out to its managers so they can act on it—and although the outside or external user gets a report in summary form, management accounting wants to produce information that is detailed so the manager can act upon it.

Financial Accounting Criteria

Financial accounting results must contain data that are relevant and reliable. In addition, they must also be comparable, understandable, and timely. In summary, data must be:

- *Relevant* to decisions that are made, and *appropriate* for the intended use
- *Reliable* in that data can be *verified* and are *objectively* presented
- *Comparable* to some standard (such as a regulatory agency)
- *Understandable* to the user
- *Timely* in that the importance to the user has not diminished

The two major criteria are relevancy and reliability. Relevancy supports (or perhaps corrects) the user's expectations about the organization and also informs the user about the outcome of events (past, current, or future) affecting the organization. Reliability involves the assurance that the data are error free to a reasonable degree and therefore, an independent third party would arrive at the same results. Reliability also involves the assurance that the data are presented objectively with a lack of bias.

Of the three remaining criteria, comparable to some standard implies there is an existing benchmark that can be used for comparison. The comparable criteria also assumes consistency across time periods. The understandable to the user criteria assumes a straightforward presentation that does not require additional interpretation. The timely criteria assumes no extraordinary time lag in release of the results that would render the data virtually useless.

Financial Accounting Assumptions

There are four basic assumptions found in all financial accounting. They are separateness, continuity (or going concern), uniform measures, and periodicity.

SEPARATE ENTITY The organization is assumed to have a specific area of accountability as a separate entity. This means a clear boundary must exist between the organization and any of its participants. No matter how large or how small, the organization is accounted for separately. Its transactions are not mixed with the transactions of another entity.

GOING CONCERN   The organization is assumed to have ongoing continuity; thus, the organization is a "going concern" and is assumed to have no definite point of termination in its operations. Therefore, the organization will continue to exist into the future.

UNIFORM MEASURES   All financial data are measured in a single uniform unit of measure with a monetary basis. In the United States, the single uniform unit of measure is the dollar (or to be very specific, dollars and cents). The general assumption is that this unit of measure with a monetary basis has been uniform for a long period of time—but rare instances and unusual circumstances can overturn this assumption. For example, in France, this single uniform unit of measure used to be the franc, but now should be the euro.

PERIODICITY   The organization's life can be subdivided into specific time periods such as a month or a quarter or a year for the purposes of reporting. The financial accounting reporting period for reports released to external users is often a 12-month period. This period could be a calendar year or a fiscal year. A *calendar year* always begins on the first of January and ends on the last day of December. (The accounting abbreviation is "CY.") A *fiscal year* is also 12 months long, but it begins on the first of a month other than January and ends 12 months later on the last day of a month other than December. (The accounting abbreviation is "FY.") An annual reporting period that begins on July 1 and ends on the next June 30 would be a fiscal year.

REPORTING FINANCIAL RESULTS

Financial accounting reports may be issued at various points in time. The extent of the reports will vary according to their use. For example, quarterly interim reports may be required by a bond-financing trustee. These quarterly reports may be prepared in accordance with GAAP but may be aggregated and presented in a short summary form. The year-end report for a 12-month operating period would be a much longer report, containing a great deal of disclosure, appendices, and exhibits. Annual reports are definitely intended for outside, or external, distribution. Annual reports must be prepared according to GAAP. These reports may be prepared by an outside accounting firm, generally a certified public accounting firm.

Financial Reports Prepared Within the Organization

If financial reports are prepared internally (within the organization), there is generally no opinion rendered to accompany the financial statements. The financial reports may be prepared exactly in accordance with GAAP, but they are still created internally. This means the user needs to understand that no outside party has had a part in preparing the financial reports. In the example of the bond-financing trustee just described, it may be acceptable for the quarterly reports to be prepared within the organization, but the trustee will almost surely require that the year-end report be prepared by an outside firm.

Financial Reports Prepared by an Outside Firm

An outside accounting firm may be called upon to issue financial statements. The outside accounting firm may report upon the results of the financial statements in one of three ways: (1) a compilation; (2) a review; or (3) an audit. The three types of statements reflect three levels or degrees of responsibility undertaken by the outside accounting firm.

COMPILATIONS AND REVIEWS   The compilation merely presents the information in report format, and no opinion is rendered by the outside accounting firm. A letter from the firm is placed at the front of the report that clearly states this fact.

The review is an intermediate degree of responsibility. A letter from the outside firm is placed at the front of the report that states the report has been reviewed for its adherence to GAAP. No responsibility is taken that the information is accurately presented.

AUDITS   The audit report contains an opinion placed at the front of the report. The accounting firm attests that, in their opinion, the financial statements are presented in accordance with GAAP. This opinion is the highest level of attesting to the statements.

A number of third-party users can and will require that audited financial statements be filed with them at least annually. Audited statements are a common requirement to support bank loans or bond financing. Publicly held companies are required to file audited statements with the SEC. The publicly held organization will probably issue an annual report to its stockholders, and the audited statements will appear in its annual report.

Accounting Principles

To begin a discussion of accounting principles, we must first define revenue and expense. *Revenues* are the amounts earned by an organization when the organization is going about its business. In the case of a health care organization, most revenues are earned from delivering services. Other revenues are earned by selling medical supplies and drugs. *Expenses* represent the costs that are necessary to earn the revenue. In other words, expenses are the costs of doing business. Examples of expenses in a health care organization include labor (nurses' wages and payroll taxes, for example) and the cost of medical supplies and drugs.

Three principles are at work in financial accounting:

1. time period
2. revenue
3. matching

The Time Period Principle

The time period principle is a concept that requires accounting data to be reported at *regular intervals*. These regular intervals (commonly month end, quarter end, or year end) are "mileposts" where the accountants will update the organization's books. Therefore, for example, at the end of the month, the revenue accounts and the expense accounts will be updated. If this process is repeated at the end of each month, the time period principle has been upheld, because the updates have occurred at regular stated intervals. The time period principle works alongside the revenue principle and the matching principle.

The Revenue Principle

The revenue principle informs the accountant about *when* to record revenue; that is, revenue must be recorded when it is earned and not before it has been earned. The revenue principle also informs the accountant about *how much* revenue to record; that is, revenue must be recorded that is equal to the cash value of the service rendered or the item (supplies or drugs, for example) transferred in the transaction.

The Matching Principle

The matching principle informs the accountant about when to record expenses. The matching principle occurs in three steps: (1) identify, (2) measure, and (3) match. The accountant is supposed to first *identify* the expenses that have been incurred during the accounting period that is being updated, then the accountant must *measure* the expenses. Finally, the accountant must *match* the expenses to the revenues that have been earned during the accounting period that is being updated.

The final step of the matching principle is to subtract the expenses from the revenues for the period being updated in order to obtain the net income or the net loss. This net income or net loss is then reported for the period being updated.

ACCOUNTING METHODS: ACCRUAL BASIS VERSUS CASH BASIS

The difference in accounting methods revolves around whether financial information is accumulated and reported on the accrual basis or the cash basis. Each is described in this section.

Accrual Basis

When the accrual basis is used, management records revenues when they are earned (that is, when the service, drug, or medical supply item is provided), and records expenses when they are incurred. The accrual basis uses the revenue principle to record revenue and the matching principle to match expenses to revenue in the same period; that is, the period being updated. GAAP require that an organization use the accrual basis.

Cash Basis

When the cash basis is used, revenues are not recorded until the cash payment is received and expenses are recorded when they are paid for in cash. This means the revenue might be in one fiscal period and the related expense might be in another fiscal period, because one transaction happened considerably before or after the other transaction. The cash basis accounting method does not meet the requirements of GAAP.

Modified Cash Basis

When the modified cash basis is used, revenues are not recorded until the cash payment is received, but expenses receive one of two types of treatment. Most expenses, such as salaries and wages, are not recorded until they are paid for in cash. However, some expenses—particularly supplies, insurance, and equipment—are handled differently. These expenses are spread over the time period (fiscal period) when they are being used. Thus, supplies are spread over time until they are used up and insurance is spread over time until it has expired. Equipment is spread over its useful life (generally 3, 7, or 10 years, depending on the type of equipment). The modified cash basis is also known as the *hybrid method* because it uses elements of both the cash basis and the accrual basis. The modified cash basis accounting method does not meet the requirements of GAAP.

Exhibit A-2 sets out the financial accounting assumptions for the accrual basis, the cash basis, and the modified cash basis accounting methods.

Exhibit A-2 **Comparison of Cash Basis and Accrual Basis**

Accounting Basis	Revenue	Cost
Accrual Basis for service entity	Revenues earned at the point *when service is provided.*	Cost of the service is equal to the value of resource given up. Recognized at the point *when service is provided.*
Cash Basis for service entity	Revenues earned at the point *when cash is received* (aka cash inflow).	Cost of the service equals the amount of cash spent. Recognized at the point *when cash is disbursed* (aka cash outflow).
Modified Cash Basis for service entity	Revenues earned at the point for *when cash is received* (aka inflow).	Cost of most services equals the amount of cash spent. But some items (such as supplies, insurance, and equipment) are recognized at the point when the service is provided.

FINANCIAL STATEMENTS

This section introduces financial statements contents and their presentation. It concludes with an example.

Financial Statement Presentation

Management accounting reports can take many forms because they are intended for internal use, but financial accounting reports for external use appear in a required format. For example, certain common usage is expected for the treatment of time periods and of comparative statements.

Time Periods

The time periods reported in financial statements will generally be annual. Therefore, the reports contain year-end time periods. Sometimes reports will be quarterly and therefore contain time periods of 3 months apiece rather than the 12-month annual period.

Comparative Statements

Many statements prepared for financial accounting purposes report on more than one time period. These comparative statements assume the time periods will usually be of the same length (12 months, for example). The figures will be set side-by-side in two columns. The most recent reporting period is generally reported in the left-hand column, while the older period is reported in the right-hand column.

Financial Statement Titles Vary

Although financial statement titles may vary between and among different organizations, the financial accounting principles remain the same. Exhibit A-3 illustrates some examples of the variations in titles that often occur.

The Three Primary Financial Statements

There are three financial statements that will always be present in financial accounting. They are the balance sheet, the statement of income, and the statement of cash flow. A fourth financial statement can be presented in alternative ways that influences whether it becomes a separate statement or not. All are discussed in this section.

Balance Sheet

The balance sheet is also known as the *statement of financial position* (see Exhibit A-3). It presents the organization's assets (also known as *resources*) and its liabilities, and the difference between the assets and liabilities at a particular point in time. This difference is known as *equity* in for-profit organizations and as *fund balance* in not-for-profit organizations. A balance sheet does what its name implies; it balances. Therefore, assets, on one side of the balance sheet, equal liabilities plus equity (or fund balance) on the other side. The equation is expressed as follows:

For-Profit

$$Assets = Liabilities + equity$$

Not-for-Profit

$$Assets = Liabilities + fund\ balance$$

Exhibit A-3 **Comparison of Report Titles**

Report Title Used in This Book	Commonly Called	May Also Be Called
Balance sheet	Balance sheet	Statement of financial condition
		Statement of financial position
Statement of income and changes in equity	Income statement	Operating statement
		Earnings statement
		Activity statement
		Statement of revenue and expenses
Statement of cash flow	Cash flow statement	Statement of change in financial position
		Funds statement

The balance sheet is like a snapshot, because it freezes these accounts on a particular date (the last day of the year, for instance). Exhibit A-4 illustrates the usual format. Assets are divided into "current" and "noncurrent." Current assets will be converted into cash during the next accounting period—typically a 12-month period. Noncurrent, or long-term, assets will have an expected benefit that lasts more than a single year.

Statement of Income

The income statement, also known as the *operating statement* (see Exhibit A-3), presents the organization's financial performance. The income statement includes revenues, expenses, and the difference between the revenues and expenses. This statement covers certain period of elapsed time (1 year, for example).

Exhibit A-5 illustrates the usual format. Operating revenue is presented, followed by operating expenses. The difference is income or loss, then nonoperating gains or losses are presented. This difference is either net income (loss) before taxes (for-profit version) or excess of revenue over expenses (not-for-profit version). For-profit organizations can take a number of legal forms, the most common of which are corporations and partnerships. Although corporations pay a corporate tax in the United States, partnerships do not. Because Exhibit A-5's: example is a corporation, two more lines are present on the income statement; income tax and net income (loss) after taxes.

Exhibit A-4   **Two Balance Sheet Examples**

Corporate For-Profit Balance Sheet		Not-for-Profit Balance Sheet	
Assets		**Assets**	
Current assets	$ xxx	Current assets	$ xxx
Noncurrent assets	xxx	Noncurrent assets	xxx
Total assets	$ xxx	Total assets	$ xxx
Liabilities and Equity		Liabilities and Fund Balance	
Current liabilities	$ xxx	Current liabilities	$ xxx
Noncurrent liabilities	xxx	Noncurrent liabilities	xxx
Total Liabilities	$ xxx	Total liabilities	$ xxx
Stockholders' equity	xxx	Fund balance	xxx
Total liabilities and equity	$ xxx	Total liabilities and fund balance	$ xxx

Exhibit A-5 **Two Income Statement Examples**

Corporate For-Profit Income Statement		Not-for-Profit Operating Statement	
Operating revenue	$ xxx	Operating revenue	$ xxx
Operating expenses	xxx	Operating expenses	xxx
Operating income (loss) before taxes	$ xxx	Excess of operating revenue over operating expenses	$ xxx
Other nonoperating gains (losses)	$ xxx	Other nonoperating gains (losses)	$ xxx
Net income (loss) before taxes	$ xxx	Excess of revenue over expenses	$ xxx
Income tax	xxx		
Net income (loss) after taxes	$ xxx		

Statement of Cash Flow

The statement of cash flow, also known as the statement of changes in financial position (see Exhibit A-3), presents how the organization's resources were used. The statement of cash flow summarizes the causes of cash inflows and cash outflows. This statement covers the same period of elapsed time as does the income statement.

Exhibit A-6 illustrates the usual format. Cash flows are presented from operating activities, investing activities, and financing activities. The business of the organization is thus sorted into these three categories. Operating activities arise from the normal business of the organization. An example of investing activities would be cash flow resulting from interest income. An example of financing activities would be a business loan. The net cash flow resulting from the combination of all three types of activities represents "net increase (decrease) in cash and cash equivalents," the last line on the statement.

The Fourth Financial Statement

A fourth financial statement can be presented in alternative ways that influences whether it becomes a separate statement or not. This statement's purpose is to

Exhibit A-6 **Two Statements of Cash Flow Examples**

Corporate For-Profit Statement of Cash Flow		Not-for-Profit Statement of Change in Financial Position	
Cash flows from operating activities	$ xxx	Cash flows from operating activities	$ xxx
Cash flows from investing activities	xxx	Cash flows from investing activities	xxx
Cash flows from financing activities	xxx	Cash flows from financing activities	xxx
Net increase (decrease) in cash and cash equivalents	$ xxx	Net increase (decrease) in cash and cash equivalents	$ xxx

provide a picture of changes in the equity (or the fund balance) of the organization. The explanation, or reconciliation, of changes in equity can be treated in one of two ways in the financial statements. It can either appear in a fourth statement, or it can be combined with the income statement (in which case there will be only three statements instead of four).

Exhibit A-7 illustrates the usual format for a fourth statement. In Exhibit A-7, the beginning balance appears first, followed by the net income (loss) for the period. The ending balance is the last line of the statement.

Exhibit A-8 illustrates the alternative combined format. In Exhibit A-8, the changes in equity are hooked onto the end of the income statement. Therefore, net income (loss) for the period, the last line of the regular income statement, also serves as the first line of the changes in equity portion of the combined statement. The beginning equity balance becomes the second line. The two are added together to arrive at the ending equity balance on the final line.

Compare Exhibit A-5 with Exhibit A-8 to see the difference in treatment. Then compare Exhibit A-7 with Exhibit A-8 to see that the information remains the same, even though the order has been rearranged.

APPLICATION

The following situation illustrates all four statements for the Woods Group Medical Practice. The statements cover a 1-year period, from January 1 to December 31, and are prepared on the accrual basis.

Balance Sheet

Exhibit A-9 includes assets, liabilities, and partners' equity. The balance sheet heading shows the single date of December 31 because this statement is a snapshot on one particular day. For December 31, 2005, the balance sheet balances show total assets equal to $132,600 balanced by total liabilities and partners' equity of $132,600.

Exhibit A-7 Stand-Alone Statements of Changes in Equity: Two Examples

Corporate For-Profit Statement of Change in Equity		Not-for-Profit Statement of Change in Fund Balance	
Beginning balance stockholders' equity	$ xxx	Beginning fund balance	$ xxx
Net income (loss) after taxes	xxx	Excess of revenue over expenses	xxx
Ending balance stockholders' equity	$ xxx	Ending fund balance	$ xxx

Exhibit A-8   **Statement of Changes in Equity Combined with the Income Statement: Two Examples**

Corporate For-Profit Income Statement and Changes in Equity		Not-for Profit Income Statement and Changes in Fund Balance	
Operating revenue	$ xxx	Operating revenue	$ xxx
Operating expenses	xxx	Operating expenses	xxx
Operating income (loss) before taxes	$ xxx	Excess of operating revenue over operating expenses	$ xxx
Other nonoperating gains (losses)	$ xxx	Other nonoperating gains (losses)	$ xxx
Net income (loss) before taxes	$ xxx	Excess of revenue over expenses	$ xxx
Income tax	xxx	Beginning fund balance	$ xxx
Net income (loss) after taxes	$ xxx		
		Ending fund balance	$ xxx
Beginning balance stockholders equity	$ xxx		
Ending balance stockholders equity	$ xxx		

CURRENT ASSETS   Remember that current assets are cash or are expected to be turned into cash within the coming year. Current assets in this example include cash, accounts receivable, and medical supplies inventory. The accounts receivable shown on the statement are net of a reserve for bad debts. The medical supplies inventory represents supplies purchased but not yet used; under the accrual system, they are assets (inventory) rather than supplies.

LONG-TERM ASSETS   Long-term assets include equipment. The purchase price of the equipment is reduced by its accrued depreciation. Depreciation is the way that assets are charged to expense. Each year's depreciation is accumulated into and shown as *accrued depreciation* on this balance sheet. The accrued depreciation accumulated by year end ($20,000) is subtracted from the total equipment cost ($77,500) to arrive at the net long-term assets of $57,500.

CURRENT LIABILITIES   Remember that current liabilities represent liabilities that are expected to be paid within the coming year. Current liabilities in this example include accounts payable, wages payable, and interest payable. The accounts payable shown on the statement represent bills to be paid for regular operating expenses such as copy paper and utilities. Wages payable represent salaries that are owed but not yet paid. Interest payable represents interest that is owed but not yet paid. Under the accrual system, these items are liabilities, or debts, because the equivalent expense has been recorded as an expense in this period, but the equivalent debt has not yet been paid.

Exhibit A-9   **Woods Group Medical Practice**

Balance Sheet
December 31, 2005 and 2004

	12/31/2005	12/31/2004
Assets		
Current Assets		
Cash	$22,200	$21,000
Accounts receivable, net	50,000	43,000
Medical supplies inventory	2,900	2,500
Total Current Assets	**$75,100**	**$66,500**
Long-Term Assets		
Equipment	$77,500	$70,000
Less accrued depreciation	(20,000)	(10,000)
Net Long-Term Assets	**57,500**	**60,000**
Total Assets	**$132,600**	**$126,500**
Liabilities		
Current Liabilities		
Accounts payable	$3,400	$2,500
Wages and payroll taxes payable	10,600	8,000
Interest payable	100	200
Total Current Liabilities	**$14,100**	**$10,700**
Long-Term Liabilities		
Notes payable	7,500	10,000
Total Liabilities	**$21,600**	**20,700**
Partners' Equity		
Partners' equity	111,000	105,800
Total Liabilities and Partners Equity	**$132,600**	**$126,500**

LONG-TERM LIABILITIES   Remember that long-term liabilities are not expected to be paid within the coming year. This statement shows notes payable of $7,500. The figure is actually a net figure, as some amount has been paid, but additional money has been borrowed. (See the statement of cash flow for further details.)

PARTNERS' EQUITY   Remember that assets equal liabilities plus equity. The partners' equity represents their ownership interest in the medical practice. The $111,000 is actually a net figure, because it includes both income earned and monies withdrawn from the practice by the partners. (See the statement of changes in the partners' equity for further details.)

Income Statement

Exhibit A-10 includes revenues, operating expenses, and operating income. The line following the income statement heading shows the period that the statement covers. It covers a 12-month period or a year of operations. The total operating revenues of $640,000 less the total operating expenses of $422,750 plus the other revenue of $5,250 equal the net income of $222,500.

OPERATING REVENUES   Some medical practices divide their revenues by partner and that is how this statement reports revenue. Partner A earned gross revenue (before expenses) of $420,000 and Partner B earned $220,000, for a total of $640,000.

Exhibit A-10   **Woods Group Medical Practice**

	Income Statement For Year Ending 12/31/2005		
Operating Revenues			
Partner A	$420,000		
Partner B	220,000		
Total Operating Revenue			**$640,000**
less:			
Operating Expenses			
Partner A			
Salaries and wages	$140,000		
Fringe benefits	35,000		
Supplies used	25,000	$200,000	
Partner B			
Salaries and wages	$35,000		
Fringe benefits	8,750		
Supplies used	6,000	$49,750	
Office Administration			
Salaries and wages	$81,000		
Fringe benefits	20,250		
Insurance expense	24,550		
Interest expense	1,200		
Depreciation expense	10,000		
Rent and utilities	36,000	173,000	
Total Operating Expenses			422,750
Operating Income			217,250
Other Revenue			5,250
Net Income			$222,500

OPERATING EXPENSES   Expenses are expensed as the full amount used in the year, because these statements have been prepared on the accrual basis. Certain operating expenses are divided by partner, because these are the expenses that can be directly attributed to their individual revenues. In this example, these include salaries and wages, fringe benefits, and supplies used. The salaries are for clinical labor that directly assist the individual doctor.

The remainder of the expenses are shared by the partners and are grouped as "office administration." These include clerical labor that is shared by the doctors, and other general office expenses such as rent and utilities. The three sets of operating expenses on this statement ($200,000, $49,750, and $173,000) are added to arrive at total operating expenses of $422,750.

OTHER REVENUE   The other revenue classification means revenue earned that is outside the definition of operating revenues. In this case, one of the doctors received honorariums for two speeches he made. This income did not have to go into the partnership—he could have kept it personally—and it did not directly have to do with providing medical services. Therefore, the accountant recorded the $5,250 as other revenue.

Statement of Cash Flow

Exhibit A-11 includes the three types of cash flow along with the net increase in cash during the year. The line of the statement heading following the title shows the period that the statement covers. It covers the same 12-month period or a year of operations. The statement of cash flow essentially converts the accrual basis entries back to their net cash effects for the period. The cash flow from the three types of activities ($228,500, − $7,500, and − $219,800) are combined to arrive at the overall cash increase of $1,200.

CASH FLOW FROM OPERATING ACTIVITIES   This section of the statement begins with the net income of $222,500 and converts accrual operations to cash basis operations. To review this statement, you will need to refer to the balance sheet. The five figures (both positive and negative) in the left column, ranging from minus $7,000 to 1,000, net out at a negative figure of $6,500. The $6,500 is subtracted from the accrual net income figure of $222,500 to arrive at cash flow from operating activities of $16,000.

But how did the accountant arrive at the five figures in the left column that net out to ($6,500)? The depreciation figure of $1,000 is added back in its entirety to the accrual net income, because depreciation is a "paper figure" and does not actually represent cash expenditures of that amount. Depreciation expense is the value of assets such as equipment "used" during the period. The equipment will last a certain number of years, and its total cost is spread over the total number of years of its useful life. The amount attributable to each year is entered by an adjusting entry; in this case, the adjusting entry for the year was $1,000.

Exhibit A-11   **Woods Group Medical Practice**

Statement of Cash Flow For the Year Ending 12/31/2005		
Cash Flow from Operating Activities		
Net income		$222,500
Accounts receivable increase	(7,000)	
Supplies inventory increase	(4,000)	
Depreciation expense	1,000	
Accounts payable increase	900	
Accrued wage payable increase	2,600	
Cash flow adjustment to net income	(6,500)	
Cash flow from operating activities		$216,000
Cash Flow from Investing Activities		
Purchase of property, plant, and equipment		(7,500)
Cash Flow from Financing Activities		
Accrued interest payable increase	(100)	
Long-term debt payment	(10,000)	
Long-term debt borrowing	7,500	
Cash withdrawals by partners	(217,300)	($219,900)
Increase (Decrease) in Cash During Year		(11,400)

The accounts receivable increase and the supplies inventory increase both represent increases in balance sheet current asset items. For example, the balance sheet (see p. xxx) shows that the accounts receivable at the end of the previous year was $43,000, while the accounts receivable at the end of the current year was $50,000. Thus, the increase is $7,000 as shown on the statement of cash flow. Notice that both these items are decreases on the cash flow statement. This is because on the accrual basis, an increase in an asset means a decrease in cash. When the accounts receivable rose $7,000, that represented extra cash that was tied up and not available for use during the year. Therefore, when the accrual figures convert to show overall cash flow for the year, the $7,000 has to be a decrease.

The accounts payable increase and the accrued wage payable increase both represent increases in balance sheet current liability items. For example, the balance sheet shows that the accounts payable at the end of the previous year was $2,500, while the accounts payable at the end of the current year was $3,400. Thus the increase is $900 as shown on the statement of cash flow. Notice that both these items are increases on the cash flow statement. This is because on the accrual basis, an increase in a current liability means an increase in cash. When the accounts payable rose $900, that represented extra cash that was not tied up in payable—this much more cash was available during the year. Therefore, when the accrual figures convert to show overall cash flow for the year, the $900 has to be an increase.

CASH FLOW FROM INVESTING ACTIVITIES   This section of the statement has a single amount of $7,500. The single amount represents the purchase of property, plant, and equipment, which is an investing activity. The appropriate entry is a negative, or "minus," entry. In the case of the Woods Group, there was a $7,500 purchase, so the $7,500 purchase price is shown as a negative figure on the cash flow statement.

CASH FLOW FROM FINANCING ACTIVITIES   This section of the statement contains four items, three of which are negative and one of which is positive. To review this statement you will need to refer to the balance sheet. The four items net to a total negative amount of $219,900 in the far right column.

The first three items all have to do with debt. The interest payable item decreased $100, which results in a negative adjustment on the cash flow statement as explained earlier in this section. The long-term debt of $10,000 that was shown on the statement at the first of the year was paid off early. (It was shown properly as long-term debt, but the doctors decided to pay it off before the due date.) This debt payment used cash, so the $10,000 is a negative, or "minus" item on the cash flow statement. The doctors also borrowed $7,500 to buy the new equipment previously discussed. This debt is a long-term debt, and it is properly shown on the statement as a positive figure of $7,500.

The fourth and last item in the cash flow from financing activities is cash withdrawals by partners. This amount represents the partners' draws from the partnership. It is obviously a reduction of cash, so the $217,300 is shown on the cash flow statement as a negative figure.

Statement of Changes in Partners' Equity

Exhibit A-12 includes the equity beginning balance, the operating income, the partners' draws, and the equity ending balance. The line of the statement heading after the title shows the period that the statement covers. It covers the same 12-month period or a year of operations. To review this statement, you will need to refer to the balance sheet, the income statement, and the cash flow statement (see pp. 416, 417, and 418). The beginning balance of $105,800 is adjusted by two line items to arrive at an ending balance of $111,000.

The beginning balance at the first of the year can be seen on the balance sheet. The net income of $222,500 comes from the last line of the income statement. The partners' cash withdrawal amount of $217,300 can be seen on the cash flow statement. The net of these two items is $5,200. Thus, the $105,800 beginning balance plus $5,200 equals the ending balance of $111,000.

Exhibit A-12   **Woods Group Medical Practice**

Statement of Changes in Partners' Equity		
for the Year Ending 12/31/2005		
Beginning balance January 1, 2004		$105,800
Plus net income	$222,500	
Less partners cash withdrawals	(217,300)	
		5,200
Ending balance 12/31/2005		$111,000

BASIC CONCEPTS IN STATISTICAL ANALYSIS

This appendix is a review of basic concepts for readers who have not recently dealt with statistical processes. For those without course work in statistics, it can serve as an introduction to concepts related to analysis approaches used in this book. It discusses the probabilistic nature of phenomena, distributions of attributes of phenomena, descriptions of those attributes, and the general methodology of using linear statistical models to make inferences from quantitative data.

VARIATION AND PROBABILITY

In decision analysis, we frequently act as if we know exactly what the amount of independent variables considered in our decision will be. In budgeting for a laboratory, we might say that the number of tests that will be demanded will be 4,000 per month. This is called a *deterministic* estimate. We know, however, that the number of such tests varies from month to month, even when there is not a stable trend in the variation. Though 4,000 may be a good estimate, we do not expect the test count to be exactly 4,000. If we are budgeting expenses for a future month, we would like an idea of how small or large the demand might be because of random influences we cannot predict. The nature of this variation is referred to as its *distribution*. If we plot the monthly test count for a number of previous months (say to the nearest hundred tests), we create a frequency distribution of the monthly

427

workload. Table B-1 shows such a data set. Figure B-1a and Figure B-1b both illustrate frequency plots of that data. We describe the distribution by computing measures of *central tendency* and measures of *variability*.

Measures of Central Tendency

Measures of central tendency produce a single statistic that is meant to represent the whole distribution of measures on the attribute of interest. It indicates the

Table B-1 Frequencies of Monthly Test Counts for a 2-Year Period

Count	3,600	3,700	3,800	3,900	4,000	4,100	4,200	4,300	4,400	4,500	4,600
Frequency	1	1	2	3	4	4	3	2	2	1	1
Mean = 4,087					Mode = 4,050				Median = 4,075		

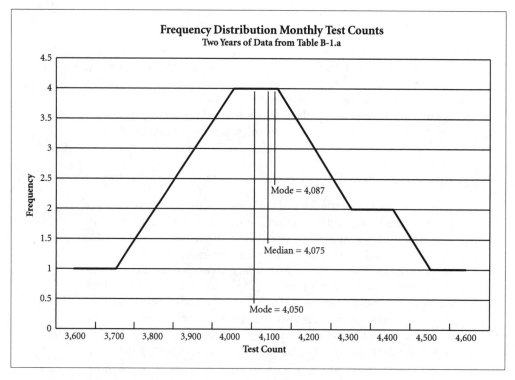

Figure B-1a **Frequency Distribution Monthly Test Counts**

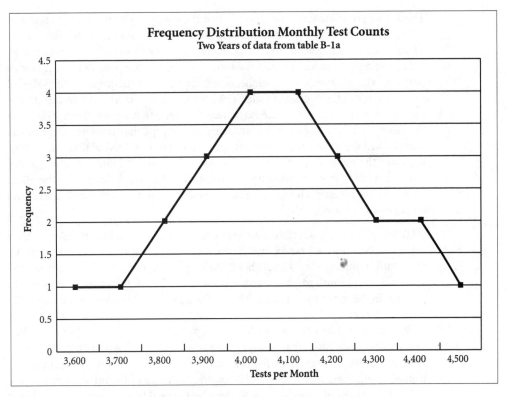

Figure B-1b   **Frequency Distribution Monthly Test Counts**

general amount of the attribute, but says nothing about the degree with which it varies from observation to observation.

ARITHMETIC AVERAGE (OR MEAN)   The *arithmetic average* is the sum of all the measures divided by the number of items measured. The formula is:

$$\mu - \sum_{i=1}^{N} (x_i)/N$$

Where:

μ = the arithmetic mean

i = a specific observation

x_i = the measurement on a specific observation

N = the number of observations

Σ = The sum from the first (i = 1)
through the last (N) observation

The arithmetic average is commonly called the *mean* or just the *average*. It is also called the *expected value*, because it is the most probable amount that will occur in a future situation if there is no change in what is known about the causes of the attribute being measured; that is, if the future will be like the past. When one takes a deterministic approach to decisions, one generally uses the mean as the value of each attribute in the decision model. The mean, however, can be greatly affected by a few events whose measures are extremely high or extremely low. Table B-2 shows the same distribution as the one in Table B-1 except that the test count in the month with the most tests is changed from 4,600 to 6,000. Note that this change increases the mean from 4,079 to 4,146 even though the central location of the test-counts for the great majority of months is unchanged. To reduce the effect such outlying measures have on the mean, two other statistics that indicate central tendency can be used.

MEDIAN The *median* is the quantity at which half the observations have a higher value and half have a lower value. In the data in Exhibit B-1, there is no middle observation among the 24 months. In this case, the value halfway between the 12th and 13th month in a rank ordered list of the monthly measurements would be used. In the monthly test count, the median, measured this way, would be 4,100 tests per month.

When the median item falls within a group of observations with the same value, to say that the median is that measure does not reflect the division of scores as precisely as one might wish. Table B-2 is a rank order array of each monthly count. Intuitively, with more measures of 4,100 on the high side of the middle point of the array, the concept of a median would seem best served by a value in the lower part of the cluster of the scores of 4,100. The computation to adjust the median statistic to 4,075, in order to make this correction, is also shown in Exhibit B-1.

Now look at Table B-2. Because the month with the highest count of tests (6,000 tests) was much higher than the other months, it raised the arithmetic mean to a higher value than it would have been if that score had been 4,600, as it is in Table B-1. However, the size of the test count in this outlier month does not change the median. It is still 4,075 tests per month. Note that changing scores at either end of the distribution in Exhibit B-1 would not change the computation of the median.

MODE Another statistic that can indicate central tendency is the mode. The mode is simply the value that exists most often in the group of measurements

Table B-2   **Frequencies of Monthly Test Counts for a 2-Year Period with an Outlier**

Count	3,600	3,700	3,800	3,900	4,000	4,100	4,200	4,300	4,400	4,500	6,000
Frequency	1	1	2	3	4	4	3	2	2	1	1

Mean = 4,146   Mode = 4,050   Median = 4,075

Exhibit B-1   **Median Computation when the Middle Point Lies Within Multiple Observation with the Same Value**

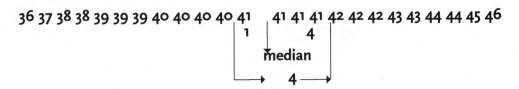

1. The middle observation lies within a group of scores of 41.
2. The score of 41 ranging from a lower boundary or 40.5 to its upper boundary of 41.5.
3. The median score lies between the 12th and 13th month.
4. That point is 1/4 (or 25 percent) of the distance from 40.5 to 41.5.
5. This measure is $40.5 + 0.25(41.5 - 40.5) = 40.75$ or 4,075 tests per month.

being analyzed. In the distribution show in Table B-1, the mode is said to be 4,050 tests. Both the 4,000 and the 4,100 values have the same frequency, so one would use their midpoint. Modes can also reveal the clustering of measures at different levels of the attribute being measured. Suppose, in examining the relationship of bone fractures per thousand population by age groups, we found much high frequencies in people in their late teens and those in their early seventies. This would be a *bimodal situation*. If the modal frequency of breaks in the older people was greater than that among the teenagers, we could say that there was a *major mode* at the older age group. Breaks in teenagers would be called the *minor mode*.

If a distribution has only one mode, it may reflect the location of the highest frequency of scores but not reflect the whole array of scores well. Figure B-1 shows such a situation. The mode is at 4,050, but many more of the items have measures above the mode than below it. Figures B-2a and B-2b show a symmetric and a skewed distribution. *Skewness* refers to the creation of a *tail* on one end of the distribution caused by more observation to that end of the mean than to the other. These two figures also show the effect of skewness on the relationships among the mean, median, and mode. In a symmetric distribution, these three statistics are the same. In a skewed distribution, the median is moved from the mode in the direction of the long tail or toward the higher volume of observation. The mean is drawn still farther in that direction because the outlying measures in the long tail pull the average in their direction.

USE OF MEAN, MEDIAN, OR MODE   When the mean fails to adequately indicate where most of the measures are centered because it has been distorted by "averaging in" some very high or very low measures, the mode or median may give a

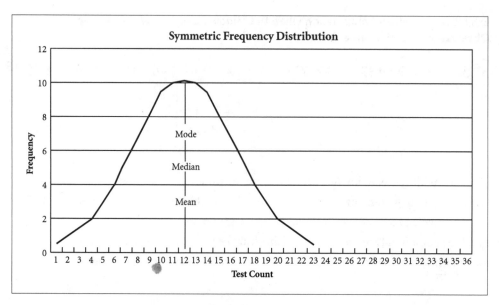

Figure B-2a **Symmetric Frequency Distribution**

better indication of central tendency. The mode is useful because it is easily picked out when the frequency distribution is plotted. In a symmetric distribution it is unaffected by outlier scores. However, like the mean, it does not represent the central tendency well if the distribution is greatly skewed. Modes will not represent a central tendency at all if the distribution has more than one of them.

In cases where there are significant outliers or skewness in the distribution, the median presents a better indication of the center of the distribution as a whole. Again, the purpose of statistics on central tendency is to have a single number that represents the array of measures of the attribute of concern. This statistic, however, only tells about the center of the distribution. This does not tell about the variability of the measured attribute.

Measures of Variability

To understand a distribution of measures of an attribute, we want to know where the measures rest on the measurement scale used. We can learn this from statistics on the central tendency. We also want to know the degree to which they cluster near the central tendency.

We want a statistic that informs us of the distance that the measures might be from the central value. For the measure from a single observation, this distances is called the *deviation* of the data point, or measurement. The formula is:

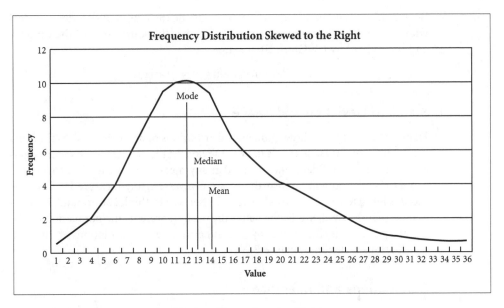

Figure B-2b   **Frequency Distribution Skewed to the Right**

$$\text{Deviation} = (x_i - \mu)$$

Where: x_i = the value of a specific observation

μ = the mean of the attribute value in the total number of observations

The average deviation is, therefore:

$$\sum_{i=1}^{N} (x_i - \mu)/N$$

Where: N = total number of observations

However, because any x_i can be above or below the mean, negative deviations can cancel out positive ones, and the sum will not indicate the total of these absolute distances. To avoid this problem, use the square of the deviations, all of which are positive numbers. These squared deviations also have helpful mathematical qualities that are beyond the scope of this appendix. It is enough to say that analyses will generally use the squared deviations. The average squared deviation is called the *variance*. Its formula is:

$$\text{Variance} = \left(\sum_{i=1}^{N} (x_i - \mu)^2 \right) / N$$

Because of its mathematical qualities, the statistic most used to describe and deal with variability is the *standard deviation*, which is the square root of the variance and abbreviated by the Greek letter sigma, σ.

$$\text{Standard deviation} = \sigma = \sqrt{\text{variance}}$$

Standard Deviation and Shape

Figures B-3a and B-3b show frequency distributions of an attribute with the same mean but different standard deviation. Obviously, the smaller the standard deviation, the more confident one can be that any measure of the attribute from the subject population will be near the mean. Conversely, any measure far from the mean is less likely to occur by chance. Another way to think about standard deviation is that the smaller it is, the better the mean represents the population of observations. This is illustrated by the superimposed presentation of the two distributions is shown in Figure B-3c.

Distributions and Inference

Mathematical formulae have been developed whose plotted curves closely match the shape of many distributions found in real-world phenomena. One that con-

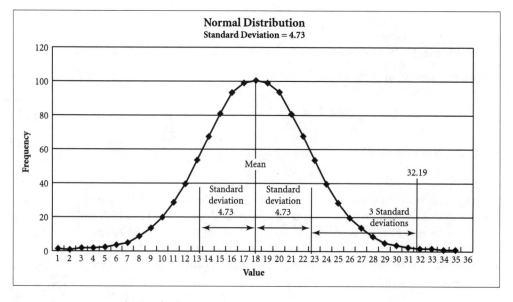

Figure B-3a   **Normal Distribution**
Standard Deviation = 4.73

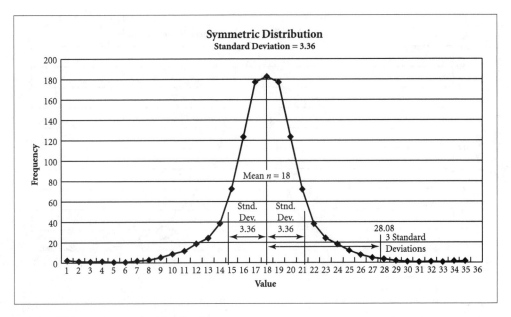

Figure B-3b   **Symmetric Distribution**
Standard Deviation = 3.36

forms to the distribution of many phenomena is called the *normal distribution*. It is a symmetric, bell-shaped curve whose location and shape is completely determined by knowing its mean and standard deviation.

Areas Under the Curve

Some general characteristics of frequency curves are basic to statistical inference. Figure B-4 shows the same data that is in Figure B-2a, but in the form of a column chart. Note that the values of measurements on an attribute are on the x-axis, ranging from 1 to 23. Note also that the columns are of equal width, so that the area covered by any column is proportional to its height. The height of each column is determined by the frequency of observations with its values. This means that the area covered by each column is proportional to the number of times the measure associated with the column occurred. Because all measurement values observed are plotted, the total area covered by the columns represents the entire population of observations. We can say that the proportion of the total area covered by the columns to the left of any given value represents the proportion of observations whose measurement was lower than that value. We can also say that the proportion of the total area covered by columns representing any range of values on the x-axis is the proportion of observations in that range.

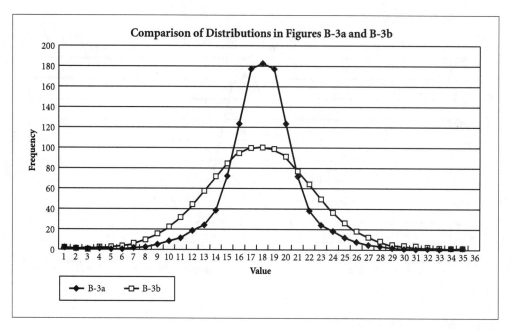

Figure B-3c   **Comparison of Distributions in Figures B-3a and B-3b**

Now, if we connect the center point of the tops of each column, the resulting line will have the same shape as the curve in Figure B-2a. More important, the proportions among areas under the curve will have the same relationships as the areas in Figure B-4. If the curve is mathematically defined, we know what those relationships are. For instance, in a normal curve, 34.13 percent of the area will fall between the mean and one standard deviation from the mean. The area between the mean and any multiple of the standard deviation from the mean is known. For instance, 49.87 percent of the area under the curve in a normal distribution will fall between the mean and three standard deviations from it. The areas for an array of mathematical curves of frequency distributions found in the world are known. These are given in common mathematical tables. Even better, they are imbedded in statistical software so that the software can determine the areas under the appropriate curve and probabilities that a score larger or smaller or in a given range can be found in a given population.

As an example, suppose we want to know if throughput time is being controlled in jobs whose normal distribution of time conforms to the distribution in Figure B-2a. We pick a job at random, measure its throughput time, and find that it was 25. We can say that the process is out of control because the chance of getting that level of the attribute when the process is in control (operating at its historic throughput times) is virtually zero. There is virtually no area under the curve at a score of 25 or higher. Knowing the area under the frequency distribution

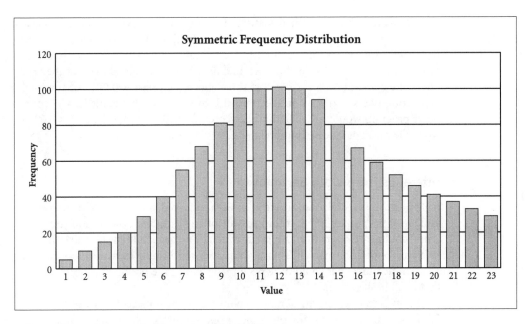

Figure B-4   **Symmetric Frequency Distribution**

curve that falls between the mean of the scores of the attribute and the score in question allows us to make a statement about the probability that any given observation that came from the population that formed the distribution.

We can use a common human attribute, body temperature, to further illustrate the use of the normal distribution of frequency curves to make decisions. Assume that throughout the world body temperatures of healthy people form a normal distribution with a mean of 98.6°F and a standard distribution of 0.8°F. If a person has a temperature of 101.0°F, is the person within the population of healthy people or is the person sick? In this case, the mean of the population to which we hope the person belongs is 98.6. The person's temperature of 101.1°F deviates from the mean by 2.4°F, (101.0 − 98.6). This is three standard deviations above the mean, (2.4/0.8). As just mentioned, the observations between the mean and three standard deviations make up 49.87 percent of the total observations in a normal distribution. Because 50 percent of the observations are above the mean in any symmetric distribution, only 0.13 percent are at or above three standard deviations from the mean—or, there is only a 0.13 percent chance that the person is in the population of healthy people. Most probably, based on the attribute of temperature, the person is sick. This inference is based on our opinion that, because the probability of finding a healthy person with a temperature of 101.0°F is only 13 out of 10,000, we believe this temperature is caused by some sort of illness.

In statistical literature, the deviation of a score divided by the standard deviation of the population from which the score is thought to come is called a *z-score*. In this example, we would say that the temperature of 101.0°F had a z-score of three. The probability tables for a normal distribution would show that the area under the curve outside a z-score of three above the mean is 0.0013 of the total area. Computer solutions would express this by showing a $p <$ statistic. The computer program would indicate that the score of 101.0 or higher had a p<0.0013 when the mean of its distribution is 98.6.

Inference from Data Samples

In the previous section, we inferred something about the health of a person by looking at the probability that the measure of an attribute of the person (temperature) could have come from a healthy person. The probability was so low that we inferred the person was sick. This analysis involved a single measure compared to all such measures that could have been made within the population of interest—that is, all healthy people.

We often want to make inferences about groups of subjects from a population. We may want to know if the outcomes from one protocol are better than those from another, or if the cost of one production process is less than that of another. In these situations, we take samples from the different groups and compare their measurements on the attributes of interest. Though we often speak of comparing groups, we actually compare measurements of attributes. When samples are taken at random from a population, variation of the attribute within the sample exists. This creates the question of what score to use as the measure of the attribute in the sample and how to compare these sample scores to a distribution of scores from other groups. The following steps are used to do this:

1. The mean of the sample scores on the attribute is used to represent the sample's value. It is indicated by the symbol, $\bar{x}$ (called x-bar).
2. The standard deviation is computed in the same way the standard deviation of a population is computed, except:

$\bar{x}$ is used instead of μ.
n is used instead of N, where n is the number of observations in the sample.
The symbol, s^2, is used for the variance of the sample, instead of σ^2.

$$s^2 = \sum_{i=1}^{N} (x_i - \bar{x})^2 / (n - 1)$$

Note that s (the sample standard deviation) is to s^2 as σ is to σ^2 in a whole population.

The denominator (n − 1) is used to compute the variance (or average of squared deviations) rather than the total number of observations. This adjusts for the fact that a sample will not have as large a variance as the population from which it is drawn. This is because some of the outlying observations that could come from the whole population will not be in the sample. This means that the variance of the total population of subjects will be larger than the variance of the sample. We want to use the variance of the sample as an estimate of the variance of the population. Using (n − 1) in the denominator makes s^2 larger than it would be if the denominator were n, corrects for the possible underestimation, and serves as an estimate of the attribute's variance in the population from which the sample was taken.

When we select a sample of a specified size and compute its mean, our observation is of the sample, not an individual subject in the sample. If we want to know the probability of the sample coming from a population by using the technique for making inferences about individual observations, we must compare our sample mean to a frequency distribution of similar observations. This would be a distribution of means of the population of similar samples. This is an important fact and makes dealing with samples more complex than dealing with individual observations hypothesized to come from a population whose mean and standard deviation we already know.

The frequency distribution of mean scores of all the samples of a given size that could come from a population is called the *distribution of sample means* or the *sampling distribution*. Some helpful characteristics of this distribution and its relationship to a given sample are noted.

1. The mean of this distribution will be the same as the mean of the population from which the samples are taken.
2. For large samples (generally considered samples of 50 or more observations), it is close to a normal distribution no matter what the shape of distribution of the underlying population.
3. For smaller samples, the shape of the distributions is also symmetric. Their shape and standard deviations depend on the size of the samples. They are called *t-distributions*.

A little qualitative explanation of *degrees of freedom* (*df*) may be helpful at this point. The shape of a t-distribution depends on the *df*s available in the computation of the estimate of the standard error, s. In order to compute s, the mean of the sample must first be computed. If we know the mean of the sample and all but one of its observation values, the last value can only be that which would produce the mean when combined with the values that are known. So, if we know the mean of the sample, the value of one observation no longer furnishes additional information; it has no freedom to vary. Computations requiring sample values have lost one *df*.

When we do not know the value of the population's standard deviation, we are forced to estimate it using the variance of the sample. Because computing the variance of the sample demands computing the sample's mean, we have used a *df*. We now have only (n − 1) degrees of freedom remaining. Because the standard error of the sample distribution is dependent on s, computations involving s also have (n − 1) degrees of freedom. This difference changes the shape of the distribution of sample meant to what are called t-distributions. A t-distribution is symmetric like a normal distribution but has thicker tails. Each t-distribution depends on the *df* of the sample. The smaller the sample (and hence the smaller the *df*), the thicker are the tails. As sample sizes and *dfs* get larger, the t-distribution becomes more like a normal distribution. At sample sizes above 50, they are practically the same and the distribution of the means is considered to be a normal distribution.

4. The standard deviation of a distribution of sample means is the standard deviation of the population from which the samples were taken divided by the square root of the sample size. It uses the symbol, $s_{\bar{x}}$:

Where:

$$s_{\bar{x}} = \frac{\sigma}{\sqrt{n}}$$

and is called the *standard error of the means* or simply the *standard error*. Here σ is the standard deviation of the population from which the samples have been drawn. As discussed, σ is estimated to be s, where:

$$s = \left[\sum_{i=1}^{n} \frac{x_i - \bar{x}}{n - 1} \right]^{1/2}$$

Note: $\sqrt{z}$ and $(z)^{1/2}$ are both expressions for the square root of z.

Given these relationships, we can

- Select a sample of a given size n.
- Compute its variance $s^2 = \sum_{i=1}^{n} (x_i - \bar{x})^2 / (n - 1)$
- Use the square root of this variance as an estimate of the standard deviation of the population from which the sample was drawn
- Divide s by the square root of the sample size to estimate the standard error of the means $s_{\bar{x}} = \dfrac{s}{\sqrt{n}}$

The mean of the distribution of sample means is also the mean of the population from which the sample is taken. Because the distribution of sample means for large samples is a normal distribution and we now also have a good estimate of that distribution's standard deviation (the standard error), we know everything we need to know in order to infer the probability that a given sample came from a population with a given mean.

We make inferences about the sample in the same way we made inferences about a single observation using the population's mean and standard deviation—except, in the case of a sample, we use the distribution of the sample means and its standard error. We compute how many times the distance between the hypothesized mean and the mean of our sample can be divided by the standard error. For a large sample forming a normal distribution, this is a z-score. For a small sample, this is called a t-score and is interpreted using the t-distribution appropriate to the *df* of the sample. The areas under the curves on either side of these scores are known and indicated in z-score or t-score tables as appropriate.

AN APPLICATION

We have initiated a new procedure that has, in the past, taken on average 62 minutes to complete. We have taken a sample of 60 applications of the new procedure. The times taken by these applications are shown in Table B-3.

- The mean of the sample is 60.633 minutes.
- The sum of squared deviations is 1,257.431.
- The estimate of the variance of the population, s^2, is 21.312. It is the sum of squared deviations divided by $(n - 1)$ where $n = 60$.
- The estimated standard deviation of the population, s, is the square root of the estimated variance. It computes to 4.617.
- The standard error of the distribution of sample means is the estimated standard deviation of the population divided by the square root of the sample size. This computes to 0.596, $(4.617/\sqrt{60})$.
- Because the comparison population has a mean of 62 minutes, the z-score for the sample is $-2.294 = (62.000 - 60.633) / 0.596$.
- Tables for a normal distribution (60 is considered a large sample) or computer software show that the probability of a score this low in a population whose mean 62 minutes is less than 0.88 percent. This is expressed in the statistic, $p < 0.0088$.

The question posed by this example is: Does the fact that the mean of the sample is 60.63 indicate that the population from which it was drawn has a mean less than that of the old procedure, which was 62 minutes? We have determined that the mean of our sample is $62.000 - 60.633 / 0.596 = -2.294$ standard errors from the mean of the old procedure. Another way to say this is that the sample mean has a z-score of -2.294. Either tables for a normal distribution or computer software will tell that the area under the distribution's curve for scores at or lower than a z-score of -2.294 is 0.0088 of the total area. This means that there is only a 0.88 percent chance that the sample could have a mean as low as 60.633 if the population it came from had a mean of 62.000. We would infer from this that the new procedure was, indeed, faster than the old one. Because we believe that a randomly selected sample with a probability that small would not be picked by chance, we

Table B-3 Process Time Data and Descriptive Statistics Work Sheet

Procedure Time in Minutes	Quantity of Procedures	Σ Minutes	Deviation	Deviation²	Σ Deviations²	
50	1	50	−10.633	113.061	113.061	Mean = total minutes / total procedures
51	2	102	−9.633	92.795	185.59	= 3,638/60
52	2	104	−8.633	74.529	149.085	= 60.633 minutes
53	2	106	−7.633	58.263	116.526	
54	2	108	−6.633	43.997	87.994	s^2 = sum of deviations² / (n − 1)
55	2	110	−5.633	31.731	63.426	= 1,257.431 / 59
56	3	168	−4.633	21.465	64.395	= 21.312
57	3	171	−3.633	13.199	39.597	$s = \sqrt{s^2} = \sqrt{21.312}$
58	3	174	−2.633	6.933	20.799	= 4.617
59	3	177	−1.633	2.667	8.001	
60	4	240	−0.633	0.401	1.604	Standard error of means = $s/\sqrt{n}$
61	5	305	0.367	0.135	0.675	= $4.617/\sqrt{60}$
62	5	310	1.367	1.869	9.480	= 0.596
63	5	315	2.367	5.603	28.015	
64	4	256	3.367	11.367	45.468	z-score = (x − μ) / standard error
65	3	195	4.367	19.071	57.213	with hypothesized μ = 62
66	3	198	5.367	28.805	86.415	
67	2	134	6.367	40.539	81.087	z-score for sample = $\dfrac{60.633 - 62.000}{0.596}$
68	2	136	7.367	54.273	108.564	
69	2	138	8.367	70.007	140.014	
70	1	70	9.367	87.741	87.741	p < .0088
71	1	71	10.367	107.475	107.475	
Sums	60 Procedures	3,638 Minutes			1,257.431	

say that the difference between the mean of the hypothesized population (the old procedure) and our sample of the new procedure is *statistically significant*. The time taken by the new procedure really is shorter than the time taken by the old one.

Statistics texts, when determining whether a difference is statistically significant, often refer to establishing a critical probability. If the probability that the sample is different from the hypothesized mean or mean of another sample is less than this preestablished threshold, we would say that the differences are statistically different. The area outside the t-score, which represented the preset probability for stating that a difference exists, was called the *critical region*. When researchers were dependent on tables of areas under frequency distribution curves to find the probability of differences existing, this was rather necessary. Because many experiments are conducted with a small sample and the distribution of each sample is dependent on its *df*, there would have to be separate tables for each *df* and each threshold probability. The alternative would be for the analyst to compute the $p<$ value, which is not a simple task. In this approach, the analysis would set the $p<$ threshold before the analysis. These thresholds could be set at common levels, usually 0.1000, 0.0500, 0.0100, or 0.0005. If, after analyzing the data, $p<$ was smaller than the preset threshold, the conclusion was that a difference did exist; this approach demanded only four different t-distribution tables. Now that computer software can give a $p<$ statistic for any sample size, setting a $p<$ statistic before analysis is no longer necessary. However, analysts must be careful not to state that there is a statistical difference when many decision makers would not agree that the $p<$ statistic justifies that belief.

Operational significance is also important in decision making. Although there is a statistically significant difference in the time taken by the two procedures, whether the difference of 1.367 minutes makes any difference to the operation of the clinic is a critical management question. If not, we would say that the difference is statistically significant but not operationally significant.

A logical question in this example situation still is unanswered. If there is only a 0.88 percent probability that the population from which the sample was drawn has a mean of 62 minutes, what is the mean of that population? Our sample mean is only an estimate of the mean of the population from which it came. We would like to at least be able to state a range of scores for the population mean in which we have a 98 percent chance of being correct. From our knowledge of normal distributions (available from distribution tables), we know that there is a 98 percent probability that an observation will be within $z = 2.33$ of the population mean. This means that, given a sample mean, the population mean (at a probability of 98 percent) will fall within $z = 2.33$ from it. In this example, the population would then fall within 1.39 minutes, 2.33 (0.5960), of the sample mean of 60.633 minutes. This is the range between 59.24 and 62.02 minutes.

Correlation, Regression, and Prediction

The term *correlation* refers to how one variable changes in response to the change of another variable. If two variables are perfectly correlated and we know how one will change, we can predict the change in the other. If we also know the starting point from which each has been changing and we know the future value of one, we can predict the future value of the other.

For instance, assume that the total variable cost per period is perfectly correlated with output per period. If we know the last period's units of output and we know the change in output from the last period to the next, we can predict the total of variable costs for the next period. This assumes that there are no changes in prices of resources or efficiency of production from period to period that would change the variable cost per unit of output. If we could accurately forecast output for future periods, we could forecast any period's total variable cost, because the two are perfectly correlated.

However, perfect correlation rarely exists. There is almost always more than one variable that affects the dependent variable from period to period. In the example, these would be resource prices and production efficiency. However, if these changes are relatively small compared to changes in output, knowing the output allows predicting total variable costs more accurately than simply assuming it will remain at its historic average. Because of the array of factors that affect the variable cost, correlation with any one related variable will be less than perfect. Therefore, the predictive power of any one correlated variable will be limited. For the amount of one variable to be used to predict that of another, there are three necessary conditions:

1. There should be a theoretical, or rational, reason the variables are related. This allows one to determine if an outside variable differing in the future, will change the correlation.
2. There is stability in the relationship between the variables so that past correlation will hold into the future.
3. The correlation should be large enough to justify using one to predict the other.
4. Occurence of the causal variable must precede the dependent variable.

It is helpful to view the relationship between two variables graphically. This is done by plotting the values of each variable for each observation. If we are examining the relationship between cost and output in operating periods, we can plot those two variables for a number of past periods. Figures B-5a through B-5c show generalized examples of such plots. In Table B-5a, there is little or no correlation between the variables. Knowing the value of one variable does not tell much about the other. Across the range of x variable, many y scores range from 2 to 13. In Figure B-5b, there is some relationship between the variable. It is obvious that as x increases so does y. Also the variation of y values at any given level of x is much

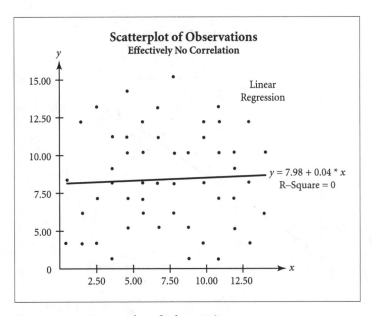

Figure B-5a   **Scatterplot of Observations**

less than in Figure B-5a. In Figure B-5c, there is a perfectly predictive relationship between the two variables. If we know the value of x, we also know the value of y for any observation. Figure B-5c depicts a perfect linear correlation between x and y. Such a relationship can be expressed by the equation $y = a + b(x)$, the equation of a straight line. If we believe such a relationship exists, the amount of the correlation can be expressed by the Pearson product moment correlation, r. Where:

$$r = \frac{\sum\limits_{i=1}^{n} (x_i - \bar{x})(y_i - \bar{y})}{\left[\left(\sum\limits_{i=1}^{n} (x_i - \bar{x})^2\right)\left(\sum\limits_{i=1}^{n} (y_i - \bar{y})^2\right)\right]^{1/2}}$$

Note: $\sqrt{z}$ and $(z)^{1/2}$ are both expressions for the square root of z.

The numerator of this formula is often referred to as SP, the *sum of products*. The denominator is the square root of the sum of squared deviations of the x values (SS_x) times the sum of squared deviations of the Y values (SS_Y). The formula can be restated as:

$$r = \frac{SP}{\sqrt{SS_x \, SS_Y}}$$

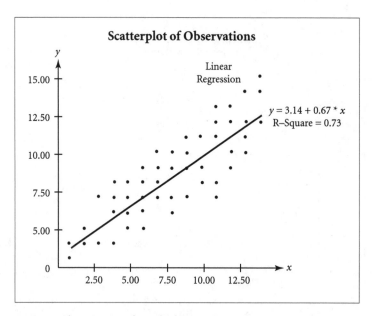

Figure B-5b   **Scatterplot of Observations**

Notice that the numerator will be positive if both x and y values of observations are above or below their mean, because both factors will have the same sign. The size of the numerator will be large if observations with either large or small values of x are accompanied by large or small values of y, respectively. Intuitively, large values of the numerator indicate strong correlation between x and y, because they will result from large deviations of x being multiplied by large deviation of y. If large values of x occur with small values of y, and vice versa, the sign of the numerator will be negative.

Concurrently the denominator will always be positive, because it is determined by squared deviations. Additionally, the denominator is the product of the total squared deviations of the x and the y variables. Therefore, if r is positive, y increases as x increases. If r is negative, y decreases as x increases.

Though it is beyond the scope of this book, several other important characteristics of r can be proved:

1. If there is no correlation between the two variables, the numerator will be zero; hence r will be zero.
2. When there is perfect correlation, the denominator will equal the numerator and r will be 1.
3. When r is squared the resulting number, r^2, will indicate the portion of the variation in the y variable that is explained by the x variable.

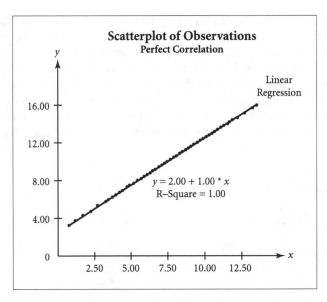

Figure B-5c   **Scatterplot of Observations**

Simple Regression

Figure B-5c is a plot of data in which there is a perfect correlation between x and y. If the value of x is known, there is only one corresponding y value; hence the value of y is also know. In Figure B-5b, there appears to be a positive correlation between x and y, but knowing x does not give a single corresponding value for y. However, knowing x does limit our possible predictions of y and improves the prediction over simply using the expected value of y.

Simple regression analysis gives a linear model with which to predict y if we know x. It draws a straight line through the data in such a way that the sum of the squares of the vertical distances between the line and each data point is a minimum. The process is called the *least squares approach*. Realize that the line drawn through the data can also be represented by the equation of a straight line:

$$y = a + b(x).$$

In this equation, a represents the intercept on the y axis and b is the slope of the line. The computations are:

$$b = SP / SS_x$$
$$a = \overline{y} - b\,\overline{x}$$

The value of y on the line corresponding to an x value represents the central tendency of y values that occur with that value of x. The vertical distance between the regression line and each point is the amount of error in the regression model's prediction of the y-score for that observation. This means that if we had used the regression line to predict that point, the prediction would have been off by that amount. These errors in the value of *y* for specific *x*s are analogous to deviations from the mean in an analysis of a single variable. The y-value on the regression line associated with an x-value is the estimated value of y, called y-hat: Its symbol is $\hat{y}$.

The sum of squares error is $\displaystyle\sum_{i=1}^{n} (y_i - \hat{y}_i)^2$ *and is abbreviated* SS_{error}.

The standard error of these estimates is $(SS_{error} / df)^{1/2}$.

In this case, because the means for both the x and y scores must be computed to define the regression line, df = n − 2.

Just as with the other sample distributions, the smaller the standard error, the closer the observations are to their mean. Inspection of Figures B-5a through B-5c indicates that as *r* increases, the standard error decreases. Both a high *r* and a small standard error of the estimate indicate that the regression line fits the data well and can be used to make fairly accurate predictions of *y*. In regression analysis, the squared value of *r* is usually reported as R^2. It has the same meaning as r^2, discussed earlier. It indicates the fraction of the variation in y that is predicted by variations in *x*. If $R^2 = 1$, *y* can be predicted with perfect accuracy. If it is zero, we cannot make predictions about *y* from knowing *x*.

Because the data used to construct the regression line is really a sample of population of all the observation that could be made of the phenomenon being analyzed, it is possible that the R^2 in the sample is impressively high even when it is zero in the population.

The report of results from a computerized regression analysis will give the following statistics:

a: The y intercept on a graph of the regression line. It is the constant in the equation of the regression line.
b: The slope of the regression line. It is the coefficient of x in the equation for of the regression line.
R^2: The square of the Pearson product moment coefficient for the correlation between *x* and *y*, gives the fraction of the variation of *y* that is predicted by

x and indicates the goodness of fit of the regression line to the sample data.
p< The probability that, even though the sample data produced a regression analysis with a positive R^2, the R^2 in the population is zero.

In this book, simple regression analysis is used to analyze cost behavior and establish trends, changes, and attributes over time.

INDEX